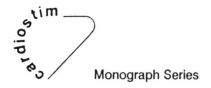

Monograph Series

NEW
PERSPECTIVES
IN
CARDIAC PACING, 3

Edited by

S. SERGE BAROLD, M.B., B.S., FRACP, FACP, FACC, FESC

Chief, Division of Cardiology
Department of Medicine
The Genesee Hospital
Professor of Medicine
University of Rochester
School of Medicine and Dentistry
Rochester, New York

and

JACQUES MUGICA, M.D.

Chief, Department of Cardiac Pacing and Electrophysiology
Centre Chirurgical Val D'Or
Saint Cloud, France

FUTURA

Futura Publishing Company, Inc.
Mount Kisco, NY

Library of Congress Cataloging-in-Publication Data

New perspectives in cardiac pacing, 3 / edited by S. Serge Barold,
  Jacques Mugica
      p.   cm.
    Includes bibliographical references and index.
    ISBN 0-87993-542-1
    1. Cardiac pacing.   I. Barold, S. Serge.   II. Mugica, Jacques.
    [DNLM: 1. Arrhythmia—complications.   2. Cardiac Pacing,
Artificial.   3. Pacemaker, Artificial.   WG 168 N53132]
RC684.P3N483   1992
617.4′12059—dc20
DNLM/DLC
for Library of Congress   92-49196
                                                                        CIP

Copyright 1993
Futura Publishing Company, Inc.

Published by
Futura Publishing Company, Inc.
2 Bedford Ridge Road
Mount Kisco, New York 10549

LC #: 92-49196
ISBN #: 0-87993-542-1
Every effort has been made to ensure that the information in this
book is as up to date and as accurate as possible at the time of
publication. However, due to the constant developments in medicine,
the authors, the editors, or the publisher cannot accept any legal or
any other responsibility for any errors or omissions that may occur.

Printed in the United States of America.

This book is printed on acid-free paper.

To our wives—
Jennie and Catherine

Contributors

Eckhard Alt, M.D.
Associate Professor of Internal Medicine, Technical University of Munich, Rechts der Isar Medical Center, Munich, Germany

Lucia Ansani, M.D.
Assistant Cardiologist, S. Anna Hospital, Ferrara, Italy

Giovanni Enrico Antonioli, M.D., Ph.D.
Chief of Cardiology, S. Anna Hospital, Ferrara, Italy

Antonio Asso, M.D.
Research Fellow, Cardiac Electrophysiology, University of Minnesota, Minneapolis, Minnesota

Dario Barbieri, M.D.
Assistant Cardiologist, S. Anna Hospital, Ferrara, Italy

S. Serge Barold, M.B., B.S., FRACP
Chief, Division of Cardiology, Department of Medicine, The Genesee Hospital, Professor of Medicine, University of Rochester School of Medicine and Dentistry, Rochester, New York

David G. Benditt, M.D.
Professor of Medicine, Director, Cardiac Arrhythmia Service, University of Minnesota, Minneapolis, Minnesota

Johan Brandt, M.D., Ph.D.
Senior Resident, Department of Cardiothoracic Surgery, Lund University Hospital, Lund, Sweden

Jeffrey A. Brinker, M.D.
Associate Professor of Medicine, Director, Interventional Cardiology and Adult Pacemaker Laboratory, Johns Hopkins Medical Institutions, Baltimore, Maryland

Charles L. Byrd, M.D.
Clinical Professor of Surgery, University of Miami School of Medicine, Miami; Attending Surgeon, Florida Medical Center, The Heart Institute of Florida, Ft. Lauderdale, Florida

Serge Cazeau, M.D.
Cardiologist, Department of Cardiac Pacing and Electrophysiology, Centre Chirurgical Val d'Or, Saint Cloud, France

Elizabeth Ching, R.N.
Section of Cardiac Electrophysiology, Department of Cardiology, Cleveland Clinic Foundation, Cleveland, Ohio

Derek T. Connelly, M.B., Ch.B.
Fellow in Cardiology, Royal Brompton National Heart and Lung Hospitals, London, United Kingdom

Claude Daubert, M.D.
Professor of Cardiology, Chief, Department of Cardiology, University Hospital, Rennes, France

Kenneth A. Ellenbogen, M.D.
Director, Electrophysiology and Pacing, Medical College of Virginia, and McGuire V.A. Medical Center, Associate Professor of Internal Medicine/Electrophysiology, Medical College of Virginia, Richmond, Virginia

Svein Faerestrand, M.D., Ph.D.
Consultant, Department of Cardiology, University School of Medicine, Haukeland Sykehus, Bergen, Norway

Jerry C. Griffin, M.D.
Professor of Medicine, Division of Cardiology, University of California, San Francisco, California

Gabriele Guardigli, M.D.
Assistant Cardiologist, S. Anna Hospital, Ferrara, Italy

Ronell Hansen, M.D.
Research Fellow, Cardiac Electrophysiology, University of Minnesota, Minneapolis, Minnesota

David L. Hayes, M.D.
Consultant, Division of Cardiovascular Diseases and Internal Medicine, Mayo Clinic and Mayo Foundation, Associate Professor of Medicine, Mayo Medical School, Rochester, Minnesota

Nancy B. Hedin, R.N.
Physician Technical Assistant, Florida Medical Center, The Heart Institute of Florida, Ft. Lauderdale, Florida

Chu-Pak Lau, M.D.
Senior Lecturer and Chief, Cardiology Division, Department of Medicine, The University of Hong Kong, Queen Mary Hospital, Hong Kong

Christophe Leclercq, M.D.
Assistant Professor of Cardiology, University Hospital, Rennes, France

Paul A. Levine, M.D.
Vice President and Medical Director, Siemens Pacesetter, Inc., Sylmar; Clinical Professor of Medicine, Loma Linda University Medical Center, Loma Linda, California

Keith Lurie, M.D.
Assistant Professor of Medicine, University of Minnesota, Minneapolis, Minnesota

Phillipe Mabo, M.D.
Professor of Cardiology, University Hospital, Rennes, France

James D. Maloney, M.D.
Co-Director, Section of Cardiac Electrophysiology, Director, Electrophysiology Laboratory, Department of Cardiology, Cleveland Clinic Foundation, Cleveland, Ohio

Rick McVenes, B.S.
Staff Scientist, Medtronic, Inc., Minneapolis, Minnesota

Harry G. Mond, M.D., FRACP
*Physician to the Pacemaker Clinic, Royal Melbourne Hospital,
Victoria, Australia*

Jacques Mugica, M.D.
*Chief, Department of Cardiac Pacing and Electrophysiology, Centre
Chirurgical Val d'Or, Saint Cloud, France*

Gianfranco Percoco, M.D.
Assistant Cardiologist, S. Anna Hospital, Ferrara, Italy

Sergio L. Pinski, M.D.
*Fellow in Cardiac Electrophysiology, Department of Cardiology,
Cleveland Clinic Foundation, Cleveland, Ohio*

Stephen Remole, M.D.
*Assistant Professor of Medicine, University of Minnesota, Minneapolis,
Minnesota*

Anthony F. Rickards, M.B., B.S., FRCP
*Consultant Cardiologist and Director of Pacing and Electrophysiology,
Royal Brompton National Heart and Lung Hospitals, London, United
Kingdom*

Philippe Ritter, M.D.
*Cardiologist, Department of Cardiac Pacing and Electrophysiology,
Centre Chirurgical Val d'Or, Saint Cloud, France*

Massimo Santini, M.D.
*Chief, Cardiology Department, San Filippo Neri Hospital, Rome,
Italy*

Susan J. Schwartz, M.S.
*Biomedical Engineer, Florida Medical Center, The Heart Institute of
Florida, Ft. Lauderdale, Florida*

Hans Schüller, M.D.
Associate Professor of Cardiothoracic Surgery, Consultant Cardiothoracic Surgeon, Department of Cardiothoracic Surgery, Lund University Hospital, Lund, Sweden

Elena B. Sgarbossa, M.D.
Clinical Research Fellow in Cardiac Electrophysiology, Department of Cardiology, Cleveland Clinic Foundation, Cleveland, Ohio

Bruce S. Stambler, M.D.
Co-Director, Electrophysiology, McGuire V.A. Medical Center, Assistant Professor of Internal Medicine/Electrophysiology, Medical College of Virginia, Richmond, Virginia

Ken Stokes, B.Chem.
Senior Research Fellow, Medtronic, Inc., Minneapolis, Minnesota

Tiziano Toselli, M.D.
Assistant Cardiologist, S. Anna Hospital, Ferrara, Italy

Corinne Varin, M.D.
Cardiologist, Department of Cardiology, University Hospital, Rennes, France

Mark A. Wood, M.D.
Co-Director, Electrophysiology and Pacing, Medical College of Virginia, Assistant Professor of Internal Medicine/Electrophysiology, Medical College of Virginia, Richmond, Virginia

Preface

This book was conceived as a companion to the monographs *New Perspectives in Cardiac Pacing* 1 and 2, published four and two years ago. Cardiac pacing has grown so fast over the last few years that assimilation of new knowledge and its clinical application have become major challenges even for experts involved in the field on a day-to-day basis. We tried in this book to present a proper balance of technical and clinical material to provide, like its predecessors, many of the answers to the question, "What's new in cardiac pacing?" with emphasis on progress in rate-adaptive pacing which constitutes over half of the contents. Chapters reevaluating old subjects such as the pacemaker syndrome, effect of drugs on the pacing threshold, natural history of the sick sinus syndrome after pacemaker implantation, etc., bring new life and excitement into what is often taken for granted, while other chapters such as single lead VDD pacing, automatic mode switching, etc., focus on important new concepts and developments.

We thank the contributors for their superb work and Futura Publishing Company (Ms. Linda Shaw, Editor, and Mr. Jacques Strauss, President) for their continued efforts in producing books that are not out of date when published. This book would not have been possible without the total devotion of Mrs. Wilma Shaughnessy who by now we suspect knows more about cardiac pacing than we do.

S. Serge Barold
Jacques Mugica

Contents

PART III
Selection of Pacing System and Follow-Up

PART I

Basic Concepts, Indications, and Consequences of Cardiac Pacing

Chapter 1

Indications for the Use of Implanted Arrhythmia Devices: Comments on the 1991 ACC/ AHA Task Force Report

JERRY C. GRIFFIN

Introduction

*I*n the early 1980s, major concerns were voiced regarding the overutilization of pacemakers.[1] The American College of Cardiology and the American Heart Association responded by developing and publishing guidelines for the use of permanent pacemakers in patients with bradyarrhythmias. These were developed under the auspices of the Joint Association Task Force on Assessment of Cardiovascular Procedures. A subcommittee was convened under the chairmanship of Dr. Robert Frye, and included adult and pediatric cardiologists, electrophysiologists, and surgeons. Importantly, the group included members not working predominantly in cardiac pacing as well as those who were. The guidelines were published in 1984[2] and rapidly became the standard by which medical practice was judged in the United States. It was adopted by many professional review organizations as their benchmark for professional performance.

By the late 1980s, sufficient new information in the field necessitated updating the 1984 document. A second subcommittee was formed under the chairmanship of Dr. Leonard Dreifus, a member of the original committee. In 1991, the updated and revised guidelines were published.[3]

New Perspectives in Cardiac Pacing, Vol. 3, edited by S. Serge Barold and Jacques Mugica, Mount Kisco, NY, Futura Publishing Co., © 1993.

TABLE *1*
ACC/AHA Guidelines Report 1991: Classification System Used for 1984 and 1991 Guidelines[3]

Class I
Conditions for which there is general agreement that permanent pacemakers or antitachycardia devices should be implanted.

Class II
Conditions for which permanent pacemakers or antitachycardia devices are frequently used but there is divergence of opinion with respect to the necessity of their insertion.

Class III
Conditions for which there is general agreement that pacemakers or antitachycardia devices are unnecessary.

Format and Definitions

The two documents share a common approach to the problem of codifying a large and complex body of medical literature and decision making. All indications are assigned to one of three classes (Table 1). The classes are distinguished largely by the uniformity of opinion of the validity of the indication. Of course, other factors have significant weight and may affect the decision process in real-life situations. These are recognized by the committee and some of the more common ones discussed. Many of the indications rest on the presence or absence of symptoms. The document provides a list of those symptoms commonly associated with significant bradycardia. It also recognizes the very real problem that some of the more subtle ones, such as fatigue or congestive heart failure, may be appreciated only in retrospect, after bradycardia is relieved.

Overview: Indications for Pacing in Bradycardias

Pacing in Acquired AV Block in Adults (Table 2)

The guidelines separate the acquired AV blocks into two groups, those with and those without chronic infra-His conduction abnormalities. In the absence of chronic infra-His block, the guidelines confer class I status only on those indications where AV block is associated with

TABLE *2*

ACC/AHA Guidelines Report 1991: Indications for Permanent Pacing in Acquired AV Block in Adults[3]

Class I
   A. Complete heart block, permanent or intermittent, at any anatomic level, associated with any one of the following complications:
      1. Symptomatic bradycardia. In the presence of complete heart block, symptoms must be presumed to be due to the heart block unless proved to be otherwise.
      2. Congestive heart failure.
      3. Ectopic rhythms and other medical conditions that require drugs that suppress the automaticity of escape pacemakers and result in symptomatic bradycardia.
      4. Documented periods of asystole ≥3.0 sec or any escape rate <40 beats/min in symptom-free patients.
      5. Confusional states that clear with temporary pacing.
      6. Post-AV junction ablation, myotonic dystrophy.
   B. Second degree AV block, permanent or intermittent, regardless of the type or the site of block, with symptomatic bradycardia.
   C. Atrial fibrillation, atrial flutter, or rare cases of supraventricular tachycardia with complete heart block or advanced AV block, bradycardia, and any of the conditions described under I.A. The bradycardia must be unrelated to digitalis or drugs known to impair AV conduction.

Class II
   A. Asymptomatic complete heart block, permanent or intermittent, at any anatomic site, with ventricular rates of 40 beats/min or faster.
   B. Asymptomatic type II second degree AV block, permanent or intermittent.
   C. Asymptomatic type I second degree AV block at intra-His or infra-His levels.

Class III
   A. First degree AV block.
   B. Asymptomatic type I second degree AV block at the supra-His (AV node) level.

symptoms. The block may be of second or third degree, associated with atrial fibrillation, or at any anatomic level. Pacing in asymptomatic patients with third degree block at any level and a rate <40 bpm, or second degree block of type II is considered a class II indication. Also considered class II is asymptomatic type I AV block, if the site is intra- or infra-His; however, type I block above the His bundle is considered class III.

TABLE *3*

ACC/AHA Guidelines Report 1991: Pacing in AV Block Associated with Myocardial Infarction[3]

Class I
   A. Persistent advanced second degree AV block or complete heart block after acute myocardial infarction with block in the His-Purkinje system (bilateral bundle branch block).
   B. Patients with transient advanced AV block and associated bundle branch block.

Class II
   A. Patients with persistent advanced block at the AV node.

Class III
   A. Transient AV conduction disturbances in the absence of intraventricular conduction defects.
   B. Transient AV block in the presence of isolated left anterior hemiblock.
   C. Acquired left anterior hemiblock in the absence of AV block.
   D. Patients with persistent first degree AV block in the presence of bundle branch block not demonstrated previously.

Pacing in AV Block Associated with Myocardial Infarction (Table 3)

A variety of forms of AV and intraventricular conduction abnormalities occur in the aftermath of acute myocardial infarction (MI). Patients with persistent high grade or complete block should be paced if the block is in the His-Purkinje system. The necessity for pacing persistent block in the AV node is uncommon if one waits a sufficient time. In addition, the guidelines now accept pacing after transient high grade or complete block if associated with development of bundle branch block.

Pacing in Chronic Bifascicular and Trifascicular Block (Table 4)

In the presence of chronic bundle branch block, intermittent type II AV block is regarded more seriously. In this setting, it is a class I indication for pacing. In the absence of bundle branch abnormalities, it is considered only a class II indication. The management of patients with

TABLE 4

ACC/AHA Guidelines Report 1991: Pacing in Bifascicular and Trifascicular Block (Chronic)[3]

Class I
- A. Bifascicular block with intermittent complete heart block associated with symptomatic bradycardia (as defined).
- B. Bifascicular or trifascicular block with intermittent type II second degree AV block without symptoms attributable to the heart block.

Class II
- A. Bifascicular or trifascicular block with syncope that is not proved to be due to complete heart block, but other possible causes for syncope are not identifiable.
- B. Markedly prolonged HV (>100 ms).
- C. Pacing-induced infra-His block.

Class III
- A. Fascicular block without AV block or symptoms.
- B. Fascicular block with first degree AV block without symptoms.

intermittent, undocumented symptoms and bifascicular block is often difficult and the cause of symptoms is frequently not distal conduction system block. This setting is one of the few where electrophysiologic (EP) testing can be helpful, and three class II indications are based at least in part on the results of EP study. Findings of an H-V interval >100 ms or pacing induced infra-His block at abnormal rates suggest advanced His-Purkinje disease and pacing is indicated at a class II level. Finally, the use of EP study and other diagnostic testing to eliminate other causes of syncope allows one to proceed with pacing as a therapeutic trial.

Pacing in Sinus Node Dysfunction (Table 5)

While more concise than for AV block, the indications for pacing in sinus node dysfunction syndrome are also more nebulous. The guidelines stress the necessity for demonstrating the temporal correlation between symptoms and bradycardia. The mere observation of symptoms and bradycardia at separate times is not an indication for pacing. At the same time, it is recognized that sinus node dysfunction often results from drug therapy. When such drugs are necessary for the control of other problems, pacing is indicated to prevent symptomatic bradycardia.

TABLE 5

ACC/AHA Guidelines Report 1991: Pacing in Sinus Node Dysfunction[3]

Class I
  A. Sinus node dysfunction with documented symptomatic bradycardia. In some patients, this will occur as a consequence of long-term (essential) drug therapy of a type and dose for which there are no acceptable alternatives.

Class II
  A. Sinus node dysfunction, occurring spontaneously or as a result of necessary drug therapy, with heart rates <40 beats/min when a clear association between significant symptoms consistent with bradycardia and the actual presence of bradycardia has not been documented.

Class III
  A. Sinus node dysfunction in asymptomatic patients, including those in whom substantial sinus bradycardia (heart rate <40 beats/min) is a consequence of long-term drug treatment.
  B. Sinus node dysfunction in patients in whom symptoms suggestive of bradycardia are clearly documented not to be associated with a slow heart rate.

Pacing in Hypersensitive Carotid Sinus and Neurovascular Syndromes (Table 6)

In hypersensitive carotid sinus syndrome, the emphasis is on the identification of triggering or provocative factors. In the presence of such factors, symptomatic episodes constitute a class I indication for pacing. In the absence of provocative factors, but with an abnormal carotid sinus reflex response, the indication is only class II. A role for tilt-table testing is now recognized (see below) in the determination of the need for pacing in some patients. This area is undergoing rapid evolution and further changes in indications for pacing in neurovascular syndromes will likely occur.

Pacing in Children (Table 7)

Children provide a number of variations on the themes set forth above. These are delineated in Table 7. In particular, the problems of congenital and postsurgical AV block are detailed.

TABLE *6*

ACC/AHA Guidelines Report 1991: Pacing in Hypersensitive Carotid Sinus and Neurovascular Syndromes[3]

Class I
  A. Recurrent syncope associated with clear, spontaneous events provoked by carotid sinus stimulation; minimal carotid sinus pressure induces asystole of >3 sec duration in the absence of any medication that depresses the sinus node or AV conduction.

Class II
  A. Recurrent syncope without clear, provocative events and with a hypersensitive cardioinhibitory response.
  B. Syncope with associated bradycardia reproduced by a head-up tilt with or without isoproterenol or other forms of provocative maneuvers and in which a temporary pacemaker and a second provocative test can establish the likely benefits of a permanent pacemaker.

Class III
  A. A hyperactive cardioinhibitory response to carotid sinus stimulation in the absence of symptoms.
  B. Vague symptoms, such as dizziness or light-headedness, or both, with a hyperactive cardioinhibitory response to carotid sinus stimulation.
  C. Recurrent syncope, light-headedness or dizziness in the absence of a cardioinhibitory response.

Changes in the Guidelines: 1984 to 1991

Special Forms of Acquired AV Block

The 1991 guidelines include two new conditions under the broad heading of symptomatic complete heart block. The first is AV block resulting from catheter ablation of the AV conduction system. Though this procedure may leave the patient with a junctional or lower rhythm of reasonable rate, its reliability and long escape times make pacing mandatory. The association of myotonic dystrophy and AV block is well established. It is now clear that such blocks usually occur in the His-Purkinje system, therefore pacing is indicated.

TABLE 7

ACC/AHA Guidelines Report 1991: Use of Pacemakers in Children[3]

Class I
- A. Second or third degree AV block with symptomatic bradycardia, as defined.
- B. Advanced second or third degree AV block with moderate to marked exercise intolerance.
- C. External ophthalmoplegia with bifascicular block.
- D. Sinus node dysfunction with symptomatic bradycardia, as defined.
- E. Congenital AV block with wide QRS escape rhythm or with block below the His bundle.
- F. Advanced second or third degree AV block persisting 10–14 days after cardiac surgery.

Class II
- A. Bradycardia–tachycardia syndrome with need for an antiarrhythmic drug other than digitalis or phenytoin.
- B. Second or third degree AV block within the bundle of His in an asymptomatic patient.
- C. Prolonged subsidiary pacemaker recovery time.
- D. Transient surgical second or third degree AV block that reverts to bifascicular block.
- E. Asymptomatic second or third degree AV block and a ventricular rate <45 beats/min when awake. Complete AV block when awake, with an average ventricular rate <50 beats/min.
- F. Complete AV block with double or triple rest cycle length pauses or minimal heart rate variability.
- G. Asymptomatic neonate with congenital complete heart block and bradycardia in relation to age.
- H. Complex ventricular arrhythmias associated with second or third degree AV block or sinus bradycardia.
- I. Long QT syndrome.

Class III
- A. Asymptomatic, postoperative bifascicular block.
- B. Asymptomatic postoperative bifascicular block with first degree AV block.
- C. Transient surgical AV block that returns to normal conduction in <1 week.
- D. Asymptomatic type I second degree AV block.
- E. Asymptomatic congenital heart block without profound bradycardia in relation to age.

The Problem of AV Block and Acute Myocardial Infarction

Controversy continues to surround many of the indications for permanent pacing in patients with conduction abnormalities associated with an acute myocardial infarction. The committee raised pacing for transient AV block occurring in the setting of bundle branch block after acute MI from a class II to a class I indication. Pacing for persistent advanced second degree or third degree block was separated according to the site of block. Origination in the His-Purkinje system remains a class I indication, while origination in the AV node has been downgraded to class II. It is also considered that first degree block occurring in conjunction with various bundle branch blocks does not constitute an indication for pacing.

Asymptomatic Patients with Chronic Bi- and Trifascicular Block

The 1991 guidelines are somewhat more aggressive with this group of patients. If asymptomatic, the 1984 guidelines listed intermittent type II block occurring in the setting of chronic fascicular disease as a class II indication for pacing. In the 1991 guidelines, this has been upgraded to a class I indication, in recognition of the risk of catastrophic bradycardia associated with infra-His block. Marked prolongation of the H-V interval is now recognized as a class II indication.

Head-Up Tilt Testing and Indications for Pacing

Our understanding of the various neurovascular syndromes causing bradyarrhythmias has expanded significantly since 1984. Provocative testing by passive head-up tilt is now a commonly used modality for the evaluation of patients with syncope and near-syncope. The 1991 guidelines recognize the use of tilt-table testing in the evaluation of the need for pacing. They also stress the importance of repeat testing with a demonstration that pacing prevents previously provoked symptoms.

Ambulatory Monitoring and Pacing for Children

The timing of pacemaker implantation in patients with congenital third degree AV block is difficult. In the past, symptoms, wide-complex escape rhythms, or severe bradycardias were the principal indicators. More recent studies suggest that ambulatory ECG monitoring provides other useful signs such as awake average ventricular rates <50 bpm, double or triple cycle length pauses, or minimal heart rate variability. Each of these is now recognized as a class II indication.

Overview: Indications for Different Modes of Pacing

Since 1984 several new modes of cardiac pacing have come into widespread use. The current guidelines feature a greatly expanded review of mode and device selection for patients receiving permanent pacemakers.

Overview: Indications for Pacing in Tachycardias

The section on pacing for tachyarrhythmias is also significantly expanded. Indications are grouped by type of device. Devices are in turn grouped according to whether they automatically recognize and act to terminate the tachycardia, must be manually activated to terminate tachycardia, or pace persistently for the prevention of tachycardia. Automatic pacemakers are indicated for drug-resistant supraventricular tachycardia and in recurrent VT if a defibrillator is also implanted. Manually activated devices may be used to terminate VT under monitoring in patients who are not candidates for an ICD. Overdrive dual chamber pacing may be useful in some patients with atrioventricular and AV node reentry tachycardias resistant to drug therapy. Overdrive pacing may also be used in patients with ventricular arrhythmias as well as torsade de pointes resulting from the congenital long QT syndrome. These indications were judged to be more controversial and therefore class II.

Overview: Indications for Use of the ICD

Certain requirements are stressed for evaluation of candidates for implantation of an ICD. The arrhythmia must be life-threatening and remediable causes must be ruled out. In general, indications for the device derive from one of three situations: less invasive therapies are predicted to be ineffective (or found to be toxic), a therapy predicted effective fails clinically, or the efficacy of other therapies cannot be assessed (most often because the patient is not inducible during EP study). These circumstances usually provide class I indications for the device. The use of the ICD as an alternative to drug therapy or serial drug testing is deemed a class II indication. Recurrent syncope without documentation of a concurrent arrhythmia is a common problem. If appropriate arrhythmias are inducible in the EP laboratory and the patient falls into one of the situations above, the level of indication is class II. However, if ventricular arrhythmias are not induced in the EP laboratory, the device is thought not to be indicated.

References

1. Greenberg A, Kowey PR, Bargmann E, Wolfe SM. Permanent pacemakers in Maryland. Report by Health Research Group, Washington, DC, July 1982.
2. Frye RL, Collins JJ, DeSanctis RW, et al. Guidelines for permanent cardiac pacemaker implantation, May 1984. Circulation 1984;70:331A–339A.
3. Dreifus LS, Fisch C, Griffin JC, et al. Guidelines for implantation of cardiac pacemakers and antiarrhythmia devices. JACC 1991;18:1–13.

Chapter 2

Cardiac Pacing for Carotid Sinus Syndrome and Vasovagal Syncope

DAVID G. BENDITT, STEPHEN REMOLE,

ANTONIO ASSO, RONELL HANSEN,

KEITH LURIE

Introduction

Carotid sinus syndrome (CSS) and "vasovagal" syncope are perhaps the best known of the various neurally mediated syncopal syndromes (Table 1). The former, although a relatively infrequent clinical condition, may be considered the prototype of these syndromes and has been the subject of study for many years.[1-7] Vasovagal syncope, on the other hand, despite being quite common, has proven to be elusive to study until the recent application of tilt-table testing techniques.[8-11]

The pathogenesis of the neurally mediated syncopal syndromes remains incompletely understood. Current concepts suggest that afferent impulses from a variety of peripheral receptors (e.g., mechanoreceptors, chemoreceptors) in any of a number of organ systems (e.g., ventricular myocardium, bladder, airways), as well as inputs from higher central

Dr. Asso is supported by the Fondo Investigacion, Sanitaria, Spain. Dr. Remole is a recipient of a grant-in-aid from the American Heart Association, Minnesota Affiliate. Ronell Hansen was supported in part by a grant from the Howard Hughes Medical Institute. Dr. Lurie is a recipient of a grant from the National Institutes of Health, Bethesda Maryland.

New Perspectives in Cardiac Pacing, Vol. 3, edited by S. Serge Barold and Jacques Mugica, Mount Kisco, NY, Futura Publishing Co., © 1993.

TABLE *1*

Neurally Mediated Syncopal Syndromes

Emotional syncope (common or "vasovagal" faint)
Carotid sinus syncope
Gastrointestinal stimulation
  swallow syncope, defecation syncope
Micturition syncope
Cough syncope
Sneeze syncope
Glossopharyngeal neuralgia
Airway stimulation
Raised intrathoracic pressure
  trumpet-playing, weight-lifting

nervous system sites, impinge on vasomotor control areas in the medulla and result in efferent neural signals that cause both bradycardia and peripheral vasodilatation.[8,11] In the case of carotid sinus syndrome, the principal source of afferent neural activity is presumably the carotid baroreceptors. In vasovagal syncope, although cardiopulmonary mechanoreceptors appear to be the principal source of the neural afferent signals required to trigger the episode in susceptible subjects, precipitating factors are also needed in order to set the stage (e.g., anxiety, pain, dehydration, exercise).

In patients with neurally mediated syncope, symptoms may be due to either marked bradycardia or peripheral vasodilatation. However, in most cases, both phenomena are critical. Consequently, clinical differentiation of "cardioinhibitory," "vasodepressor," and "mixed" forms is important in order to establish effective treatment strategies. Thus, patients with severe bradycardia alone may be candidates for pacing, those individuals with predominant vasodepressor responses are managed primarily pharmacologically, while those with "mixed" forms require a combination of techniques.

Efficacy of Pacing in Carotid Sinus Syndrome

A number of reports have focused on both the overall effectiveness of cardiac pacing and the optimal pacing mode for treatment of patients with carotid sinus syndrome.[5,12–23] Understandably, these studies have dealt primarily with the "cardioinhibitory" or "mixed" forms of the syndrome (i.e., cases with demonstrable bradyarrhythmias).

In a retrospective report, Sugrue et al.[5] assessed treatment and follow-up in 56 syncope patients who met criteria for CSS. The diagnosis was based on demonstration during carotid sinus massage of either an asystolic pause of 3 seconds or greater, or a vasodepressor response of greater than 50 mm Hg. Forty-seven patients (84%) were diagnosed as primarily exhibiting a cardioinhibitory response, while three patients (5%) had predominantly vasodepressor findings, and six (11%) were of the mixed type. Thirteen patients (group 1) received no treatment, 20 received anticholinergic drug therapy (group 2), and 23 received pacemakers (group 3). Follow-up data were available in 53 cases (11 group 1, 19 group 2, and 23 group 3), with a mean duration of follow-up of 40 months (range 6–120 months). Overall, although baseline findings were substantially similar in the three groups of patients, a greater proportion of group 3 paced patients tended to be asymptomatic during follow-up compared to the other groups (group 1, 7/13 [54%]; group 2, 15/20 [75%]; group 3, 16/23 [80%]). Furthermore, dual chamber pacing was effective in 9/9 cardioinhibitory patients and 2/3 vasodepressor patients, while VVI pacing was effective in 8/10 of the former and 0/1 of the latter. Therefore, since most physicians find chronic anticholinergic drug therapy to be impractical in these patients due to side effects, findings in this study support the utility of cardiac pacing for prevention of symptom recurrences in CSS patients. On the other hand, the applicability of the study is limited by its retrospective nature, and the probability that thorough electrophysiologic assessment and tilt-table testing for identification of other causes of syncope were not routinely performed during the 1974–1983 time period encompassed by the patient population.

The report by Morley et al.[12] provides one of the most detailed assessments of the efficacy of cardiac pacing and the impact of mode selection in CSS patients, and established the model for subsequent studies of this issue. Seventy paced CSS patients (50 men, 20 women, mean age 68 years) were followed for a mean of 18 months after pacemaker implantation. A positive carotid sinus massage in these patients was defined as asystole (62 patients) or complete AV block (8 patients) exceeding 3 seconds' duration. Permanent cardiac pacing was based on symptom suppression during carotid sinus massage in the presence of temporary ventricular pacing. During subsequent follow-up of mean duration 18 months, 89% of patients were rendered asymptomatic by cardiac pacing. However, as is noted below, several patients required pacing mode and/ or device changes in order to achieve this excellent result.

The benefits of cardiac pacing in CSS are also evident from the report by Blanc et al.,[15] which details treatment and follow-up in 54 patients. Thirty-three patients (group 1) were initially untreated, while 21 patients (group 2) were treated with cardiac pacemakers. During follow-up, 58% of group 1 patients had syncope recurrences by 5 years, while only one patient in group 2 had symptom recurrence. Over a 10-year period in our own laboratory, detailed clinical and electrophysiologic studies resulted in a diagnosis of CSS in 13 patients with recurrent syncope. Two patients with end-stage malignancies were treated medically (ephedrine) and remained asymptomatic until succumbing to their underlying disease at 5 months and 16 months, respectively. Two other patients were also initially treated with ephedrine alone. However, despite initial apparent symptom suppression, both ultimately required cardiac pacing due to syncope recurrence. They have since remained asymptomatic for more than 5 years. One patient refused all therapy, and continues to experience dizzy spells, but has used conservative measures (avoidance of tight collars, rapid neck movements, etc.) to avert frank syncope. The remaining eight patients underwent pacemaker implantation (in conjunction with ephedrine therapy in four individuals) and have been without syncope recurrence for more than 5 years. Thus cardiac pacing alone (six patients, dual chamber pacing in all but one patient with chronic atrial fibrillation) or in conjunction with ephedrine (four patients) has been highly effective in all 10 individuals treated, with complete prevention of symptom recurrences during 5 years of follow-up.

Optimal Pacing Mode Selection for Carotid Sinus Syndrome

The overall value of implantable cardiac pacemakers for symptom relief in CSS patients appears to be well established. However, the optimal pacing mode for such patients often remains a source of debate.

In the study referred to earlier by Morley et al.,[12] the impact of pacing mode on efficacy of pacemaker therapy in CSS patients was carefully assessed. Among this study's most important conclusions is the now well-accepted fact that single chamber atrial pacing (AAI or AAIR) is contraindicated in CSS patients due to their high incidence of paroxysmal AV block. Additionally, the findings revealed that among patients initially paced in the VVI mode (55 patients) or later converted to the VVI mode, even if transiently (two patients), symptoms persisted in 10/57 (18%). Among patients originally paced in a dual chamber mode (seven patients) or later converted to dual chamber pacing (nine patients), two (2/16, 13%) remained symptomatic. Thus, while residual symptoms may not have clearly differed between single chamber and dual chamber modes in this study (the frequency and/or severity of symptoms was not addressed), there appeared to be a trend in favor of dual chamber pacing.

In a further analysis designed to clarify the basis for persistence of symptoms in some patients, Morley et al.[12] evaluated hemodynamic responses during carotid sinus massage using intra-arterial pressure monitoring and 40° head-up tilt. Findings in three groups of individuals were reported. Group 1 included 12 CSS patients with persistent symptoms despite ventricular pacing; group 2 included 14 CSS patients who were asymptomatic after ventricular pacing; group 3 was made up of 11 non-CSS patients who were undergoing evaluation for dizziness or syncope. As summarized in Figure 1,[12] the vasodepressor response was greater in CSS patients (groups 1 and 2) than in non-CSS patients (group 3), and was significantly greater in CSS patients with persistent symptoms (group 1) than in group 2 patients. Additionally, ventricular "pacing effect" (i.e., susceptibility to induction of clinically significant hypotension by ventricular pacing alone) was greater in patients with persistent symptoms (group 1) than in the others. Consequently, careful assessment of individual hemodynamic responses during carotid sinus massage, during ventricular pacing, and during both together should be an integral part of the evaluation of all CSS patients.

Others have also assessed the utility of hemodynamic evaluation prior to selection of pacing mode in CSS patients.[18,20–23] For instance, Brignole et al.[20] evaluated pacing therapy prospectively in 60 consecutive CSS patients presenting with syncope or presyncope. Dual chamber pacing was selected in 26 patients based on findings of: (1) cardioinhibitory CSS with symptomatic "pacemaker effect," (2) mixed type CSS with VA conduction or orthostatic hypotension, or (3) presence of severe sinus bradycardia. VVI pacing was selected in the remaining 34 patients. During follow-up (the duration of which averaged 1 year), only two patients experienced syncope or presyncope recurrence (one in each group) for

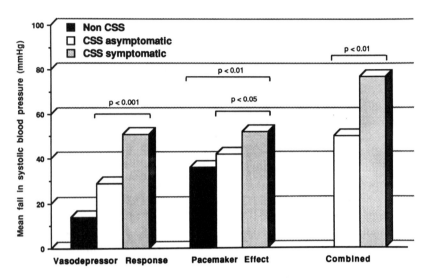

Figure 1. Histograms modified after Morley et al.[12] illustrating results of arterial pressure studies in three groups of patients (non-CSS group [n = 11], CSS-asymptomatic group [n = 14], CSS-symptomatic group [n = 12]). The ordinate indicates the mean fall of systemic pressure in each group associated with the vasodepressor response alone (left), "pacemaker effect" alone (middle), or both together (right). It is apparent that those CSS patients who remained symptomatic despite pacing showed both the most prominent vasodepressor and pacemaker effects. See text for further discussion.

an overall symptom suppression of 97% (58/60 patients). Minor symptoms did recur in approximately 35% of patients in each group. To further assess the accuracy of their selection criteria for dual chamber pacing in CSS patients, the authors introduced crossover periods in which patients with dual chamber pacemakers were paced for 2 months in the VVI mode. The VVI period resulted in significant worsening of symptoms in these individuals compared to dual chamber pacing (syncope recurrence in 8% vs. 0%; presyncope 31% vs. 0%; minor symptoms 58% vs. 31%; cardiac failure 19% vs. 0%). Consequently, careful selection of pacing mode based on hemodynamic findings was extremely useful in this set of patients, permitting the effective use of VVI pacing in 57% of patients and identifying the need for dual chamber systems in the remainder.

Deschamps et al.[22] also examined efficacy of VVI pacing in CSS patients in an attempt to define those individuals in whom it is adequate, and clarify the setting in which dual chamber pacing is recommended. Twenty-seven symptomatic CSS patients comprised the study group. During an average follow-up of 34 months, 3/27 (11%) VVI paced patients remained symptomatic. One of the latter three cases had a significant vasodepressor response, a second had marked "pacemaker effect," while the third was not characterized. Similarly, Stryjer et al.[17] observed satisfactory clinical response to VVI pacing in patients with "pure" cardioinhibitory CSS (defined as <25 mm Hg drop in arterial pressure with carotid sinus massage in the presence of cardiac pacing). Follow-up of 20 patients for 2 to 54 months was unassociated with symptom recurrence in this select set of patients. Nonetheless, the authors go on to state that "in patients with mixed forms of carotid sinus syncope . . . VVI mode . . . may indeed be accompanied by a symptomatic fall in blood pressure and cardiac output, and dual chamber pacing should be considered."

Other reports emphasize the potential clinical utility of selecting dual chamber pacing modes for CSS patients. For example, Madigan et al.[14] examined hemodynamic responses in both supine and upright posture during DVI and VVI pacing in CSS patients. Patients selected for this study were those having a history of dizziness or syncope, and evidence during carotid sinus massage of a pause of 3 seconds or longer. Eleven patients met these criteria (mean age 65.4 years). All patients had dual chamber pacemakers implanted which could be programmed to VVI mode. An AV interval of 150 ms was chosen for testing in the dual chamber mode, and the pacing rate was set to just above the patient's native heart rate. Thus, five patients were studied at 70 beats/min, four at 60 beats/min, and two at 50 beats/min. Eight of the 11 patients exhibited predominantly a cardioinhibitory form of CSS (vasodepressor response <30 mm Hg), while the remaining three patients had a "mixed" form. Findings revealed a clear-cut hemodynamic advantage for the dual chamber mode during carotid sinus massage in terms of both diminishing the magnitude and rate of blood pressure fall as well as the extent of symptoms induced. The latter findings were especially evident when testing was conducted with the patient in the upright posture (Fig. 2). Similarly, Morley et al.[13] examined long-term efficacy of dual chamber and single chamber pacing modes in 21 CSS patients using a double-blind crossover method (6 weeks in each pacing mode). Daily symptoms were recorded by each patient during follow-up. Six patients could not

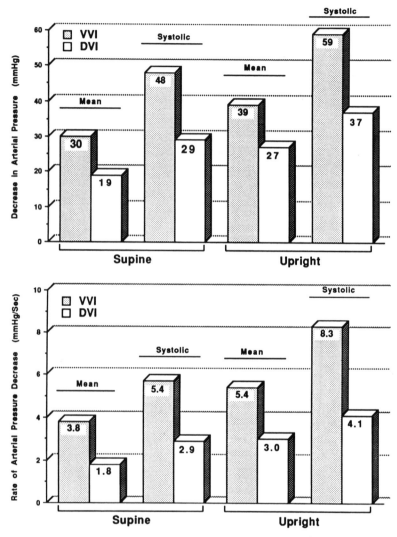

Figure 2. Data adapted from the report by Madigan et al.[14] See text for discussion. Top panel: Histograms comparing the magnitude of the fall of arterial pressure (systolic and mean values) associated with carotid sinus massage during VVI and DVI pacing. Findings with patients in the supine posture are shown at left, while those obtained with patients upright are provided on the right. Bottom panel: The format is the same as the top panel. In this case the rate of fall of arterial pressure is indicated on the abscissa for each of the two pacing modes (DVI, VVI).

tolerate the change from dual chamber to single chamber pacing and were removed from the study (all six exhibited pacemaker syndrome associated with 1:1 VA conduction). Among the remaining 15 patients, there was no apparent difference in terms of symptom frequency between the two pacing modes. However, there was a clear-cut overall patient preference for the dual chamber mode (62% preferred dual chamber, 38% reported no preference, and none favored single chamber pacing). The only factor that correlated with patient preference was the presence of VA conduction in 13/13 (100%) patients preferring dual chamber pacing versus 3/8 (38%) of those individuals with no preference.

In summary, single chamber ventricular pacing has proved effective for treatment of selected CSS patients. Typically, these have been the individuals with predominantly "cardioinhibitory" CSS in whom hemodynamic studies show no evidence of hypotension induced by ventricular pacing (i.e., minimal so-called ventricular "pacing effect"). On the other hand, dual chamber pacing appears to be more effective than ventricular pacing in "mixed" CSS (i.e., clinically significant cardioinhibitory and vasodepressor components) and in patients with more severe ventricular "pacing effect." Our own experience tends to support these conclusions, with the additional proviso that low-dose ephedrine (or similar vasoconstrictor) may be needed in patients with a critical vasoactive contribution to their hypertension.

Cardiac Pacing in Neurally Mediated ("Vasovagal") Syncope

Currently, cardiac pacing plays a much smaller role in treatment of individuals susceptible to so-called vasovagal syncope than it does in CSS patients. In fact, for the most part, the literature contains only occasional case reports describing the use of pacemakers for treatment of patients with this syndrome.[24–26] In our own experience, cardiac pacing has been utilized (in conjunction with pharmacologic treatment) in only two individuals out of more than 150 cases of vasovagal syncope evaluated by tilt-table testing during the past 5 years. Furthermore, in two other patients in whom pacemakers were placed prior to referral (both VVI mode), symptoms recurred despite pacing.[9]

A number of factors may account for the relative infrequency with which cardiac pacing is utilized in vasovagal syncope. First patients with recurrent vasovagal symptoms tend to be younger than their CSS counterparts; consequently, there is a reasonable reluctance among physicians to recommend implantable devices. Second, despite occasional reports to the contrary,[9,27] vasovagal syncope is generally accorded a benign prognosis, while symptomatic CSS is associated with greater potential for physical injury among frail elderly patients. Third, recent clinical studies employing upright tilt-table testing techniques have substantiated both the importance of vasodilation in most patients with vasovagal syncope and the inability of conventional pacing techniques alone to reverse symptomatic hypotension. On the other hand, a number of recent studies have demonstrated the effectiveness of pharmacologic interventions in such cases.[8,28,29] Finally, unlike the case with CSS patients, there has been little in the way of published reports with follow-up attesting to the benefits of cardiac pacing in vasovagal syncope.

Recently, Fitzpatrick et al.[26] highlighted the limitations of single chamber ventricular pacing in two patients who originally received devices in an attempt to prevent recurrent syncope of unknown origin. Symptoms recurred in both patients, and subsequent tilt-table testing revealed neurally mediated hypotension-bradycardia which was actually aggravated by onset of ventricular pacing. Both pacing systems were then converted to dual chamber (DDI mode with 50/80 hysteresis). Following this change, one patient became asymptomatic and one continued to experience symptoms. More recently, these same investigators[30] reported results of the hemodynamic assessment of dual chamber pacing with 50/90 rate hysteresis in seven patients with recurrent syncope who underwent paired tilt-table testing, and in whom vasovagal reactions occurred on the two successive days. Findings revealed that pacing was beneficial. In five patients, syncope was prevented despite evident onset of a vasovagal reaction as attested to by both hemodynamic recordings and development of sufficient bradycardia to initiate pacing. Two other patients remained as symptomatic as they had been during the baseline tilt test. The duration of tilt tolerated following onset of vasovagal reactions was extended by pacing (unpaced, 0.9 ± 1.2 min vs. paced 3.2 ± 1.6 min, $p < 0.01$). Nonetheless, while pacing may have prevented sudden hemodynamic collapse, eventually marked hypotension did occur despite pacing (mean arterial pressure at 3 minutes following onset of pacing, 41 ± 6 mm Hg).

The reports by Fitzpatrick et al.[26,30] provide important insight into the usefulness and limitations of cardiac pacing for patients with severe recurrent vasovagal syncope. It seems clear that, at present, pacing can only be employed in those individuals in whom onset of a vasovagal reaction is marked by substantial bradycardia (bearing in mind that many susceptible patients exhibit only a "relative" bradycardia with heart rates never falling into a slow enough range to trigger conventional rate detection algorithms). Therefore, careful evaluation is an essential requirement if an implantable pacing system is contemplated. Furthermore, the choice should be restricted to dual chamber systems with "vasovagal" hysteresis capability (long cycle length, onset rapid continuous pacing, search function for termination). Unfortunately, such systems are not yet widely available. Ultimately, hemodynamic sensors may prove helpful for both establishing the need for pacing onset and determining the appropriate time to discontinue pacing and revert to native rhythm.

Conclusion

Cardiac pacing has a clearly established role in treatment of those patients with symptomatic hypersensitive CSS in whom bradycardia can be clearly demonstrated to participate in the clinical picture. Given the reasonable goals of avoiding premature pacing system replacement or unnecessary "upgrades" during follow-up, all CSS patients should undergo careful hemodynamic assessment in both the supine and the upright postures. In those instances where findings support a truly pure cardioinhibitory form (i.e., those rare cases where no vasodepressor element is evident) or where the vasodepressor component is minimal even with the patient in the upright posture (i.e., <25 mm Hg fall in systolic pressure), and where the ventricular "pacing effect" is similarly minimal, single chamber ventricular pacing may be sufficient. However, where hemodynamic testing results are equivocal or lack reproducibility, or where prominent vasodepressor components or "pacemaker effect" coexist with demonstrable bradycardia, dual chamber pacing (optimally DDDR mode with rate hysteresis) would be the prudent pacing mode choice.

In patients with recurrent vasovagal syncope, cardiac pacing is only rarely indicated. Currently, there is no evidence to suggest that even those individuals with long asystolic pauses should be paced. However, although substantial device development is needed before an optimal pacing solution is available, device therapy may become quite helpful for those individuals who fail, cannot tolerate, or do not wish to consider pharmacologic management.

Acknowledgment: The authors wish to thank Renee Maugh and Barry L.S. Detloff for valuable technical assistance, and Stephanie Wiebke and Wendy Markuson for preparation of the manuscript.

References

1. Weiss S, Baker JR. The carotid sinus reflex in health and disease: its role in the causation of fainting and convulsions. Medicine 1933;12:297–354.
2. Lown B, Levine SA. The carotid sinus: clinical value of its stimulation. Circulation 1961;23:766–789.
3. Sugrue DD, Wood DL, McGoon MD. Carotid sinus hypersensitivity and syncope. Mayo Clin Proc 1984;59:637–640.
4. Brown KA, Maloney JD, Smith HC, Hartzler GO, Ilstrup DM. Carotid sinus reflex in patients undergoing coronary angiography: relationships of degree and location of coronary artery disease in response to carotid sinus massage. Circulation 1980;62:697–703.
5. Sugrue DD, Gersh BJ, Holmes DR, Wood DL, Osborn MJ, Hammill SC. Symptomatic "isolated" carotid sinus hypersensitivity: natural history and results of treatment with anticholinergic drugs or pacemaker. J Am Coll Cardiol 1986;7:158–162.
6. Almquist A, Gornick C, Benson DW Jr, Dunnigan A, Benditt DG. Carotid sinus hypersensitivity: evaluation of the vasodepressor component. Circulation 1985;71:927–936.
7. Strasberg B, Sagie A, Erdman S, Kusniec J, Sclarovsky S, Agmon J. Carotid sinus hypersensitivity and carotid sinus syndrome. Prog Cardiovasc Dis 1989;31:379–391.
8. Almquist A, Goldenberg IF, Milstein S, Chen M-Y, Chen X-C, Hansen R, Gornick CC, Benditt DG. Provocation of bradycardia and hypotension by isoproterenol and upright posture in patients with unexplained syncope. N Engl J Med 1989;320:346–351.
9. Milstein S, Buetikofer J, Lesser J, Goldenberg IF, Benditt DG, Gornick CC, Reyes WJ. Cardiac asystole: a manifestation of neurally mediated hypotension bradycardia. J Am Coll Cardiol 1989;14:1626–1632.
10. Grubb BP, Gerard G, Roush K, Temesy-Armos P, Elliott L, Hahn H, Spann C. Differentiation of convulsive syncope and epilepsy with head-up tilt testing. Ann Intern Med 1991;115:871–876.
11. Benditt DG, Remole S, Bailin S, Dunnigan A, Asso A, Milstein S. Tilt-table testing for evaluation of neurally-mediated (cardioneurogenic) syncope: rationale and proposedprotocols. PACE 1991;14:1–10.
12. Morley CA, Perrins EJ, Grant P, Chan SL, McBrien DJ, Sutton R. Carotid sinus syncope treated by pacing. Analysis of persistent symptoms and role of atrioventricular sequential pacing. Br Heart J 1982;47:411–418.

13. Morley CA, Perrins EJ, Chan SL, Sutton R. Long-term comparison of DVI and VVI pacing in carotid sinus syndrome. In: Steinbach K (ed). Cardiac Pacing. Proceedings of the VIIth World Symposium on Cardiac Pacing, Steinkopff Verlag, Darmstadt, 1983, pp 929–935.
14. Madigan NP, Flaker GC, Curtis JJ, Reid J, Mueller KJ, Murphy TJ. Carotid sinus hypersensitivity: beneficial effects of dual-chamber pacing. Am J Cardiol 1984;53:1034–1040.
15. Blanc JJ, Boschat J, Penther PH. Hypersensibilité sino-carotidienne. Evolution a moyen terme en fonction du traitment et des symptomes. Arch Mal Coeur 1984;77:330–335.
16. Peretz DI, Abdulla A. Management of cardioinhibitory hypersensitive carotid sinus syncope with permanent cardiac pacing: a seventeen year prospective study. Can J Cardiol 1985;2:86–91.
17. Stryjer D, Friedensohn A, Schlesinger Z. Ventricular pacing as the preferable mode for long-term pacing in patients with carotid sinus syncope of the cardioinhibitory type. PACE 1986;9:705–709.
18. Brignole M, Sartore B, Barra M, Menozzi C, Lolli G. Is DDD superior to VVI pacing in mixed carotid sinus syndrome? An acute and medium-term study. PACE 1988;11:1902–1910.
19. Brignole M, Menozzi C, Lolli G, Sartore B, Barra M. Natural and unnatural history of patients with severe carotid sinus hypersensitivity: a preliminary study. PACE 1988;11:1628–1635.
20. Brignole M, Sartore B, Barra M, Menozzi C, Lolli G. Ventricular and dual chamber pacing for treatment of carotid sinus syndrome. PACE 1989;12: 582–590.
21. Brignole M, Menozzi C, Lolli G, Oddone D, Gianfranchi L, Bertulla A. Pacing for carotid sinus syndrome and sick sinus syndrome. PACE 1990;13: 2071–2075.
22. Deschamps D, Richard A, Citron B, Chaperon A, Binon JP, Ponsonaille J. Hypersensibilité sino-carotidienne. Evolution a moyen et a long terme des patients traites par stimulation ventriculaire. Arch mal Coeur 1990;83:63–67.
23. Brignole M, Menozzi C, Lolli G, Oddone D, Gianfranchi L, Bertulla A. Validation of a method for choice of pacing mode in carotid sinus syndrome with or without sinus bradycardia. PACE 1991;14:196–203.
24. Sapire DW, Casta A. Safley W, O'Riordan AC, et al. Vasovagal syncope in children requiring pacemaker implantation. Am Heart J 1983;106:1406–1411.
25. Kus T, La Londe G, de Champlain J, Shenasa M. Vasovagal syncope: management with atrioventricular sequential pacing and beta-blockade. Can J Cardiol 1989;5:375–378.
26. Fitzpatrick AP, Travill CM, Vardas PE, Hubbard WN, Wood A, Ingram A, Sutton R. Recurrent symptoms after ventricular pacing in unexplained syncope. PACE 1990;13:619–624.
27. Engel GL. Psychologic stress, vasodepressor (vasovagal) syncope and sudden death. Ann Intern Med 1978;89:403–412.

28. Grubb BP, Temesy-Aromos P, Hahn H, Elliott L. Utility of upright tilt-table testing in the evaluation and management of syncope of unknown origin. Am J Med 1991;90:6–10.
29. Sra JS, Anderson AF, Sheikh SH, Avitall B, Tchou PJ, Troup PJ, Gilbert CJ, Akhtar M. Unexplained syncope evaluated by electrophysiologic studies and head-up tilt testing. Ann Intern Med 1991;114:1013–1019.
30. Fitzpatrick A, Theodorakis G, Ahmed R, Williams T, Sutton R. Dual chamber pacing aborts vasovagal syncope induced by head-up 600 tilt. PACE 1991;13;13–19.

Chapter 3

Lead Extraction: Techniques and Indications

Charles L. Byrd, Susan J. Schwartz,

Nancy B. Hedin

Introduction

Extraction of chronically implanted pacemaker (and now defibrillator) leads has become a more frequent and demanding task. The challenge is to safely free the lead from scar tissue that encases the electrode at the fixation site and entraps the lead body against the vein and heart wall. Many techniques for lead extraction have been employed and reported in the literature. The primary limitation of all extraction techniques is the risk of a cardiovascular accident associated with the force required to free the lead from the scar tissue. Initially, the only options for removing an incarcerated lead were traction or a major cardiac surgical procedure. Traction was sometimes successful but significant complications were reported. Cardiac surgery is successful, but has high associated risk and morbidity and is not always an option for the ill, elderly patient. The intravascular techniques described in this chapter were devised in an attempt to develop one technique applicable to all patients, with all types of leads, and with a very low complication rate. Today, for the rare failures of intravascular countertraction, limited surgical techniques offer low morbidity alternatives. Consequently, the indications for lead extraction have expanded as the risks have diminished.

New Perspectives in Cardiac Pacing, Vol. 3, edited by S. Serge Barold and Jacques Mugica, Mount Kisco, NY, Futura Publishing Co., © 1993.

Why Leads Are Difficult to Extract

Leads are difficult to extract because of scar tissue formation at sites along the lead body and at the electrode.[1,2] Without scar tissue, extraction would not be an issue. It would be easy to overpower a chronically implanted, passive fixation device by the same manipulation and traction used during the initial implant. The same would be true for active fixation devices; counterclockwise rotation of the lead would release the fixation device and consistently allow uncomplicated lead removal.

In general, the increased difficulty in removing leads is attributed to the use of passive fixation devices, longer implant durations, and a greater number of leads being implanted per patient. Passive fixation devices (tines, fins, flanges, etc.) promote scar tissue at the electrode. Advances in pacemaker and lead technology have resulted in leads remaining functional and in situ for much longer periods of time. In addition, since more patients are receiving dual chamber pacing systems, more leads are being implanted.

Scar tissue formation is part of the maturation process. It seems to form at sites where physical stress is applied by the lead to the endothelial tissue within the vein and heart wall. Frequently, two leads contact the wall in close proximity and the scarring encompasses both leads. Scar tissue also forms at sites of traumatic tissue disruption, commonly found at venous introducer entry sites. Canine data show scar tissue in the same predictable points of contact as found clinically (Fig. 1A,B).[3] Lead properties such as stiffness and diameter seem to determine the magnitude of tissue injury and resultant scar tissue.

Scar tissue may be extensive enough to obliterate the venous channel. The tensile strength of scar tissue increases as it matures, initially by increasing the cross linkages of chemical bonds, and later by calcification. After 5 to 6 years, some of these areas begin to calcify, and after 8 to 10 years, circumferential bands of calcified tissue are frequently found. The most difficult leads to remove are those implanted for 8 years or longer. Leads implanted less than 1 year tend to be most easily removed.

Lead Extraction Techniques

Traction

Lead extraction techniques can be grouped into three categories: traction, intravascular countertraction, and cardiac surgery (Table 1).[4]

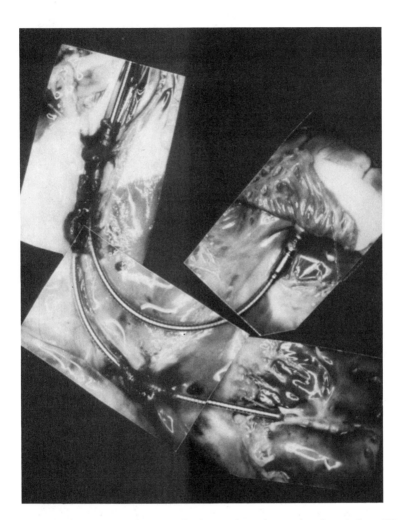

Figure 1A,B. Scar tissue. These leads, implanted in a dog for 42 days (A), and 365 days (B), show the formation of scar tissue at sections where the leads contact the endocardium. (Courtesy of Medtronic, Inc.)

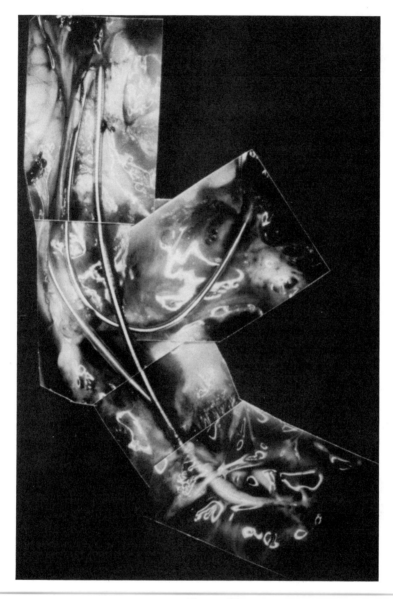

Figure 1B.

TABLE *1*
Techniques for Lead Extraction

Traction
    External traction – exerted on exteriorized portion of lead
        manual (pulling)
        sustained (weights, adhesive tape, etc.)
    Internal traction – exerted on device that has grasped lead inside ve-
        nous system
        manual (pulling on device)
        sustained (weights, etc.)
Intravascular Countertraction
    SVC approach (locking stylet and dilator sheaths)
    IVC approach (tip deflecting wire guide, Dotter basket, and sheaths)
Surgical Approaches
    Limited surgical approach
    Ventriculotomy
    Cardiopulmonary bypass

Traction, the act of exerting a pulling force, can be applied to the lead externally, or internally using a snare or catheter.[5-13] Frequently, a physician will pull on a lead to see if it can be removed without a more extensive procedure; this approach may be successful in the first few months after an implant, but should be abandoned promptly if significant resistance is met. Persistence may tear the vessel or heart or damage the lead, making subsequent traction attempts with other techniques more difficult. To exert traction on leads that have retracted into the venous system, a variety of internal traction techniques using snares, forceps, or other retrieval catheters have been reported. Even if the lead is accessible, some prefer internal traction because the traction is exerted closer to the heart. External or internal traction can also be sustained for longer periods of time (minutes to days), gradually increasing the force until the lead is freed.[14,15] With all traction methods, the force of traction needs to be enough to feel rhythmic tugging of the lead, but less than that which causes arrhythmias, hypotension, chest pain, or avulsion.

Traction, in general, is uncontrolled; the extraction force is diffused, with the weakest area giving first. The variables include duration of traction and magnitude of the tractional force. In the past, traction for extraction of leads that lacked passive fixation devices and were implanted for short periods of time (1 to 2 years) was frequently successful. However, following the introduction of passive fixation devices, traction has had limited success.[16,17] Reports of lead extractions using traction are typically limited to small series of patients (1 to 17). Complications include breaking the lead with subsequent migration,[18] myocardial avulsion,[19] avulsion of tricuspid valve leaflet,[20] myocardial rupture and tamponade,[21] and death.[22] In addition to these attendant complications, the lead may be damaged (distorted or broken), making further extraction attempts using other techniques more difficult. Also, if the traction pulls the ventricular wall to the tricuspid valve, it creates a low cardiac output; failure of the lead to return to its original position can cause a cardiovascular emergency. Therefore, a conscious effort should be made to ensure that all traction maneuvers are reversible.

Intravascular Countertraction

Intravascular countertraction techniques allow controlled and directed application of traction force to specific areas of scar tissue in the veins and heart. The goal is to break through the various areas of scar tissue restraining the lead without tearing vascular or cardiac structures. Countertraction is defined as traction on the lead and/or electrode countered by dilator sheaths advanced over the lead. Ideally, to extract a lead using the countertraction principle, the dilator sheaths are passed over the lead and close to the scar-encased electrode (approximately 1 cm from the heart wall) (Fig. 2). At this point, traction is applied to the lead. The force of the traction is contained within and countered by the circumference of the distal end of the dilator sheaths (Fig. 3). The electrode is pulled free from the scar tissue and into the sheaths; the heart wall falls away (Fig. 4). The lead and sheaths are then removed together, preventing the tip of the lead from attaching to the tricuspid valve or to the vein during its withdrawal. The traction force applied is primarily limited by the tensile strength of the lead. If the tensile strength of the scar tissue is greater than that of the lead, and if too much force is applied, the lead will break.

Since the extraction forces used are confined to a small area (the circumference of the sheaths), a second lead positioned next to the extracted lead can be left undisturbed. Leads implanted less than 1 week

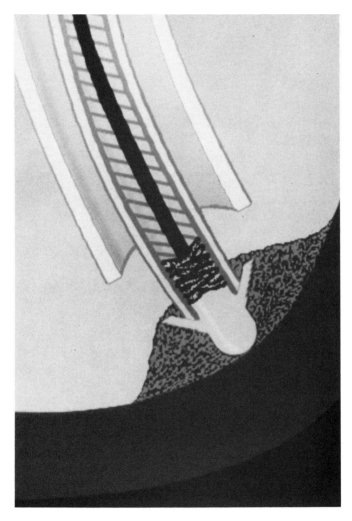

Figure 2. Preparing for countertraction at the electrode. After advancing sheaths through vascular scar tissue, the larger sheath is advanced as close to the electrode as possible (about 1 cm away from the myocardium). (Courtesy of Cook Pacemaker Corporation.)

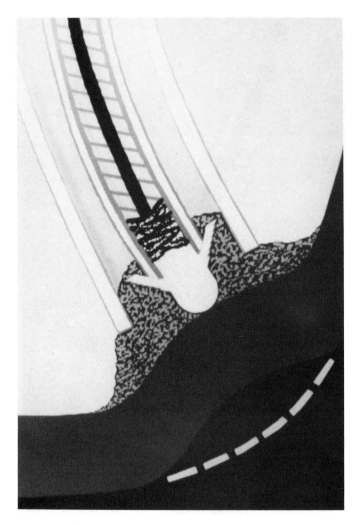

Figure 3. Countertraction. With the sheath held in place, traction is applied to the lead. The traction force is confined within the diameter of the sheath, which counters the traction and supports the myocardium to prevent invagination. The force is controlled and directed against the scar tissue. (Courtesy of Cook Pacemaker Corporation.)

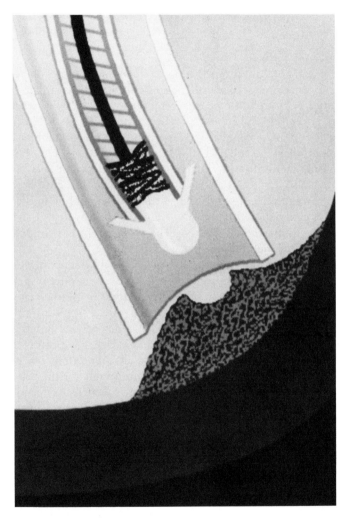

Figure 4. Results of countertraction. After the electrode has broken free from the scar tissue, the lead is removed through the sheaths. (Courtesy of Cook Pacemaker Corporation.)

have been left functioning and in position, during and after removing specific chronic leads.

General Preparation

The extractions are performed in an operating room equipped with fluoroscopy, pacing paraphernalia, and defibrillator. A cardiac surgery team should be on call in case of an emergency. The quality of the fluoroscopy is crucial, and its use is required throughout the entire procedure. It is extremely beneficial to have magnification capabilities. Monitoring equipment includes ECG, arterial blood pressure line, and fingertip oximeter. The anterior chest wall and the right and left groin are prepped and draped in a sterile fashion for simultaneous access. As additional precautions, a pericardiocentesis tray should be in the room, echocardiography should be readily available, and the patient should be typed and cross-matched for blood. The procedure is not simplistic and training in this technique is strongly advised.

Intravascular countertraction can be used with a superior vena cava (SVC) approach via the implantation vein, or with an inferior vena cava (IVC) approach.[23-27] A system of extraction tools is commercially available (Cook Pacemaker Corporation, Leechburg, PA). With either approach, the procedure can be performed under general anesthesia, or under local anesthesia with mild sedation. Initially, we routinely used local anesthesia; however, unless there is a contraindication, general anesthesia is now our preference. It is more comfortable for the patient and facilitates the procedure. In patients who were pacemaker-dependent and required all leads to be removed, an active fixation, temporary pacing lead must be implanted.

SVC Approach

The SVC approach is the initial approach when the leads are accessible in the subcutaneous tissue. The basic technique is to secure a locking stylet inside the conductor coil lumen of the lead and advance dilator sheaths over the lead.

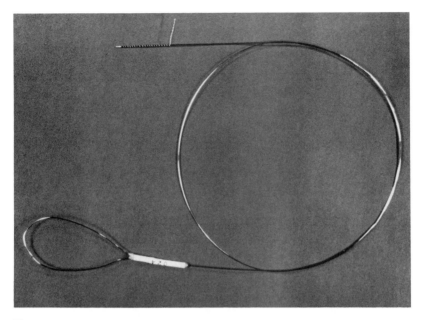

Figure 5.   The locking stylet. The locking stylet is a relatively stiff 60-cm wire with a loop handle and a fine wire wound clockwise and attached to the distal tip. The stylet is advanced to the tip of the lead, where the stylet is locked in place with counterclockwise rotation. (Courtesy of Cook Pacemaker Corporation.)

Locking Stylet: The purpose of the locking stylet (Fig. 5) is to reinforce the lead, to serve as a guide for the dilator sheaths, and to deliver extraction force to the tip of the lead. The appropriate locking stylet is selected by first exposing the coil lumen of the pacing lead and carefully sizing it using gauge pins.

Using fluoroscopy, the selected locking stylet is passed down the lead and locked as near to the electrode as possible. If the coil has been distorted to the degree that no locking stylet of any size can be advanced to the tip and locked, the stylet should be locked at the furthest possible point and used as a lead extender to facilitate sheath passage and traction. If the lead has been previously damaged to the extent that it precludes the use of the locking stylet, a large suture is secured near the proximal end of the lead and used as a lead extender. When the locking stylet cannot be passed to a site near the tip, leads have a much higher incidence of breaking. Once a lead begins to break, the SVC approach may have to be abandoned.

Management of Dilator Sheaths: Dilator sheaths are an integral part of the countertraction technique. These telescoping sheaths are used to break apart the scar tissue binding the lead to the vein wall, heart wall, and in some cases, one lead to another using countertraction principles. The telescoping sheaths may dilate the scar tissue, tear through it, and in some cases, strip the scar tissue from the vein or heart wall, actually pulling it into the sheaths. In the latter case, if the sheath's diameter is not large enough, a larger sheath capable of sliding over the circumferential band of scar tissue must be used.

Dilator sheaths are available in stainless steel and plastic. Stainless steel dilator sheaths are used to access the vein (Fig. 6). While maintaining tension on the locked stylet, two telescoping dilator sheaths (one inside the other) are passed over the lead. Fluoroscopic monitoring is essential during advancement and manipulation of the sheaths. Care must be taken to ensure that the sheaths follow the original lead path. Creating a new path with the sheaths can tear the venous structures. The first major area of scar tissue is generally found under the clavicle at the lead entrance into the vein. The scar tissue is dilated and/or ruptured by manipulating (advancing and twisting) the inner and outer sheaths in a telescoping rnanner. Once in the vein, the stainless steel sheaths are advanced no further than the first curvature in the vein (the level of the brachiocephalic vein).

After achieving venous entry, the stainless steel sheaths are interchanged with the more flexible telescoping plastic dilator sheaths (Fig. 7). Again, tension is maintained on the locking stylet at all times while advancing the sheaths, so that the sheaths follow the curvature of the lead within the venous system. The sheaths are passed down the lead through areas of scar tissue to a site near the electrode. At this point, countertraction is applied, and the lead and electrode are removed.

Maneuvering the smaller and larger sheaths in a telescoping manner is the most effective method of passing through the scar tissue. In maneuvering an acute turn, the smaller, more flexible sheath is advanced around the turn first, followed by the larger, stiffer sheath. In some cases,

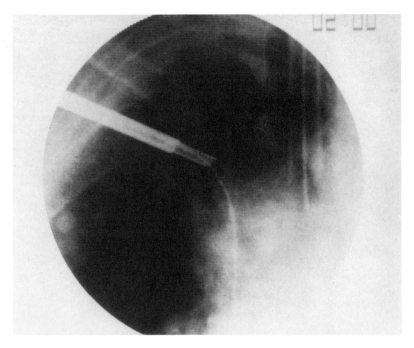

Figure 6. The SVC approach under fluoroscopic monitoring. While maintaining tension on the locked stylet, stainless steel dilators are advanced over the lead to break through scar tissue at the site of entry and access to the vein.

the smaller sheath can be first forced into the scar tissue and then the larger sheath is used to dilate or tear the scar tissue in a controlled fashion using the countertraction principle.

One critical aspect of this technique is "how hard to pull" on the lead (locking stylet) while advancing the sheaths. If insufficient traction is placed on the lead, the sheaths may not be sufficiently guided within the vein. If too much traction is placed on the lead, the method is no longer countertraction; it is reduced to direct traction with the attendant risks. In general, the traction should be adequate to support the maneuvering of the dilator sheaths and no more. This is the rationale for using the more supple Teflon sheaths. The stiffer the dilator sheaths, the more traction required and consequently, the greater the risk of tearing a vein or heart wall.

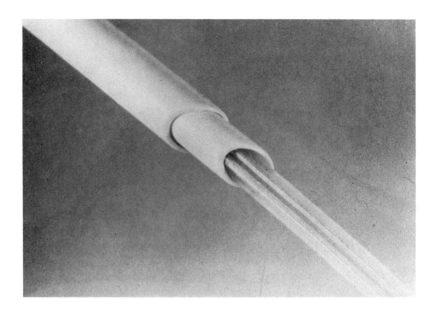

Figure 7. Plastic sheaths. After accessing the vein, the stainless steel sheaths are exchanged for flexible plastic sheaths made of radiopaque Teflon or poly- propylene. The suppleness of the Teflon sheaths permits advancement in areas with extreme curvature. While maintaining tension on the locked stylet, the sheaths are advanced in a telescoping manner. A single sheath provides more flexibility for advancing; the double layer provides the rigidity necessary to break through stubborn areas of scar tissue.

An old, large–diameter lead is sometimes encountered over which only one large sheath can be used. The advantages of telescoping are lost and the incidence of failure to pass through the scar tissue increases. Another cause for failure to pass through the scar tissue is the "snow plow" effect. In this situation, the scar tissue is peeled from the wall and pushed in front of the sheaths. Once sufficient bulk is formed, the sheaths cannot be advanced further. If the scar tissue is too severe to advance the dilator sheaths safely, if the lead breaks during attempted extraction, or if the lead is inaccessible via the SVC approach, removal via the IVC approach is indicated.

IVC Approach: Although the equipment is different, in principle, the IVC approach is similar to the SVC approach. A workstation is inserted into a femoral vein. The workstation consists of a 16F Teflon sheath with a check-flow valve at the proximal end and supplied with two inserts. One is a tapered dilator for inserting the workstation. The other is an 11F dilator sheath that allows the workstation to be manipulated in a telescoping fashion as described above. After inserting an 18-gauge needle into a femoral vein, a guidewire is passed into the right atrium. Usually the femoral vein is cannulated on the side the leads were placed; however, the right side tends to be a less circuitous route. Fluoroscopy is used throughout. The workstation with the tapered dilator inserted is passed over the guidewire and into the atrium. The tapered dilator is removed and the 11F sheath is inserted. A Dotter wire basket snare and a tip-deflecting wire guide are passed through the sheaths (Fig. 8). The workstation protects the veins during insertion and manipulation of the snares. The tip-deflecting wire guide is advanced and manipulated to hook the lead and position it for entanglement in the more substantial Dotter wire basket snare. Once grasped by the snare, the lead is pulled into the sheaths and the sheaths are advanced over the lead to apply countertraction. Once the electrode has been freed from the embedding scar tissue, the lead is withdrawn inside the sheaths and removed. For multiple lead extractions,

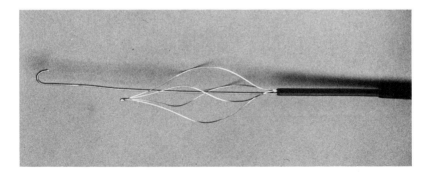

Figure 8. Equipment for the IVC approach. The tip-deflecting wire guide is hooked around the lead and used to position the lead for snaring by the more powerful Dotter basket. The sheaths are then advanced toward the electrode to provide countertraction. (Courtesy of Cook Pacemaker Corporation.)

the outer sheath generally remains in place until all leads have been extracted.

It is important upon removing the sheaths from the femoral vein to ensure no debris has been left behind. Any debris such as clot or scar tissue left in the femoral or iliac veins could serve as a nidus for thrombus formation. Aspiration of blood during withdrawal of the sheaths and the presence of hemorrhage from the puncture site requiring pressure to control is probably sufficient to ensure that no debris has been left behind. If the puncture site does not hemorrhage, the femoral vein should be explored.

Clinical Results Using Intravascular Countertraction

Development of intravascular countertraction techniques began in 1984.[28] Today, the techniques are well-established and specialized equipment for the procedure is commercially available. Our experience using these techniques illustrates the success of intravascular countertraction, the rare conditions under which the technique is not sufficient, and the type of complications that may be encountered. A national database of multicenter results established in 1988 allows further analysis of the intravascular techniques.[29]

Byrd Database: Our database includes 264 patients, 63% male, with an average age of 66 years (range 10 to 97 years). For the procedures performed prior to the development of the locking stylet (94), a ligature was tied to the lead as previously described. Of the 481 leads, 63% of the leads were originally positioned in the ventricle and 37% were in the atrium. The primary indications for lead extraction are listed in Table 2.

An SVC approach was used for 72%, an IVC approach for 10%, and an SVC approach followed by an IVC approach for 18%. Of 481 leads, 99% were removed using intravascular countertraction. Of these, 9% were removed except for the distal tip, which remained embedded in the scar tissue.

In all but two patients with retained tips, no problems subsequently developed. In one patient with endocarditis, the lead broke during extraction, leaving a 3-cm length embedded in the ventricle. A ventriculotomy was performed to extract the remaining portion. In one patient

TABLE *2*

Indications for Intravascular Lead Extraction, Clinical Experience

Indications	Byrd Database 264 Patients (%)	Multicenter Database 630 Patients (%)
Lead replacement	25.8	38.5
Infection	24.6	34.1
Septicemia/endocarditis	21.6	11.3
Erosion	7.6	5.2
Pain	5.7	2.1
Pre-erosion	4.5	2.4
Chronic draining sinus	4.5	1.5
Free-floating or migrating lead	2.6	1.8
Thrombosis	0.8	0.3
Tricuspid regurgitation	0.0	0.3
Other	2.3	2.2

with septicemia, the lead broke during extraction, leaving a 5-cm length embedded in scar tissue; 5 months later septicemia recurred and the remaining section was removed through a ventriculotomy.

Five leads (in four patients) were not removed with intravascular countertraction. In two patients (three leads), leads could not be removed with intravascular countertraction because of the extent of scar tissue engulfing the leads. In the first of these patients, the lead was removed with the limited surgical approach. In the latter, the leads were removed with transatrial countertraction. There were two failures because a complication occurred before lead extraction was accomplished.

There were five major complications (1.9%). One patient died from pulmonary embolism immediately following lead extraction; this septic patient had recently recovered from a pulmonary embolism, coma, and dissemination. A second patient died 3 days postoperatively from pulmonary embolism. In one patient, an evolving tamponade occurred when the atrium was torn by calcified tissue engulfing the lead. A sternotomy was performed, and the laceration, extending from the IVC onto the inferior portion of the right atrium, was repaired with a running suture. In the remaining two patients, the tears resulted from persisting beyond the point of known safety. In one patient with right mediastinal shift following a lobectomy 1 month prior to lead extraction, blood pressure dropped quickly after the final lead was removed; a small hole at the junction of the brachiocephalic vein and the SVC was repaired. In one patient with endocarditis, the lead broke, leaving bare wire and a small piece of infected insulation due to a small tear at the junction of the IVC and right atrium. Using the IVC approach, the bare wire cut the sheaths and the patient became hypotensive with tachycardia. A median sternotomy was performed to repair a small tear at the junction of the IVC and right atrium (one suture) and to complete extraction through a ventriculotomy.

Each of the patients with a tear had an emergency median sternotomy and a direct closure of the tear. The last patient had, in addition, the impacted infected lead removed through a ventriculotomy.

National Multicenter Database: As of February, 1992, the multicenter database contained data for intravascular lead extractions at 121 participating institutions; nine physicians had performed more than 10 procedures. Extraction of 1055 leads from 630 patients was attempted. The average patient age was 65 years (range 8 to 95 years). The indications are shown in Table 2.

Of the 1055 leads, 31% were initially placed in the atrium and 69% in the ventricle. The leads had been implanted for an average of 57 months (range 0.2 to 264 months). The fixation mechanisms were passive for 71%, active for 23% (helix), and 6% had either no fixation device or no fixation mechanism specified.

The SVC approach was used for 85%, the IVC approach for 5%, and the SVC approach followed by the IVC approach for 10%. Of the 1055 leads, 85% were completely extracted, 8% were extracted except for the distal tip, and 7% were not extracted. For 70% of the leads that were not extracted, the IVC approach was not tried. Major complications (hemothorax, tamponade, pulmonary embolism) occurred in 2%, with 0.5% death. Multivariate analysis has shown that success is higher for bipolar leads, higher for active fixation leads, higher for shorter implant durations, and higher for more experienced physicians.[30]

Comparison of the Databases: One hundred seventy of the Byrd patients are included in both the Byrd and multicenter national databases.

Ninety-four of our patients had leads extracted before the multicenter database was established. The Byrd database encompasses all of our extractions including the early attempts that utilized a wide variety of equipment and approaches. With time and experience, our techniques and equipment evolved and became more sophisticated. As expected, this is reflected in the trend of our success rate. Although the multicenter national database contains a significant number of our patients, it is influenced by the learning curves of each extraction center. Other differences in the two patient populations include our greater utilization of the IVC approach, our more aggressive approach due to our more extensive experience, and the fact that our patients tend to be sicker, have older leads, more leads, and/or leads that have been damaged by previous extraction attempts.

Ancillary Surgical Procedures

Transatrial Countertraction

In 1985, the limited surgical approach was first described for extracting chronic pacing leads not removable by early transvenous traction techniques.[31] It is a low morbidity surgical approach designed to avoid the more extensive thoracotomy and median sternotomy. Due to the success of intravascular countertraction techniques, extraction of leads by the limited surgical approach is now limited to special circumstances. Examples are patients requiring lead extraction secondary to superior vena cava syndrome in whom a new system is to be implanted transatrially or a failure of the intravascular countertraction technique.[32,33]

Under general endotracheal anesthesia, the skin is prepped and draped in a sterile fashion. A small incision is made over the 3rd or 4th costochondral cartilage. The decision on which cartilage bed to enter is made after viewing the heart under fluoroscopy. The incision is carried through the subcutaneous tissue, separating the muscle and exposing the perichondrium. The cartilage is removed, the pleura reflected, and the pericardium opened and suspended to the subcutaneous tissue. If an atrial lead is to be removed, a purse-string suture is placed around the implant site in the atrium. An atriotomy incision is made, the electrode grasped, and the entire lead removed retrogradely. To remove a ventricular lead, a tip-deflecting wire guide is passed through the purse-string suture into

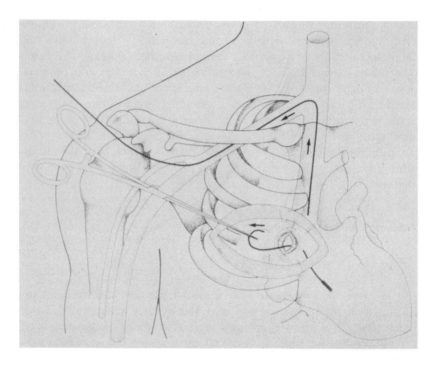

Figure 9.   Transatrial countertraction. An atriotomy incision is made. For an atrial lead, the entire lead is removed retrogradely. For a ventricular lead, the lead is pulled up to the purse-string using a tip-deflecting wire guide, grasped, and transected. The proximal end is removed retrogradely. A locking stylet is inserted into the remaining distal portion of the lead, which is then removed using countertraction techniques.

the right atrium, encircling the lead. The lead is pulled up into the purse-string, grasped with a clamp, and transected. The proximal end is pulled out retrogradely (Fig. 9). A locking stylet is inserted into the remaining portion of the lead and the distal end removed using countertraction techniques.

This transatrial countertraction technique may be the approach of choice when a transatrial implant is indicated.[32] A primary advantage of the transatrial implant technique (over an epicardial approach) is that it allows implantation of state-of-the-art bipolar pacing systems. With epicardial approaches, one is limited to the use of large, unipolar epicardial leads, pacemakers with large connector blocks, and abdominal positioning of the pacemaker.

Ventriculotomy

A right ventriculotomy is the only current method of removing infected lead segments impacted in the ventricle that are not removable using intravascular or transatrial countertraction techniques.[34] The procedure requires a median sternotomy and a small cardiomyotomy via a purse-string suture in the myocardium over the electrode. The tip of the electrode is located by palpation, triangulation using 26-gauge needles, and fluoroscopy. A purse-string suture is placed over the electrode tip, and the lead is grasped and extracted retrogradely through a small stab wound.

Cardiopulmonary Bypass

Today, the only indication for cardiopulmonary bypass to remove leads is when the patient needs a cardiac procedure for other reasons; the lead can be removed at the same time.[21,35,36] This offers the clearest operative field with the widest exposure. Dissection of points of lead entrapment is performed under direct vision, and the risk of myocardial or valvular damage is minimized.

Management of Inflammatory Tissue

To reduce patients' morbidity and exposure to antibiotic therapy, infected tissue requires special care in debridement and closure. The usual sequence of events includes percutaneous insertion of a temporary pacing lead (same side), if needed, debridement of all inflammatory tissue, extraction of leads, obtaining hemostasis, and closure of the wounds. These incisions are closed primarily using a closed drainage system, when indicated. If the patient has an acute cellulitis, the pocket should not be debrided; it should be left open to heal by secondary intention. For this technique to be successful, care must be taken to ensure hemostasis.

Emergency Surgical Approaches

Extraction-related, cardiovascular emergencies are caused by tears in the vein or heart. A median sternotomy gives exposure to these structures, including the brachiocephalic veins. Consequently, all patients are prepared for a median sternotomy and the required surgical instruments are available. The indication of a tear is a precipitous drop in systemic blood pressure as the patient develops a cardiac tamponade. Tears of the subclavian or brachiocephalic vein and pleura are rare, but have occurred and result in massive bleeding within the chest cavity. These injuries are more difficult to manage than those causing tamponade, due to the time constraints placed on controlling the hemorrhage.

Patients with a cardiac tamponade can be supported with external massage for a brief period, allowing time to prepare for a median sternotomy. Once the sternum is split, the pericardium should not be opened until instruments are available to control the hemorrhage. For example, suction must be available to expose the site of injury. Most tears are easily controlled but must be quickly found upon entering the pericardium to limit blood loss. Once the site of hemorrhage is identified, it is sutured closed using conventional techniques without cardiopulmonary bypass. These injuries have been successfully treated in our series.

Indications for Lead Extraction

The indications for lead extraction are directly related to the risk and morbidity of the extraction procedure.[25] Historically, only patients with life-threatening conditions such as septicemia have been considered candidates for lead extraction. Today, indications can be grouped into those conditions considered *mandatory, necessary, or discretionary.*

Mandatory conditions are those in which leaving the lead in place would be life-threatening or disabling. Septicemia and endocarditis are widely accepted as mandatory conditions for lead removal. Some situations involving migration of severed transvenous leads are also mandatory, such as those causing life-threatening arrhythmias. Obliteration of all usable veins, a mishap following an attempted lead extraction that leaves a broken or free-floating lead in the vascular system, and a traumatic injury to the lead-vein site may also be considered mandatory conditions.

Necessary conditions are those in which the lead should be removed to correct a problem or to prevent a life-threatening situation from developing, but the existing problem would not be considered life-threatening. An example of a necessary condition would be pocket infection; when treated by removal of the pacemaker while leaving the leads in place, the natural history is recurring infections evolving into a chronic draining sinus. Consequently, patients may require life-long medical management and in many cases, chronic antibiotic treatment.

Discretionary conditions are those in which it is preferable to remove the leads, but it would rarely be a medical necessity. Discretionary conditions include situations such as abandonment of a site because of a malignancy or chronic pain.

An infected pacing system can be considered a mandatory or necessary condition for lead extraction, depending on the clinical manifestation of the infection.[37-39] The sequelae of infected permanent pacing leads range from simple erosions resulting in a draining sinus to a life-threatening, systemic infection.[40,41] Septicemia may result from a pocket infection with infected tissue along the intravascular portion of the lead and/or drainage into the bloodstream. Pockets with negative bacteriology in the presence of potentially infected leads have only a slightly lower complication rate than those with positive bacteriology.[38] The mortality with persistent infection when infected leads are not removed can be as high as 66%.[39] Because of this statistic, it has been recommended that infected leads be removed, even in the elderly high-risk patient, using open-heart surgery if necessary.[38]

Migration of severed transvenous leads may also be considered mandatory or necessary indications, depending on the clinical manifestations. For example, if the proximal lead tip is bouncing in the right ventricle causing a ventricular arrhythmia, the indication is mandatory. A free-floating lead not causing an arrhythmia represents a necessary indication. Migrating leads have perforated the heart, causing hemorrhage or hemopericardium, and have formed vegetation, causing emboli to the lungs.[42-44] Fatality secondary to lead migration has been reported to be as high as 66%.[39]

Other situations with nonfunctional retained leads could also be considered necessary, such as those having a potential for causing vein thrombosis. Thirty to 80% of all intracardiac portions of pacemaker leads endothelialize.[45] The incidence of clinically undetected vein thrombosis has been reported to be as high as 44%,[46] suggesting that reasonable efforts be made to remove all retained leads. Consequently, removal of the old leads during lead replacement procedures may have merit, especially if the leads have been implanted less than 8 to 10 years and the patient's general medical condition would support such a procedure, and/ or it is anticipated that the patient will be requiring additional leads in the future.

Summary

Lead extraction has evolved into a well-defined, technical procedure, allowing the removal of most leads using countertraction techniques. Indications for a standard superior vein approach (SVC), a transfemoral approach (IVC), or a ventriculotomy via a median sternotomy are clear. Physicians performing lead extractions should be proficient in these techniques as well as emergency procedures in order to ensure safe removal of chronically implanted leads. In addition, the extraction devices necessary to perform these procedures are available and are clinically proven. The high success and low complication rate justify our continued efforts to perfect extraction techniques and devices in order to more efficiently remove those pacing and defibrillator leads envisioned for the future.

Acknowledgment: Sincere appreciation goes to Heidi J. Smith, PhD, MED Institute, West Lafayette, Indiana, for her assistance in the preparation of this manuscript.

References

1. Smith HJ, Fearnot NE, Byrd CL, et al. Where does scar tissue form to inhibit extraction of chronic pacemaker leads? (abstr) J Am Coll Cardiol 1992 (in press).
2. Byrd CL, Smith HJ, Fearnot NE, et al. The effect of scar tissue formation on success of intravascular lead extraction (abstr). PACE 1992;15(Apr. Pt. II):571.
3. Stokes K. Medtronic, Inc. 1992 (unpublished data).
4. Byrd CL, Schwartz SJ, Hedin NB. Lead extraction: indications and results. Cardiol Clin 1992 (in press).
5. Deutsch L, Dang H, Brandon JC, et al. Percutaneous removal of transvenous pacing lead perforating the heart, pericardium, and pleura. AJR 1991;156: 471–473.

6. Gould L, Maghazeh P, Giovanniello J. Successful removal of a severed transvenous pacemaker electrode. PACE 1981;4:713–715.

7. Kratz JM, Leman R, Gillette PC. Forceps extraction of permanent pacing leads. Ann Thorac Surg 1990;49:676–677.

8. Ramo BW, Peter RH, Kong Y, et al. Migration of a severed transvenous pacing catheter and its successful removal. Am J Cardiol 1968;22:880–884.

9. Rossi P. "Hook catheter" technique for transfemoral removal of foreign body from right side of the heart. Am J Roentgenol Radium Ther Nucl Med 1970;109:101–106.

10. Swersky RB, Reddy K, Hamby RI. Balloon catheter technique for removing foreign bodies from heart and great vessels. NY State J Med 1975; 75:1077–1079.

11. Thomas J, Sinclair-Smith B, Bloomfield D, et al. Non-surgical retrieval of a broken segment of steel spring guide from the right atrium and inferior vena cava. Circulation 1964;30:106–108.

12. Witte J, Munster W. Percutaneous pacemaker lead-transecting catheter. PACE 1988;11:298–301.

13. Zehender M, Buchner C, Geibel A, et al. Diagnosis of hidden pacemaker lead sepsis by transesophageal echocardiography and a new technique for lead extraction. Am Heart J 1989;118(5):1050–1053.

14. Bilgutay AM, Jensen NK, Schmidt WR, et al. Incarceration of transvenous pacemaker electrode. Removal by traction. Am Heart J 1969;77(3):377–379.

15. Kaizuka H, Kawamura T, Kasaagi Y, et al. An experience of infected catheter removal with continuous traction method and silicon rubber wearing. Ky Obu Geka 1983;36:309–311.

16. Madigan NP, Curtis JJ, Sanfelippo JF, et al. Difficulty of extraction of chronically implanted tined ventricular endocardial leads. J Am Coll Cardiol 1984;3:724–731.

17. Shennib H, Chiu RCJ, Rosengarten M, et al. The nonextractable tined endocardial pacemaker lead. Can J Cardiol 1989;5(6):305–307.

18. Mayer ED, Saggau W, Welsch M. Late pulmonary embolization of a retained pacemaker electrode fragment after attempted transatrial extraction. Thorac Cardiovasc Surgeon 1985;33:128–130.

19. Furman S. Removal of myocardial fragment containing a pacemaker electrode. Ann Thorac Surg 1975;19:716–718.

20. Lee ME, Chaux A, Matloff JM. Avulsion of a tricuspid valve leaflet during traction on an infected, entrapped endocardial pacemaker electrode. The role of electrode design. J Thorac Cardiovasc Surg 1977;74:433–435.

21. Jarvinen A, Harjula A, Verkkala K. Intrathoracic surgery for retained endocardial electrodes. Thorac Cardiovasc Surgeon 1986;34:94–97.

22. Garcia-Jimenez A, Alba CMB, Cortes JMG, et al. Myocardial rupture after pulling out a tined atrial electrode with continuous traction. PACE 1992;15:5–7.

23. Brodell GK, Castle LW, Maloney JD, et al. Chronic transvenous pacemaker lead removal using a unique, sequential transvenous system. Am J Cardiol 1990;66:964–966.

24. Byrd CL, Schwartz SJ, Hedin NB, et al. Intravascular lead extraction using locking stylets and sheaths. PACE 1990;13:1871–1875.
25. Byrd CL, Schwartz SJ, Hedin NB. Intravascular techniques for extraction of permanent pacemaker leads. J Thorac Cardiovasc Surg 1991;101(6):989–997.
26. Fearnot NE, Smith HJ, Goode LB, et al. Intravascular lead extraction using locking stylets, sheaths, and other techniques. PACE 1990;13(Part II):1864–1870.
27. Goode LB, Byrd CL, Wilkoff BL. Development of a new technique for explantation of chronic transvenous pacemaker leads: five initial case studies. Biomed Instrumen Technol 1991;25:50–53.
28. Byrd CL, Schwartz SJ, Sivina M, et al. Experience with 127 pacemaker lead extractions (abstr). PACE 1986;9:282.
29. Smith HJ, Fearnot NE, Byrd CL, et al. Intravascular extraction of pacing leads: complications and factors affecting success (abstr). PACE 1991;14:675.
30. Wilkoff BL, Smith HJ, Fearnot NE, et al. Intravascular lead extraction: multicenter update for 523 patients (abstr). PACE 1992;15(Apr. Pt. II):513.
31. Byrd CL, Schwartz SJ, Sivina M, et al. Technique for the surgical extraction of permanent pacing leads and electrodes. J Thorac Cardiovasc Surg 1985;89:142–144.
32. Belott PH, Byrd CL. Recent developments in pacemaker implantation and lead retrieval. In: Barold SS, Mugica J (eds.). New Perspectives in Cardiac Pacing, edition 2. Futura Publishing Co, Mount Kisco, NY, 1991, pp 105–131.
33. Hill SL, Berry RE. Subclavian vein thrombosis: a continuing challenge. Surgery 1990;108(1):1–9.
34. Dubernet J, Irarrazaval MJ, Lema G, et al. Surgical removal of entrapped endocardial pacemaker electrodes. Clin Prog Pacing Electrophysiol 1986;4:147–152.
35. Panday SR, Nanivadekar SA, Chaukar AP, et al. Broken cardiac catheter: successful removal from the heart under emergency cardiopulmonary bypass with concomitant, closure of an atrial septal defect. J Postgrad Med 1971;18(4):201–205.
36. Yarnoz MD, Attai IA, Furman S. Infection of pacemaker electrode and removal with cardiopulmonary bypass. J Thorac Cardiovasc Surg 1974;68:43–46.
37. Choo MH, Holmes DR, Gersh BJ, et al. Infected epicardial pacemaker systems. Partial versus total removal. J Thorac Cardiovasc Surg 1981;82:794–796.
38. Parry G, Goudevenos J, Jameson S, et al. Complications associated with retained pacemaker leads. PACE 1991;14:1251–1257.
39. Rettig G, Doenecke P, Sen S, et al. Complications with retained transvenous pacemaker electrodes. Am Heart J 1979;98:587–594.
40. Grogler FM, Frank G, Greven G, et al. Complications of permanent transvenous cardiac pacing. J Thorac Cardiovasc Surg 1975;69:895–904.
41. Ruiter JH, Degener JE, Mechelen RV, et al. Later purulent pacemaker pocket

infection caused by *Staphylococcus epidermidis:* serious complications of in situ management. PACE 1985;8:903–907.

42. Dalal JJ, Robinson CJ, Henderson AH. An unusual complication of the unremoved unwanted pacing wire. PACE 1981;4:14–16.
43. Davi BV, Rajani RM, Lokhandwala YY, et al. Unusual case of pacemaker lead migration. Catheterization Cardiovasc Diagn 1990;21:95–96.
44. Wolfram T, Wirtzeld A. Pulmonary embolization of retained transvenous pacemaker electrode. Br Heart J 1976;38:326–329.
45. Robboy SJ, Harthorne JW, Leinbach RC, et al. Autopsy findings with permanent pervenous pacemakers. Circulation 1969;39:495–501.
46. Lee ME, Chaux A. Unusual complications of endocardial pacing. J Thorac Cardiovasc Surg 1980;80:934–940.

Chapter 4

Effect of Drugs on Pacing Threshold in Man and Canines: Old and New Facts

S. Serge Barold, Rick McVenes,

Ken Stokes

Introduction

Studies evaluating the effect of drugs on the pacing threshold have generated conflicting data because of the following: (1) animal data cannot always be extrapolated to man, (2) a lack of uniform measurement techniques, (3) different electrode characteristics, (4) different sites of pacing (transvenous vs. epicardial), and (5) varying doses of drugs and routes of administration have further contributed to the problem.[1-3] Measurement of the pacing threshold in terms of number of variables: current (mA), voltage (volts), pulse width (ms, keeping the voltage constant), and energy (microjoules) also makes comparison of data difficult.

Human Studies

Almost all the studies in man were performed in patients with chronic transvenous pacing leads, but occasionally with temporary leads (Table 1).

New Perspectives in Cardiac Pacing, Vol. 3, edited by S. Serge Barold and Jacques Mugica, Mount Kisco, NY, Futura Publishing Co., © 1993.

TABLE 1
Effects of Drugs on Pacing Threshold*

Drug	Human Studies		
	Decrease	Increase	No Change
Quinidine Procainamide		Doenecke et al.[6] (A) SU, PT; Gay and Brown[8] (B) (TOX); Mehta and Kahn[9] (B) T (TOX)	Preston et al.[5] (?B) SU, PPE; Preston et al.[4] (A) PE; Garmardo et al.[7] (A) T
Disopyramide Lidocaine		Hayler et al.[10] (B); Mohan et al.[14] (A) T; Heinz[13] (A) T	Rydén and Korsgren[11] (A) T; Doenecke et al.[6] (A) SU PT; Young et al.[12] (A); Preston et al.[5] (A) SU, PPE; Adornato et al.[16] (A) (VENT); Adornato et al.[16] (B) (ATR and VENT)
Mexiletine		Kafka et al.[15] (C); Mohan et al.[14] (A) T; Adornato et al.[16] (A) (ATR)	
Phenytoin Flecainide		Heinz[13] (A) T; Hellestrand et al.[18,19] (A) T (A and B) P; Adornato et al.[16] (A and B) (ATR and VENT); McClelland et al.[17] (B); Walker et al.[20] (B and D); Lau et al.[26] (A) T RD	Doenecke et al.[6] (?A) SU, PT
Encainide Propafenone		Satel et al.[21] (B); Kafka et al.[15] (C); Montefoschi and Boccadomo[27] (B and D) (ATR); Adornato et al.[22] (A and B) (ATR and VENT); Bianconi et al.[23] (ATR and VENT); Cornacchia et al.[24] (B); Soriano et al.[25] (B) RD	

Drug		
Propranolol	Kubler and Sowton[31] (A) T	Creamer et al.[29] (A and B) Mohan et al.[14] (A) T Szabo and Solti[30] (A) T Preston et al.[5] (A) SU PPE
Sotalol	Kakfa et al.[15] (C)	
Amiodarone		Creamer et al.[29] (A and B) Nielsen et al.[28] (B)** Adornato et al.[16] (A and B) (ATR and VENT)
Verapamil	Doenecke et al.[6] (A) SU PT Diewitz and Baldus[33] (A) T	Mohan et al.[14] (A) T
Acetylcholine		Westerholm[32] (A) P and PE
Atropine		Preston et al.[4] (A) PE
Ouabain		Young et al.[12] (A)
Digoxin	Westerholm[32] (A) P and PE	
Lanactoside C	Haywood and Wyman[35] (A) SU PPE	Preston et al.[4] (A) PE
Isoprotenerol	Preston et al.[4,5] (A) PE Levick et al.[36] (A)	
Orciprenaline (Alupent)	Westermann et al.[34] (A) T Diewitz and Baldus[33] (A) T	
Alcohol		Westerholm[32] (C) P and PE
Enflurane, Isoflurane, Halothane		Zaidan et al.[46] TE (acute study)

* All data were obtained from chronically implanted transvenous ventricular leads unless stated otherwise.
A = acute transvenous study; B = chronic oral therapy; C = acute oral therapy; D = case report; SU = site unstated; TOX = toxic levels only; ATR = atrial; VENT = ventricular. All threshold studies are ventricular unless stated as ATR = atrial. When only VENT is indicated, there is a corresponding atrial study. T = study with temporary endocardial leads; PT = probably transvenous; TE = temporary epicardial leads; P = study with permanent endocardial leads indicated only if there is another study with temporary or other leads in the same article. PE = permanent epicardial leads; PPE = probably PE; RD = rate dependent increase in threshold.
** Acute and chronic thresholds after transvenous pacemaker implantation.

Class 1A Antiarrhythmic Agents

In therapeutic levels, Class 1A antiarrhythmic drugs do not cause clinically important changes in the ventricular pacing threshold. Preston et al.[4,5] found no change with procainamide and quinidine, while Doenecke et al.[6] found a probably insignificant 10–15% increase in the ventricular pacing threshold (in terms of energy) with procainamide. No plasma drug levels were determined in these studies.

Camardo et al. found little or no effect on the ventricular pacing threshold in late diastole using constant current pulses after the administration of 1,000 mg of procainamide intravenously[7] (50 mg/min), generating levels ranging from 6.4 to 13.56 µg/mL (mean = 10.0). The mean threshold in the control state was 0.74 ± 0.10 mA and after procainamide it was 0.93 ± 0.19 mA. Procainamide levels were obtained at the end of the strength-interval determinations, i.e., 10–15 minutes after the termination of the procainamide infusion. Only three patients exhibited an increase of threshold of 0.15 mA or greater (increments were 0.15 mA, 0.3 mA, and 1.25 mA, and corresponding procainamide levels were 11.0, 13.0, and 7.6 µg/mL, respectively). Procainamide[8,9] and disopyramide[10] toxicity may, however, cause an excessive rise in the ventricular pacing threshold with failure to capture. In this situation, pacemaker malfunction may produce, as in hyperkalemia, varying degrees of pacemaker exit block (discussed later). Drug toxicity commonly occurs in combination with hyperkalemia in patients with severe congestive heart failure.

Type 1B Antiarrhythmic Drugs

Lidocaine

Four studies found a change in the ventricular pacing threshold following the acute intravenous (IV) administration lidocaine.[5,6,11,12] In two other IV studies,[13,14] relatively small increases in the ventricular pacing threshold were observed; one study showed an almost immediate 20% increase in terms of mA dropping to less than 10% after 5 minutes,[12] and the other study produced an increase in the mean voltage threshold from 0.803 ± 0.422 V to a mean of 1.171 ± 0.808 V.[14]

Mexiletine

Mohan et al.[14] studied patients with temporary pacemakers and demonstrated an increase in the ventricular pacing threshold from 1.89 ± 0.833 V to 2.662 ± 0.990 V following IV mexiletine. Kafka et al.[15] administered a single oral dose of mexiletine and found a 19% increase in terms of pulse width (keeping the voltage constant) with individual variations as high as 100%. Adornato et al.[16] also evaluated the effect of IV mexiletine and found an increase in the atrial pulse width threshold (from 0.111 ± 0.074 to 0.140 ± 0.068 ms with fixed output voltage at 2.5 V), but the ventricular pacing threshold remained unaffected. Adornato et al.[16] also found that the oral administration of mexiletine, 600 mg/day for 15 days, did not alter atrial and ventricular pacing thresholds.

Tocainide

No data are available in man.

Phenylhydantoin

One study found no effect on the ventricular pacing threshold[6] while another IV study showed a 10% increase in the ventricular pacing threshold in terms of mA.[13]

Type 1C Antiarrhythmic Agents

Compared with other antiarrhythmic drugs, type 1C drugs cause the greatest increase in the pacing threshold, especially flecainide.

Flecainide

In man, the IV and chronic oral administration of flecainide produces marked increases in both the atrial and the ventricular pacing thresholds so that pacing failure can occur even with therapeutic concentrations of flecainide.[16-20] The threshold should be tested shortly after initiation of flecainide therapy because it begins to increase after the first dose.[17] Hellestrand et al.[18] evaluated the effect of flecainide on the ventricular pacing threshold in three groups of patients.

(1) Flecainide was administered IV in 11 patients with a temporary pacing lead in the right ventricle. Flecainide increased the ventricular threshold significantly from 0.66 to 1.4 V at 0.5 ms (117%) and from 0.55 to 1.14 V at 1.0 ms (107%) measured 10 minutes after commencing flecainide infusion.

(2) Flecainide was administered IV at the time of pulse generator replacement in 10 patients with chronically implanted endocardial right ventricular leads. The mean right ventricular pacing threshold increased significantly from a control of 1.73 V to a maximum of 2.27 V at 0.5 ms pulse width (31%) and from 1.46 to 1.89 V at 1.0 ms pulse width (29%), an increase less marked than the change seen in patients with temporary leads.

(3) Seven patients with implanted pulse generators were studied after the administration of flecainide IV and orally. When administered IV, the maximum ventricular pacing threshold increase occurred 15 minutes after the start of the infusion. At a fixed amplitude of 2.7 V, the pulse width threshold increased significantly from the control value of 0.14 ms to a maximum of 0.22 ms (57%) and at an amplitude of 4.9 V from 0.06 to 0.11 ms (83%). Flecainide IV doses ranged from 100 to 200 mg. Oral flecainide therapy was administered for 3 weeks (100 mg/day for the first week, 200 mg/day in the second week, and 400 mg/day in the third week). The mean pulse width threshold values before flecainide were 0.09 ms at 2.7 V and 0.06 ms at 4.9 V. Ventricular pacing threshold values increased significantly with increasing doses of oral flecainide to 0.28 ms at 2.7 V and 0.16 ms at 4.9 V by the end of the third week, representing increases of 200% and 164%, respectively. Measurements at least 10 days after cessation of oral flecainide therapy showed that the ventricular pacing threshold had returned to 0.13 ms at 2.7 V and 0.07 ms at 4.9 V, both values not differing significantly from the control threshold values before the administration of flecainide. In patients taking oral flecainide, there was a highly significant linear correlation between the serum flecainide level and the changes in the chronic ventricular threshold both at amplitudes at 2.7 V and 4.9 V. The most significant increase in the ventricular pacing threshold occurred after chronic oral flecainide, the average increase being 160–200% in terms of pulse width.

Adornato et al.[16] studied the effect of flecainide on the atrial and ventricular pacing thresholds in patients with chronically implanted transvenous leads. The control pulse width atrial threshold (at a fixed voltage of 2.5 V) was 0.123 ± 0.066 ms. IV flecainide (2 mg/kg over 30 min) increased the atrial pacing threshold significantly to 0.373 ± 0.206 ms at 2.5 V, an increase of 273%. Chronic administration of flecainide (orally 200 mg/day for 15 days) increased the atrial threshold significantly to 0.235 ± 0.093 ms at 2.5 V (91% increase). The control ventricular pacing threshold was 0.088 ± 0.034 ms at 2.5 V. With IV flecainide, it rose significantly to 0.195 ± 0.064 ms (113% increase), and after the chronic administration of flecainide for 15 days, the threshold also increased significantly to 0.133 ± 0.055 ms at 2.5 V (51% increase).

McClelland et al.[17] also demonstrated that the ventricular pacing threshold increased significantly in patients with temporary endocardial right ventricular electrodes, 71 hours after flecainide therapy (0.60 mA to 1.30 mA) compared with an increase from 0.6 mA to 0.92 mA over 71 hours in the control patients who received no drug therapy. In this study, flecainide, 200 mg twice daily, was administered for at least four doses, but not during the subsequent 12 hours.

Walker et al.[20] reported pacing failure in a patient with a VVI pacemaker after the administration of flecainide, 100 mg twice a day initially and then increased to 200 mg twice a day. On the fourth day of treatment, the ECG showed intermittent failure to capture. At reoperation the ventricular threshold was 5.0 V (pulse width not stated) with no evidence of lead tip displacement. Repositioning the lead at several sites could not establish consistent ventricular pacing, reflecting general refractoriness of the right ventricle. Following discontinuation of flecainide, the threshold fell abruptly over 24 hours to 1.2 V (pulse width not stated). In this case, the increase in the ventricular threshold was about 1000% (with a small contribution from the usual increase in threshold with the passage of time) and the fall in 24 hours was greater than 400% in terms of voltage.

Encainide

Encainide can also increase the ventricular pacing threshold significantly but probably not as much as flecainide. Like flecainide, encainide in relatively high therapeutic doses can cause failure to capture, as demonstrated by Satel et al.,[21] who evaluated changes in the ventricular pacing threshold in terms of energy (microjoules) in 10 patients receiving encainide. With a dose of 25 mg three times a day, the energy threshold increased by 15%, while a dose of 75 mg three times a day increased the energy threshold significantly by 75%. Changes in the duration of the QRS complex did not predict the change in the pacing threshold. Only three patients showed an increase in the ventricular pacing threshold over 100% (102%, 224%, and 556% in terms or energy).[21]

Propafenone

Kafka et al.[15] demonstrated a significant increase in the ventricular pacing threshold after a single 450 mg oral dose of propafenone in 14 patients. As a group, there was a 46% increase in pulse width threshold (voltage kept constant), with individual variations as high as 67%. Adornato et al.[22] studied the effect of propafenone on the atrial and ventricular pacing thresholds of 10 patients with dual chamber DDD pacemakers following acute administration of propafenone (30 minutes after IV injection of 2 mg/kg) and after chronic administration of 900 mg/day for 10 days. Pacing thresholds were determined in terms of pulse width at a fixed 2.5 V voltage output. The atrial pacing thresholds increased by 56.5% (acute administration) and 82.1% (chronic administration), while the ventricular pacing threshold increased by 36.0% (acute administration) and 56.5% (chronic administration). All values were statistically significant with P<0.01. Bianconi et al.[23] also evaluated the effect of oral propafenone therapy in 36 patients with permanent pacemakers (9 VVI, 15 AAI, 12 DDD). Each patient received 450 mg/day and 18 received 900 mg/day. Atrial and ventricular thresholds were measured in terms of pulse width at a fixed 2.5 V output after 7 days of therapy at a given dose. With the lower propafenone dosage, the threshold rose from 0.14 ± 0.10 to 0.21 ± 0.16 ms (55%) in the atrium and from 0.10 ± 0.08 to 0.15 ± 0.09 ms (63%) in the ventricle (all values being statistically significant). In the 18 patients who received both dosages, the atrial threshold rose to 0.31 ± 0.26 ms (120%) and the ventricular threshold rose to 0.23 ± 0.17 ms (170%). All of these values were statistically significant (P>0.0001). A threshold increment of 200% was observed in two of the 48 paced chambers (4%) with the 450 mg/day dose and in eight of the 26 paced chambers (31%) with the 900 mg/day dose. The increments of the atrial versus ventricular threshold showed no statistical significance. An increment of ≥300% was observed only with the higher dose in four cases (15%). A good linear correlation ($r = 0.76$, $P<0.001$) was found between the increment of ventricular threshold and widening of the *paced* (not the conducted) QRS complex.

Cornacchia et al.[24] also studied the effect of oral propafenone on the unipolar ventricular threshold in 70 patients (at 3 months or more after implantation) by determining threshold before and 1 week after propafenone (400–900 mg/day according to weight). The pulse width threshold was measured at 0.8, 1.6, and 2.5 V output. Propafenone increased the pulse width threshold at all voltages with the maximal changes at 0.8 V, where the pulse width threshold increased (considering all patients) from 0.33 ± 0.14 to 0.46 ± 0.22 ms ($P<0.001$). The increase at 0.8 V was 0.10 ± 0.07 ms for steroid-eluting leads and was significantly lower compared to the increase of 0.18 ± 0.21 ms for the other leads.

Soriano et al.[25] studied 18 patients with serial electrophysiologic studies before and after oral propafenone, 900 mg/day orally for 9 ± 6 days. Bipolar ventricular stimulation was perrormed at twice the diastolic threshold (threshold was defined as the lowest effective current with a rectangular pulse of 1 ms duration). The absolute values of baseline thresholds in the drug-free state and after propafenone were not published. After propafenone, intermittent rate-dependent failure of ventricular capture was repeatedly observed in five patients during right ventricular stimulation (at the apex in four and outflow tract in all) at rates ranging from 100/min to 150/min (3–9 beats were required to disclose loss of capture). The five patients (group 1) who exhibited rate-dependent capture failure were older, had longer right ventricular effective refractory periods in the baseline and after propafenone, and also exhibited significantly longer duration of the spontaneous and paced QRS complex compared to the other 13 patients (group 2) who showed no rate-dependent loss of capture. Although no blood levels of propafenone were determined, these observations suggest a more intense drug effect in group 1 patients. In four of the five group 1 patients, loss of ventricular capture was preceded by the gradual prolongation of the interval from the stimulus and the local right ventricular bipolar electrogram in a Wenckebach-like fashion. In this respect, Lau et al.[26] also reported a similar observation in a patient who developed rate-dependent failure of ventricular capture with Wenckebach exit block after the intravenous infusion of flecainide. Such rate-dependent failure of ventricular capture induced by type 1C antiarrhythmic drugs could become important in patients with DDD or rate-responsive pacemakers.

A recent single case report documented a significant increase in the atrial pacing threshold leading to loss of capture in a patient receiving propafenone, 450 mg/day.[27] In this particular case the previous threshold had been 1.8 V at 0.5 ms with an increase to beyond 5 V, 0.5 ms with propafenone therapy. Twenty-four hours after propafenone was discontinued, the original threshold of 1.8 V at 0.5 ms returned with successful atrial capture.

Amiodarone

Amiodarone has been evaluated in man in two studies.[16,28] Nielsen et al.[28] found no effect on the ventricular pacing threshold with long-term administration of amiodarone. Adornato et al.[16] found no effect on the atrial and ventricular pacing thresholds with IV administration of amiodarone; but with chronic administration of 600 mg/day for 30 days, they found a borderline statistically significant increase in the atrial (but not ventricular) pacing threshold. Although amiodarone seems to have no direct effect on pacing thresholds, an increase in the pacing threshold can occur due to amiodarone-induced hypothyroidism (discussed later).

Beta Blockers

Four reports evaluating the effect of propranolol on ventricular pacing threshold showed no change,[5,14,29,30] while another report[31] was associated with a relatively small increase in the ventricular pacing thresholds (40% in terms of energy). The effect of beta-blocker drugs on pacing threshold may be influenced by the degree of catecholamine stimulation at the time of investigation.[5] Propranolol may increase the pacing threshold if the patient has been physically active prior to testing. As a rule, propranolol does not cause clinically important changes in the ventricular pacing threshold.

Sotalol administered IV and orally produced no effect on the chronic ventricular pacing threshold in the study of Creamer et al.[29] In contrast, Kafka et al.[15] found a significant increase (19%) in the ventricular pacing threshold in terms of pulse width (keeping voltage constant) after a single

160 mg oral dose of sotalol with maximum individual threshold variations up to 100%.

Digitalis

Digitalis-like drugs do not alter the ventricular pacing threshold or may actually diminish it slightly[4,12,32] (Table 1).

Calcium Blockers

Various calcium blockers have not been studied in detail. Doenecke et al.[6] indicated in their study that verapamil administered IV caused a significant increase in the ventricular pacing threshold but provided no numerical data. Diewitz and Baldus[33] showed only a very slight increase in the ventricular pacing threshold with intravenous verapamil. On the other hand, Mohan et al.[14] were unable to detect any change in the voltage ventricular pacing threshold after IV verapamil.

Sympathomimetic Agents

Sympathomimetic agents decrease the pacing threshold, e.g., ephedrine, 25 mg q6h, IV epinephrine, or isoproterenol. However, large IV doses of these drugs given quickly may result in initial lowering of the ventricular pacing threshold followed by subsequent elevation.[4,5] Smaller doses of sympathomimetic drugs cause only a sustained threshold decrease. Alupent also reduced the pacing threshold in two studies.[33,34] Threshold alterations by sympathomimetic drugs may be abolished by IV propranolol.[5] Intravenous isoproterenol may be administered to decrease the pacing threshold in cases of pacemaker failure, though its main beneficial effect consists of an increase in the rate of the idioventricular rhythm rather than pacing threshold reduction.[35] Levick et al.[36] used an infusion of isoproterenol (4 μg/min) to successfully reverse an inability to pace the right ventricle from drug toxicity related to multiple antiarrhythmic agents.

Steroids

Glucocorticoids lower ventricular pacing threshold while mineralocorticoids (including Aldactone) increase pacing threshold. A mixed steroid such as hydrocortisone is likely to have an inconsistent effect on threshold. Prednisone, prednisolone, and dexamethasone are well known to lower ventricular pacing threshold.[4,37–42] A number of reports have indicated that large doses of steroids may temporarily reduce the high ventricular pacing threshold due to exit block with endocardial or epicardial pacemaker implantation.[37–39] Occasionally, a course of steroids may avoid pacemaker revision. Steroids may be successful early after implantation and occasionally as late as 2 years afterwards.[43,44] The reduction in ventricular pacing threshold is mostly unsustained when steroid therapy is discontinued. Steroids are now rarely used, partly because some cases of exit block may be treated noninvasively by reprogramming the pulse generator. Nagamoto et al.[45] reported endocardial exit block 2 years after pacemaker implantation (ventricular threshold greater than 7.5 V at 0.6 ms). Prednisolone, 60 mg/day, caused a decrease in the pacing threshold in a few days, and 6 months later the threshold was less than 5 V at 0.1 ms. Prednisolone was tapered and discontinued after 5 months. The ventricular stimulation threshold remained at less than 5 V, 0.1 ms for 2 years since the start of steroid therapy and over 1½ years after its discontinuation.

Miscellaneous Drugs

Volatile anesthetics such as enflurane, isoflurane, and halothane do not have any effect on the ventricular pacing threshold in patients with temporary epicardial electrodes.[46]

Hypothyroidism may cause a significant increase in the ventricular pacing threshold that may lead to failure to capture,[47,48] reversible by the administration of thyroid hormone.

Hyperkalemia

According to Hayes,[2] although potassium could be considered primarily a metabolic or physiologic variable, it could also be considered a cardioactive drug because it plays such a prominent role in the management of cardiac patients. The level of hyperkalemia at which threshold changes occur varies from patient to patient. The effect of potassium on the pacing threshold of atrial and ventricular myocardium has not been clearly defined.[49] When the serum potassium level exceeds 7.0 mEq/L, there will almost always be an increase in pacing threshold.

Latency describes the delay from the pacing stimulus to the onset of ventricular depolarization. The normal value for the interval from the pacemaker stimulus to the QRS usually measures less than 40 ms. First degree exit block (latency) and second degree type 1 (Wenckebach) exit block from the region of the pacemaker stimulus (with gradual prolongation of the interval from the pacemaker stimulus to the paced QRS complex ultimately resulting in an ineffectual pacemaker stimulus) occur mostly in terminal situations (with severe myocardial damage).[50–52] Occasionally, increased pacemaker-myocardial block is secondary to potentially reversible hyperkalemia with or without antiarrhythmic drug toxicity, particularly type 1A agents.[9] Wenckebach exit block can be produced experimentally in the laboratory by perfusion of cardiac tissue with a large concentration of antiarrhythmic agents and potassium, an effect often reversible.[53] The QRS configuration and ST-T wave abnormalities may become gradually altered during Wenckebach sequences or may remain unchanged.[51] Repolarization may be so delayed that the succeeding ventricular pacemaker stimulus falls in the refractory period of the previous beat. The pacing disturbance may progress to 2:1, 3:1 exit block, etc., and eventually to complete exit block with total lack of capture.[50–52]

Latency and exit block may be related to nonhomogeneous propagation of excitation, local changes in conduction near the electrode, failure of impulse propagation due to depression of intraatrial or intraventricular conduction, or an increase in the refractoriness.[54] Latency and exit block usually depend on the amplitude and rate of stimulation. A threshold stimulus excites the surrounding myocardium more slowly than a suprathreshold stimulus.[51] Consequently, in the presence of latency or exit block, an increase in the pacing rate leads to prolongation of the interval from the stimulus to QRS, while an increase in the amplitude of the stimulus may shorten the interval.[55] Exit block from Wenckebach periodicity is always abnormal except when exceedingly rapid nonphysiologic ventricular pacing rates are used for burst pacing during an electrophysiologic study.

Total unresponsiveness to ventricular stimulation (complete ventricular pacemaker exit block) has been reported in only three cases of hyperkalemia with plasma potassium levels of 6.6, 6.9, and 7.1 mEq/L, respectively.[50,56,57] The modest elevation of serum potassium in these cases suggests that numerous other metabolic variables may influence the sensitivity of cardiac tissue to hyperkalemia. These include other electrolyte imbalance,[58] acid base, oxygen saturation, the rate of change of plasma potassium level, the intracellular-extracellular potassium gradient,[47,59] and the etiology and severity of heart disease.[60] For this reason, the cardiac manifestations of hyperkalemia in the clinical setting tend to occur at much lower potassium levels than those measured during the experimental infusion of potassium.[52,60,61] Bashour et al.[62] reported a case of hyperkalemia-induced (K = 6.8 mEq/L) latency characterized by prolongation of the interval from the *atrial* stimulus to the paced P waves that decreased after treatment of hyperkalemia. Barold et al.[63] reported hyperkalemia-induced failure of atrial capture associated with preservation of ventricular pacing in a patient with a dual chamber DDD pacemaker when the serum K was only 6.3 mEq. This differential effect on atrial and ventricular excitability (pacing) correlates with the well known clinical and experimental observations that the atrial myocardium is more sensitive to hyperkalemia than the ventricular myocardium.

The administration of oral or intravenous potassium may decrease the ventricular pacing threshold even if the serum K level is normal,[4,5,35,59,64] a response also documented in dogs with AV block by the infusion of potassium chloride. The initial decrease is followed by an increase in pacing threshold as the potassium level rises eventually to the point of inexcitability with very high levels.[65] However, solutions tending to drive potassium into the cells, e.g., insulin and glucose, may increase the ventricular pacing threshold by altering the extracellular-intracellular potassium balance.

Animal Studies

Only a few studies have been performed in experimental animals (Table 2). Woske et al. in 1951 found that procainamide in very large doses produced a significant increase in the atrial and ventricular pacing thresholds of dogs paced epicardially from the right atrium and right ventricle.[66] These workers found that a blood level of procainamide of 20 μg/mL was essential for any increase in the pacing threshold. The threshold response to a 0.1 ms impulse increased by 50% for atrial and 70% for ventricular pacing in terms of mA. These data represent the influence of toxic levels of procainamide on the pacing threshold and

TABLE *2*

Effects of Drugs on Pacing Threshold*

	Animal Studies		
Drug	*Decrease*	*Increase*	*No Change*
Quinidine		Wallace et al.[68] (A) (ATR and VENT) RTE	
Procainamide		Woske et al.[66] (A) (ATR and VENT) RTE	Huang et al.[71] (A and B) Michelson et al.[66] (A) LE
Lidocaine			Huang et al.[71] (A)
Tocainide		Villafane et al.[69] (A) (ATR) US	Villafane et al.[69] (A) (VENT) US Huang et al.[71] (B)
Diphenylhydantoin	Bigger et al.[70] (A) (ATR and VENT) RTE**		
Flecainide		Guarnieri et al.[72] (A) T	Huang et al.[71] (A and B)
Propafenone			Present study (B) (ATR and VENT)
Moricizine		Present study (B) (ATR and VENT)	
Propranolol			Huang et al.[71] (A and B) Guarnieri et al.[72] (A) T Present study (B) (ATR and VENT)
Atenolol			Present study (B) (ATR and VENT)
Amiodarone			Huang et al.[71] (A and B)
Verapamil			Huang et al.[71] (A and B) Present study (B) (ATR and VENT)
Dilitiazem			Present study (B) (ATR and VENT)
Nifedipine			Present study (A) (ATR and VENT)
Captopril		Present study (B) (ATR)	Present study (B) (VENT)
Lithium carbonate			Present study (B) (ATR and VENT)

* All data were obtained from chronically implanted transvenous ventricular leads unless noted otherwise. A = acute transvenous study; B = chronic oral therapy. All threshold studies are ventricular unless stated as ATR = atrial. When VENT is indicated, there is a corresponding atrial study. RTE = right temporary epicardial electrodes. LE = left epicardial electrodes. T = temporary endocardial electrodes. US = unstated—site and nature of electrodes unknown.

** Without diluent. Diphenylhydantoin with diluent produced no change in pacing thresholds. Diluent alone caused a significant increase in pacing threshold.

correspond with the observations in man that only toxic levels of procainamide produce a significant increase in the ventricular pacing threshold. Michelson et al.[67] found no change in the excitability threshold in
nine dogs paced at normal or chronically infarcted ventricular sites 15–
30 minutes after the administration of intravenous procainamide: at 15
minutes the level ranged from 12.1 to 19.4 µg/mL, mean 15.0 ± 3.1,
and in 30 minutes the level ranged from 8.2 to 13.8 µg/mL, mean =
10.0 ± 2.6. After the administration of quinidine, Wallace et al.[68] showed
in dogs a relatively small but significant increase in the atrial and ventricular epicardial right ventricular pacing threshold.

Villafane et al.[69] administered tocainide intravenously in dogs to
attain therapeutic levels. This was followed by a significant increase in
the atrial pacing threshold (from 1.03 ± 0.13 V to 2.33 ± 0.61 V 1 hour
later), but no effect on the ventricular pacing threshold was observed.
Villafane et al.[69] did not indicate whether pacing was performed trans-
venously or epicardially. Bigger et al.[70] studied the influence of diphenylhydantoin on the pacing threshold in dogs with right atrial and right
ventricular epicardial electrodes. When the diluent for the drug was eliminated, Bigger et al.[70] found a slight decrease in pacing thresholds.

Huang[71] performed comprehensive pacing studies in dogs with
chronically implanted transvenous right ventricular leads. The following
drugs were administered IV and orally: procainamide, flecainide, pro-
panolol, amiodarone, and verapamil. Tocainide was administered only
orally and lidocaine was administered only intravenously. Despite adequate plasma levels of all the drugs, no changes in the ventricular pacing
threshold could be demonstrated. The lack of response to flecainide differs from the observations of Guarnieri et al.[72] in dogs as well as the
impressive augmentation of pacing thresholds seen in man. Guarnieri et
al.[72] studied the ventricular pacing threshold after defibrillation in terms
of the time required to regain ventricular capture at a given current output. In the control situation, the time required to regain ventricular capture was determined (1) at the threshold current output: 4.9 ± 1.7 sec,
compared with (2) 2.2 ± 0.9 sec at twice the current output of the pacemaker (P=0.01). After the administration of intravenous flecainide, the
time to ventricular capture increased as follows: (1) at the threshold current output from 4.9 ± 1.7 sec to 14.9 ± 2.1 sec (P=0.01); (2) at twice
the current output from 2.2 ± 0.9 sec to 5.6 ± 2.1 sec (P=0.05), indicating that in these acute dog studies flecainide increased the ventricular

pacing threshold. Guarnieri et al.[72] observed no change in the ventricular pacing threshold after IV propranolol.

Recent Animal Investigations

We recently evaluated the effect of a number of drugs on the pacing threshold of dogs. Each of five dogs (weights ranging from 19.8 to 39.6 kg) received four unipolar Medtronic (Minneapolis, MN) contemporary transvenous pacing leads. One model 4011 (Target Tip,® microporous, platinum, grooved) and one model 4023 (Capsure SP® steroid-eluting, porous, platinum, hemispherical) ventricular leads were implanted in a paired fashion in all dogs. Two transvenous unipolar atrial leads were also implanted in each dog; all received a model 6957 atrial screw-in (polished platinum active helix) and an additional lead, either model 4523 (Capsure®) or model 4511 (Target Tip®) passive fixation leads. The ventricular leads were placed at least 1 cm apart in each right ventricle. The atrial tined leads were placed in the right atrial appendage with the atrial screw-in leads in or near the appendage. All leads were associated with satisfactory pacing threshold except for one screw-in lead that became dislodged. Data from the displaced lead were therefore discarded.

Voltage thresholds were determined before and after administration of each drug with a calibrated Medtronic model 5311 pacing system analyzer (PSA—instrumental error ± 0.1 V) at pulse widths of 0.05, 0.1, 0.3, 0.5, 1.0, and 2.0 ms except for nifedipine, for which the threshold was measured only at 0.05, 0.5, and 2.0 ms. The voltage threshold after drug administration was taken as the recorded value at the maximum serum level of the drug. The voltage threshold was determined by pacing at a rate faster than sinus rhythm (usually 10 beats ppm faster) and by increasing the PSA voltage output from a low value to the minimum voltage producing consistent capture. At least two measurements were obtained, and these were often identical. When the second threshold determination differed from the first, a series of threshold measurements were obtained until a consistently repeatable value was observed. When the threshold value changed with successive trials, the maximum of six to eight iterations was accepted as threshold. A separate study at 3 and 12 weeks after implantation in the same dogs showed no change in the pacing thresholds during exercise, sleep, post-meal, and awake resting state.[73]

Pacing thresholds before and after drug administration were measured under halothane general anesthesia to facilitate percutaneous insertion of a special needle for direct access to a subcutaneous lead connection, as described by Huang et al.[71] The anesthetized state helped diminish variables such as position, alterations in heart rate due to animal excitement, etc. At 12 weeks after implantation, there was no difference in the pacing thresholds in all the dogs in the awake state versus the anesthetized state. The effect of drugs on the chronic pacing threshold was studied beginning 13 weeks after lead implantation. The following drugs were administered to all dogs: propafenone, moricizine, verapamil, diltiazem, nifedipine (not exposed to light), lithium carbonate, and captopril. Propranolol and atenolol were studied in only three dogs.

Drugs were studied under the same conditions at two or more of the following intervals after administration was started: 3–4 days, 7–8 days, and 14–15 days with the exception or intravenous nifedipine (for which pacing threshold was measured between 30 and 60 minutes after infusion) and verapamil (dosage was doubled after day 14 and the study was undertaken on day 21/22 and 28/29). The serum concentration of all drugs was measured at the time of each experiment to ensure therapeutic levels[74-90] (Table 3). If blood levels were found to be subtherapeutic, the dose was increased until a satisfactory level or significant pharmacologic effect was observed. All drugs were administered orally for a minimum of 2 weeks, except for nifedipine which was administered by IV infusion. Measurement of blood levels was problematic in the case of beta blockers, and we relied more on pharmacologic effect of a significant slowing of the heart rate, evident before and during anesthesia. Our levels for captopril varied from 0.09 to 0.54 µg/mL after 7 days and 1.0 mg/kg dose bid. After increasing to 1.5 mg/kg bid during the second week, increased levels were attained, but with most dogs showing significant decrease in blood pressure and side effects of vomiting and lethargy. Serum electrolytes showed no changes in Na^+, a decrease of K^+ from 4.5 ± 0.12 before administration to 4.08 ± 0.16 ($P<.01$) at the day 14 monitoring, and an increase in Cl^- from 109 ± 1.2 to 116 ± 1.2 ($P<.001$). (Canine normal range: K^+ 3.7–5.8, Cl^- 100–115 mEq/L).

After each drug was discontinued, another drug was administered after the greater time interval of more than three half lives of the previous drug or 7 days. The data were analyzed by conventional two-tailed paired Student's t test and $P<.05$ was taken as significant.[91]

TABLE 3
Drug Plasma Levels

DRUG (# Animals) Dosage		Published Therapeutic Levels	Max. Serum Levels Achieved Mean ± SD
Propranolol	(N = 3)	10–150 ng/mL*	11.3 ± 2.5 ng/mL
1.5 mg/kg bid		40–120 μg/mL**[74]	max = 14, min = 9
Atenolol	(N = 3)	up to 0.6 μg/mL*	0.37 ± 0.3 μg/mL
25 mg q.d.		100–200 ng/mL**[75]	max = 0.7, min 0.1
Verapamil	(N = 5)	80–400 ng/mL*	125 ± 43 ng/mL
80–160 mg bid		40–500 ng/mL**[76,77]	max = 188, min = 90
IV Nifedipine	(N = 5)	15–100 ng/mL*	25 ± 7.6 ng/mL
2.0 μg/kg/min for 10 min,		5–125 ng/mL**[76-78]	max = 39, min = 20
0.2 μg/kg/min for 30 min			
Diltiazem	(N = 5)	50–300 ng/mL*	92 ± 21 ng/mL
3.0 mg/kg tid		98–708 ng/mL**[76,79-81]	max = 125, min = 75
Captopril	(N = 5)	up to 4.0 μg/mL*	0.65 ± 0.45 μg/mL
1.5 mg/kg bid		0.19 ± 2.0 μg/mL**[82,83]	max = 1.40, min = 0.26
Propafenone	(N = 5)	0.2–3.0 μg/mL*	0.54 ± 0.31 μg/mL
300 mg tid		0.12–3.2 μg/mL†[84-86]	max = 1.0, min = 0.2
Moricizine	(N = 5)	0.25–3.0 μg/mL*[87]	1.8 ± 0.8 μg/mL
8–10 mg/kg tid		No Data Avail.**	max = 3.3, min = 1.3
Lithium Carb.	(N = 5)	0.6–1.2 mEq/L*	1.8 ± 0.8 mEq/L
12 mg/kg bid		1.26 ± 0.6 mEq/L**[88-90]	max = 3.3, min = 1.3

* Human Therapeutic Range, chronic administration values (National Medical Services, Willow Grove, PA; Medtox Laboratories, St. Paul, MN).

** Range achieved in chronic canine studies.

† No data available for chronic oral administration to canines. IV administration of single dose of 2 mg/kg has produced levels cited to 3 hours post administration.

SD = standard deviation.

Results

All drugs except for moricizine and captopril showed no significant changes in the atrial or ventricular thresholds. Moricizine showed significant increases in threshold at most pulse widths for all lead types (Table 4). Captopril exhibited increases in threshold at most pulse widths only for the atrial passive fixation devices (Table 5). We cannot explain these observations except to say that they were not due to hyperkalemia. We could not find any published data correlating serum levels and effectiveness of chronic propafenone administration in canines. Previously discussed human studies have shown significant changes in the pacing threshold after chronic propafenone administration, but our propafenone

TABLE 4

Moricizine (Threshold Voltage, Canine Data, N = 5, except for Atrial Screw-in N = 4)

Pulse Width	2.0		1.0		0.5		0.3		0.1		0.05	
	Bsln	Max	Bsln	Max	Bsln	Max	Bsln	Max	Bsln	Max	Bsln	Max
Ventricular 4023 Mean	0.34	0.40	0.44	0.52	0.58	0.70	0.78	0.92	1.48	1.96	2.34	3.32
SD	.05	.10	.05	.08	.13	.14	.16	.18	.30	.47	.60	.60
% chg	+18%		+18%		+21%		+18%		+32%		+42%	
P	NS		P < .05		P < .05		P < .05		P < .05		P < .02	
Ventricular 4011 Mean	0.48	0.58	0.62	0.74	0.80	1.12	1.04	1.36	1.98	2.78	3.24	4.82
SD	.19	.19	.25	.27	.34	.48	.30	.48	.75	1.29	1.17	2.10
% chg	+21%		+19%		+40%		+31%		+40%		+49%	
P	NS		P < .05		P < .05		P < .05		P < .05		P < .05	
Atrial Screw-in Mean	0.90	1.20	0.95	1.23	1.05	1.53	1.23	1.55	2.30	3.25	3.55	5.38
SD	.36	.48	.35	.44	.42	.68	.51	.58	1.06	1.60	1.74	2.76
% chg	+33%		+29%		+46%		+26%		+41%		+52%	
P	P < .05		P < .05		P < .05		P < .02		P < .05		P < .05	
Atrial Tined Mean	0.44	0.58	0.56	0.72	0.66	0.88	0.96	1.34	2.04	2.48	3.28	4.32
SD	.26	.41	.42	.50	.42	.52	.76	1.05	1.46	1.77	2.31	2.91
% chg	+32%		+29%		+33%		+40%		+22%		+32%	
P	NS		P < .02		P < .02		P < .05		P < .05		P < .05	

Bsln = voltage threshold prior to moricizine administration; Max = voltage threshold at maximum serum level; SD = standard deviation; % chg = % change of sample mean voltage threshold value, P = two-tailed Student's t test where P < .05 taken as significant; NS = not significant.

studies in dogs showed no significant change. This may be due to relatively low blood levels (despite aggressive dosing) and/or species variation in metabolism because the human therapeutic blood levels also show great variability.[92]

Conclusion

Many of the studies concerning the physiologic variations of the pacing threshold in man were conducted over 20 years ago with leads and pacemakers that are now obsolete. The physiologic variations of pacing threshold should be reevaluated with contemporary pacing systems to further our understanding of the effect of drugs.[73] Our animal studies with captopril and the studies of Cornacchia et al.[24] in humans

TABLE *5*

Captopril (Threshold Voltage, Canine Data, N = 5, except for Atrial Screw-in N = 4)

Pulse Width	2.0		1.0		0.5		0.3		0.1		0.05	
	Bsln	*Max*	*Bsln*	*Max*	*Bsln*	*Max*	*Bsln*	*Max*	*Bsln*	*Max*	*Bsln*	*Max*
Ventricular 4023 Mean	0.34	0.38	0.34	0.40	0.48	0.54	0.68	0.70	1.44	1.50	2.36	2.50
SD	.05	.11	.05	.08	.08	.05	.08	.10	.15	.20	.30	.39
% chg	+12%		+18%		+13%		+3%		+4%		+6%	
P	NS		NS		NS		NS		NS		NS	
Ventricular 4011 Mean	0.42	0.50	0.44	0.54	0.76	0.70	0.90	0.94	1.84	1.90	2.94	3.06
SD	.13	.16	.22	.17	.34	.24	.39	.32	.68	.66	.96	.97
% chg	+19%		+23%		−8%		+4%		+3%		+4%	
P	NS		NS		NS		NS		NS		NS	
Atrial Screw-in Mean	1.08	1.03	1.15	1.05	1.33	1.23	1.55	1.55	2.68	2.85	4.13	4.40
SD	.45	.40	.48	.40	.57	.43	.68	.57	1.18	1.31	1.84	2.20
% chg	−5%		−9%		−8%		0%		+6%		+7%	
P	NS		NS		NS		NS		NS		NS	
Atrial Tined Mean	0.40	0.48	0.42	0.56	0.60	0.72	0.74	0.94	1.56	1.84	2.60	3.06
SD	.24	.15	.19	.21	.31	.29	.31	.35	.62	.71	1.02	1.12
% chg	+20%		+33%		+20%		+27%		+18%		+18%	
P	NS		P < .01		P < .01		P < .02		P < .02		P < .05	

Bsln = voltage threshold prior to captopril administration; Max = voltage threshold at maximum serum level; SD = standard deviation; % chg = % change of sample mean voltage threshold value, P = two-tailed Student's t test where P < .05 taken as significant; NS = not significant.

suggest that lead characteristics may influence the effect of drugs on pacing threshold. Most of the data on the effect of drugs on the pacing threshold have come from human studies, and for some drugs data are scanty. For example, drugs such as tocainide, moricizine, and calcium blockers other than verapamil have not yet been studied in man. Relatively little data are available on atrial pacing thresholds. Conceivably, the atrial pacing threshold may respond to drugs differently from the ventricular pacing threshold, as suggested by the greater sensitivity of atrial myocardium to hyperkalemia. Only type 1C antiarrhythmic drugs seem to produce clinically significant increases in the pacing threshold with therapeutic doses. Our animal studies suggest that moricizine (best classified as a type 1B/1C antiarrhythmic agent) in therapeutic doses might also produce a significant increase in the pacing threshold in man similar to the other type 1C drugs (flecainide, encainide, and propafenone). In most patients with an appropriately programmed pulse generator (safety margin 2:1 in terms of voltage), the threshold increase with type 1C agents is unlikely to cause loss of capture. However, the effect of type 1C drugs is important in patients with a relatively high chronic pacing threshold, though in isolated cases with a relatively low baseline threshold, these drugs can occasionally induce a disproportionate increase in threshold and capture failure.[27] While the effect of drugs on pacing threshold has been studied mostly in patients with chronic transvenous leads, the effect of drugs on acute and chronic epicardial pacing thresholds should be examined because of the increasing popularity of implantable cardioverter/defibrillators with epicardial leads capable of antibradycardia and antitachycardia pacing.

Acknowledgment: We are grateful to Nancy Hansen, D.V.M., and Stuart Lahtinen, D.V.M., of Physiologic Research Laboratories, Coon Rapids, MN, for their contribution to the animal studies.

References

1. Dohrmann ML, Goldschlager NF. Myocardial stimulation threshold in patients with cardiac pacemakers: Effect of physiologic variables, pharmacologic agents and lead electrodes. Cardiol Clinics 1985;3:527.
2. Hayes DL. Effects of drugs and devices on permanent pacemakers. Cardio, January, 70, 1991.
3. Reiffel JA, Coromilas J, Zimmerman JM, et al. Drug-device interactions: clinical considerations. PACE 1985;8:369.
4. Preston TA, Fletcher RD, Lucchesi BR, et al. Changes in myocardial threshold. Physiologic and pharmacologic factors in patients with implanted pacemakers. Am Heart J 1967;74:235.
5. Preston TA, Judge RD. Alteration of pacemaker threshold by drug and physiologic factors. Ann NY Acad Sci 1969;167:686.
6. Doenecke P, Flothner R, Rettig G, et al. Studies of short and long term threshold changes. In: Schaldach M, Furman S (eds.). Advances in Pacemaker Technology, Springer-Verlag, Berlin-Heidelberg-New York, 1975, p 283.
7. Camardo JS, Greenspan AM, Horowitz LN, et al. Strength-interval relation in the human ventricle: Effect of procainamide. Am J Cardiol 45:856, 1980.
8. Gay RJ, Brown DF. Pacemaker failure due to procainamide toxicity. Am J Cardiol 1974;34:728.
9. Mehta J, Kahn AH. Pacemaker Wenckebach phenomenon due to antiarrhythmic drug toxicity. Cardiology 1976;61:189.
10. Hayler AM, Holf DW, Volans GN. Fatal overdose with disopyramide. Lancet 1978;1:968.

11. Rydén L, Korsgren M. The effect of lignocaine on the stimulation threshold and conduction disturbances in patients treated with pacemaker. Cardiovasc Res 1969;3:415.

12. Young MW, Meia H, Furman S, et al. Effects of lidocaine and ouabain on myocardial threshold to pacer stimuli. Circulation 1970;42(Suppl III):III-209.

13. Heinz VN. Beeinflussung der diastolischen reizschwelle des menschlichen herzens durch antiarrhythmica. Arzneim Forsch (Drug Res) 1971;8:1189.

14. Mohan JC, Kaul U, Bhatia ML. Acute effects of antiarrhythmic drugs on cardiac pacing threshold. Acta Cardiol 1984;39:191.

15. Kafka W, Hildebrand U, Städt WD. Effect of antiarrhythmic agents on chronic pacing threshold and sensing thresholds. Circulation 1985;72:111.

16. Adornato E, Catanzariti D, Casciola G, et al. Pharmacological effects on acute and chronic changes of atrial and ventricular pacing threshold. In: Santini M, Pistolese M, Alliegro A (eds.). Progress in Clinical Pacing, Excerpta Medica, Amsterdam, 1990, p 101.

17. McClelland J, Cutler J, Kudenchuk P, et al. Ventricular pacing threshold following flecainide administration. Clin Res 1989;37:150A.

18. Hellestrand KJ, Nathan AW, Bexton RS, et al. Electrophysiologic effects of flecainide acetate on sinus node function, anomalous atrioventricular connections and pacemaker thresholds. Am J Cardiol 1984;53:30B.

19. Hellestrand KJ, Burnett PJ, Milne JR, et al. Effect of the antiarrhythmic agent flecainide acetate on acute and chronic pacing threshold. PACE 1983;6:892.

20. Walker PR, Papouchado M, James MA. Pacing failure due to flecainide acetate. PACE 1985;8:900.

21. Salel AF, Seagren SC, Pool PE. Effects or encainide on the function of implanted pacemakers. PACE 1989;12:1439.

22. Adornato E, Catanzariti D, Monea P, et al. Confronto degli effetti acuti e cronici deila pentisomide e del propafenone sulla soglie di stimolazione atriale e ventricolare. Cardiostimolazione 1991;9:20.

23. Bianconi L. Boccadamo R, Toscano S, et al. Effects of oral propafenone therapy on chronic myocardial pacing threshold. PACE 1992;15:148.

24. Cornacchia O, Maresta A, Nigro P, et al. Effect or propafenone on chronic ventricular pacing threshold in patients with steroid eluting (Capsure) and conventional leads. Eur J Cardiac Pacing Electrophysiol 1992;2:A88.

25. Soriano J, Almendral J, Arenal A, et cl. Rate-dependent failure of ventricular capture in patients treated with oral proparenone. Eur Heart J 1992;13:269.

26. Lau CP, Griffith MJ, Camm AJ. Ventricular Wenckebach after intravenous therapy with Class I antiarrhythmic agents. Int J Cardiol 1988;20:141.

27. Montefoschi N, Boccadamo R. Propafenone-induced acute variation of chronic atrial pacing threshold. A case report. PACE 1990;13:480.

28. Nielsen AP, Griffin JC, Herre JM, et al. Effect of amiodarone on acute and chronic pacing thresholds. PACE 1984;7:462(Part I).

29. Creamer JE, Nathan AW, Sherman A, et al. Acute and chronic effects of sotalol and propranolol on ventricular repolarization using constant rate pacing. Am J Cardiol 1986;57:1092.

30. Szabo Z, Solti F. The significance of the tissue reaction around the electrode on the late myocardial threshold. In: Schaldach M, Furman S (eds.). Advances in Pacemaker Technology, Springer-Verlag, New York, 1975, p 273.
31. Kübler W, Sowton E. Influence of beta-blockade on myocardial thresholds in patients with pacemakers. Lancet 1970;2:67.
32. Westerholm C. Threshold studies in transvenous cardiac pacemaker treatment. Scand J Thorac Cardiovas Surg 1971;8(Suppl):1.
33. Diewitz M, Baldus O. Beeinflussung der myokardialen reizschwelle des menschen durch verschiedene antiarrhythmika und sympathikomimetika. Arzneimittel Forsch 1973;23:511.
34. Westermann KW, Geibel O, Kalmar P, et al. Das Verrholten der electrischeen reizschwelle bei stimulation mit endokardialen elektroden. Verh Dtsch Ges Kreisl Forsch 1969;35:259.
35. Haywood J, Wyman MG. Effects of isoproterenol, ephedrine, and potassium on artificial pacemaker failure. Circulation 1965;(Suppl II):II-110.
36. Levick CE, Mizgala HF, Kerr CR. Failure to pace following high dose antiarrhythmic therapy: Reversal with isoproterenol. PACE 1984;7:252.
37. Risby O, Meibom J, Nyboe, et al. The influence of prednisolone on pacemaker threshold. PACE 1981;4:A-68.
38. Thiele VG, Lachmann W, Eschmann B, et al. Zur beeinflussung des reizschwellenan nach herz schrittmacherimplantation durch prednisolon. Z Ges Inn Med 1980;35:863.
39. Rupp M, Bleifeld W, Hanrath P, et al. Glucocorticoide zur senkung der elektrishen reizschwette von schrittmachern. Dtsch Med Wachr 1973;98:858.
40. Radovsky AS, VanVleet JF. Erfects of dexamethasone elution on tissue reaction around stimulating electrodes of endocardial pacing leads in dogs. Am Heart J 1989;117:1288.
41. Preston TA, Judge RD, Lucchesi BR, et al. Myocardial threshold in patients with artificial pacemakers. Am J Cardiol 1966;18:83.
42. Benditt DG, Kreitt JM, Ryberg C, et al. Cellular electrophysiologic effects of dexamethasone sodium phosphate: Implications for cardiac stimulation with steroid-eluting electrodes. Int J Cardiol 1989;22:67.
43. Baucia JA, Marcial MB, Vargas H, et al. Tratamento do aumento cronico do limiar de estimulacao com o emprego de corticosteroides em pacientes protadores de marca-passo. Arq Bras Cardiol 1983;41:115.
44. Beanlands DS, Akyurekli Y, Keon WJ. Prednisone in the management or exit block. In: Proceedings of the VI World Symposium on Cardiac Pacing, Pacesymp, Montreal, 1979, Chap. 18-3.
45. Nagamoto Y, Ogawa T, Kunagae H, et al. Pacing failure due to markedly increased stimulation threshold 2 years after implantation: Successful management with oral prednisolone. A case report. PACE 1989;12:1034.
46. Zaidan JR, Curling PE, Craver JM Jr. Effect of enflurane, isoflurane and halothane on pacing stimulation thresholds in man. PACE 1985;8:32.
47. Basu D, Chatterjee K. Unusually high pacemaker threshold in severe myxedema. Decrease with thyroid hormone therapy. Chest 1976;70:677.
48. Schlesinger Z, Rosenberg T, Stryjer D, et al. Exit block in myxedema treated effectively by thyroid hormone therapy. PACE 1980;3:737.

49. Lyons CJ, Burgess MJ, Abildskov JA. Effects of acute hyperkalemia on cardiac excitability. Am Heart J 1977;94:755.
50. Bashour TT. Spectrum of ventricular pacemaker exit block owing to hyperkalemia. Am J Cardiol 1986;57:337.
51. Klein HO, DiSegni E, Kaplinsky E, et al. The Wenckebach phenomenon between electric pacemaker and ventricle. Br Heart J 1976;38:961.
52. Surawicz B, Chlebus H, Reeves JT, et al. Increase of ventricular excitability threshold by hyperpotassemia. Possible cause of internal pacemaker failure. JAMA 1965;191:17.
53. Klein HO, Beker B, DiSegni E, et al. The pacing electrocardiogram. How important is the QRS complex configuration? Clin Progr Electrophysiol Pacing 1986;4:112.
54. Greenspan K, Anderson GJ, Fisch C. Electrophysiologic correlate of exit block. Am J Cardiol 1981;28:197.
55. Barold SS, Falkoff MD, Ong LS, et al. Normal and abnormal patterns of ventricular depolarization during cardiac pacing. In: Barold SS (ed.). Modern Cardiac Pacing, Futura Publishing Co., Mt. Kisco, NY, 1985, p 545.
56. Sathyamurthy I, Krishnaswami S, Sukumar IP. Hyperkalemia-induced pacemaker exit block. Indian Heart J 1984;36:176.
57. O'Reilly MV, Murnaghan DP, Williams MD. Transvenous pacemaker failure induced by hyperkalemia. JAMA 1974;228:336.
58. Hughes H, Tyers F, Torman H. Effects of acid-base imbalance on myocardial pacing threshold, J Thorac Cardiovasc Surg 1975;69:743.
59. Gettes LS, Shabetai R, Downs TA, et al. Effect of changes in potassium and calcium concentrations on diastolic threshold and strength-interval relationships of the human heart. Ann NY Acad Sci 1969;167:693.
60. Fisch C. Electrolytes and the heart. In: Hurst JW (ed.): The Heart, 6th Ed., McGraw Hill, New York, 1986, p 1466.
61. Ettinger PO, Regan TJ, Oldewurtel HA. Hyperkalemia, cardiac conduction and the electrocardiogram. A review. Am Heart J 1974;88:360.
62. Bashour T, Hau I, Gorfinkel, et al. Atrioventricular and intraventricular conduction in hyperkalemia. Am J Cardiol 1975;35:199.
63. Barold SS, Falkoff MD, Ong LS, et al. Hyperkalemia induced failure of atrial capture during dual-chamber pacing. J Am Coll Cardiol 1987;10:467.
64. Walker WJ, Elkins JT, Wood LW. Effects of potassium in restoring myocardial response to a subthreshold cardiac pacemaker. N Engl J Med 1964;271:597.
65. Lee D, Greenspan K, Edmands RE, et al. The effect of electrolyte alteration on stimulus requirement of cardiac pacemakers. Circulation 1968;38(Suppl):IV-124.
66. Woske H, Belford J, Fastier FN, et al. The effect of procaine amide on excitability, refractoriness and conduction in the mammalian heart. J Pharmacol Exp Ther 1953;107:134.
67. Michelson EL, Spear JF, Moore EN. Effects of procainamide on strength interval relations in normal and chronically infarcted canine myocardium. Am J Cardiol 1981;47:1223.

68. Wallace AG, Cline RE, Sealy WC, et al. Electrophysiologic effects of quinidine. Circ Res 1966;19:960.
69. Villafane J, Katzmark S, Elbl F, et al. Effect of tocainide on pacemaker thresholds. Clin Res 1989;37:43A.
70. Bigger JT Jr, Weinberg DI, Kovalik AT, et al. Effects of diphenylhydantoin on excitability and automaticity in the canine heart. Circ Res 1970;26:1.
71. Huang SK, Hedberg PS, Marcus FI. Effects of antiarrhythmic drugs on the chronic pacing threshold and the endocardial R wave amplitude in the conscious dog. PACE 1986;9:660.
72. Guarnieri T, Datorre SD, Bondke H, et al. Increased pacing threshold after an automatic defibrillator shock in dogs: Effects of Class I and Class III antiarrhythmic drugs. PACE 1988;11:1324.
73. McVenes R, Lahtinen S, Hansen N, et al. Physiologic and drug induced changes in cardiac pacing and sensing parameters. Eur J Cardiac Pacing Electrophysiol 1992;2(Suppl 1A):A86.
74. Wilke JR. Cardiac tachyarrhythmias. In: LE Davis (ed.). Handbook of Small Animal Therapeutics, Churchill Livingstone, NY, 1985, p 267.
75. Muir WW, Sams R. Clinical pharmacodynamics and pharmacokinetics of beta-adrenoceptor blocking drugs in veterinary medicine. Compendium of Continuing Education for Practicing Veterinarians 1984;6:156.
76. Atlee JL III, Conscious state comparisons of the effects of the inhalation anesthetics and diltiazem, nifedipine, or verapamil on specialized atrioventricular conduction times in spontaneously beating dog hearts. Anesthesiology 1988;68:519.
77. Hamann SR, Kaltenborn KE, McAlister RG Jr. Pharmacodynamic comparison of verapamil and nifedipine in anesthetized dogs. J Cardiovasc Pharmacol 1985;7:224.
78. Hamann SR, McAlister RG Jr. Plasma concentrations and hemodynamic erfects of nifedipine: A study in anesthetized dogs. J Cardiovasc Pharmacol 1983;5:920.
79. Browne RK, Dimmitt DC, Miller LD, et al. Relationship between plasma diltiazem and cardiovascular responses in conscious dogs. J Cardiovasc Pharmacol 1983;5:483.
80. Bourassa MG. Haemodynamic and electrophysiologic effects of diltiazem. Acta Pharmacol Toxicol 1985;57(Suppl 11):21.
81. Yeung PKF, Mosher SJ, Quilliam MA, et al. Species comparison of pharmacokinetics and metabolism of diltiazem in humans, dogs, rabbits, and rats. Drug Metab Disposition 1990;18:1055.
82. Migdalof BH, Antonaccio MJ, McKinstry DN, et al. Captopril: pharmacology, metabolism and disposition. Drug Metab Rev 1984;15:841.
83. Singhvi SM, Peterson AE, Ross JJ, et al. Pharmacokinetics of captopril in dogs and monkeys. J Pharm Sci 1981;70:1108.
84. Puigdemont A, Lligona LL, Arboix M, et al. Pharmacokinetics of propafenone in the dog after single-dose intravenous administration. J Vet Pharmacol Ther 1987;10:351.
85. Boucher JH, Carpentier A, Duchene-Marullaz P. Propafenone in the con-

scious dog with chronic atrioventricular block: Mechanisms of chronotropic cardiac effects and plasma concentration-response relationships. J Cardiovasc Pharmacol 1986;8:885.

86. Miyazaki T, Ogawa S, Sakai T, et al. Effects of class I drugs on reentrant ventricular tachycardia in a canine model of myocardial infarction: On their antiarrhythmic and proarrhythmic mechanisms. Jpn Circ J 1988;52:254.

87. Fitton A, Buckley M. Moricizine: A review of its pharmacological properties and therapeutic efficacy in cardiac arrhythmias. Drugs 1990;1:138.

88. Leucuta S, Pop R, Kory M, et al. Pharmacokinetics and bioavailability of lithium administered to dogs as monoglutamate and carbonate. Pharm Acta Helv 1979;54:343.

89. Risch SC, Groom GP, Janowsky DS. Interfaces of psychopharmacology and cardiology. Part one. J Clin Psychiatry 1981;42:34.

90. Rosenthal RC, Koritz GD, Davis LE. Pharmacokinetics of lithium in the dog. J Vet Pharmacol Ther 1986;9:81.

91. Box G, Hunter W, Hunter J. Statistics for Experimenters, Wiley and Son, Inc., New York, NY, 1978.

92. Opie LH, Chatterjee K, Gersh BJ, et al. Drugs for the Heart, Third Ed., W.B. Saunders Co., Philadelphia, PA, 1991, p 199.

Chapter 5

Pacemaker Syndrome: Clinical, Hemodynamic, and Neurohumoral Features

KENNETH A. ELLENBOGEN,

MARK A. WOOD, BRUCE STAMBLER

Introduction

Since the first asynchronous ventricular pacemaker was implanted in 1958, pacing technology has undergone tremendous evolution. As the predominant indication for pacemaker implantation has shifted from complete heart block to sinus node dysfunction, our understanding of patient acceptance and tolerance of different pacing modes has also evolved.

To better understand the various pathophysiologic changes that occur during ventricular pacing, we will review the hemodynamic, neurohumoral, and vascular responses to ventricular pacing with special emphasis on the putative role each may play in producing the "pacemaker syndrome." In its broadest terms, pacemaker syndrome may be defined as the presence of suggestive signs and/or symptoms in the presence of AV dyssynchrony.

Clinical Features

In 1969, Mitsui and colleagues reported on a patient who complained of chest pain, dizziness, shortness of breath, cold sweats, and facial flush-

New Perspectives in Cardiac Pacing, Vol. 3, edited by S. Serge Barold and Jacques Mugica, Mount Kisco, NY, Futura Publishing Co., © 1993.

ing during ventricular pacing.[1] The authors ascribed these symptoms to an inadequate paced rate, and therefore suboptimal cardiac output. They termed this phenomenon "pacemaking syndrome." Subsequently, a number of authors reported cases of patients who experienced symptoms during ventricular pacing.[2-4,6,10-12] These patients had a wide variety of underlying cardiac conditions (including some without evidence of structural heart disease). Symptoms reported in these cases varied from mild to severe (Table 1). Some symptoms of pacemaker syndrome are fairly nonspecific. In elderly patients, these symptoms may incorrectly be attributed to a variety of other constitutional or chronic conditions common to this age group. The most commonly recorded symptoms include presyncope, frank syncope, dizziness, fatigue, dyspnea, weakness, jaw pain, headaches, vertigo, cough, dyspnea on exertion, tiredness, malaise, palpitations, venous pulsations in the neck, and chest discomfort. These symptoms have been attributed to a variety of pathophysiologic mechanisms that will be discussed more fully below.

The wide variety and often nonspecific nature of symptoms expe-

TABLE 1
Symptoms of Pacemaker Syndrome

Mild
venous or an unpleasant pulsation in neck
tiredness, weakness, malaise
fatigue
palpitations
vertigo
cough
apprehension
fullness in chest

Moderate
jaw pain
chest pain
dizziness
dyspnea on exertion
confusion/alteration of mentation
headaches

Severe
presyncope
syncope

rienced by patients with pacemaker syndrome make it difficult to arrive at an accurate estimate of the incidence of pacemaker syndrome during ventricular pacing. In one study, Nishimura and colleagues from the Mayo Clinic recorded the blood pressure and symptoms during DVI and VVI pacing in a series of 50 consecutive patients receiving dual chamber pacemakers. Ten of 50 patients (20%) experienced symptomatic dizziness during ventricular pacing. The incidence of symptoms with VVI pacing was significantly higher in patients with intact ventriculoatrial (VA conduction (9 of 23) than in those without (1 of 27). Interestingly, 13 of 14 patients with heart failure lacked VA conduction. In another study, Heldman and colleagues from the Long Beach Memorial Medical Center evaluated 40 unselected patients with DDD pacemakers during 1 week each of DDD and VVI pacing.[6] Patients were given questionnaires at the end of each week and asked to rate 16 different symptoms (e.g., shortness of breath, fatigue, dizziness, apprehension, neck pulsations, headaches, orthopnea, palpitations). Twelve of the 16 symptoms were worse during VVI than during the DDD pacing mode. The most highly significant symptomatic complaints during VVI pacing were shortness of breath, dizziness, fatigue, pulsations in the neck or abdomen, cough, and apprehension. Pacemaker syndrome (defined as exacerbation or development of one or more of the above symptoms) was clinically recognized in slightly over 80% of patients, with 65% experiencing moderate to severe symptoms. Only 17% of patients experienced no exacerbation of symptoms during VVI pacing (Fig. 1). Other investigators have presented similar data. For example, Dateling and colleagues showed in a prospective study of 217 patients, that while patients programmed to the VVIR pacing mode had better relief of symptoms than during VVI pacing, DDD pacing was superior to both (Table 2).[7] These findings were also confirmed in a smaller study with 22 patients programmed to DDD, DDDR, VVIR, and DDIR pacing modes.[8] Patients were compared based on both subjective (symptomatic, functional state, exercise tolerance, and health perception) and objective criteria (maximal exercise tolerance test time, echocardiography). In this study, five patients (all in the VVIR pacing mode) demanded early crossover to a dual chamber pacing mode because of intolerable symptoms of dyspnea, dizziness, tiredness, and/ or palpitations. These symptoms all resolved within 24 hours of being reprogrammed to a dual chamber pacing mode. In 73% of patients, the VVIR pacing mode was the least acceptable pacing modality, as measured by patient perception of general well being and exercise capacity. In

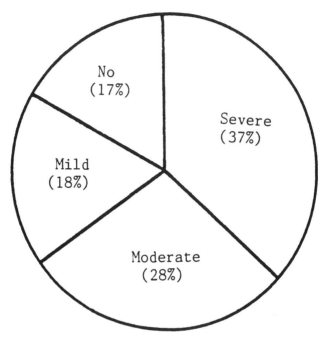

Figure 1.   Severity of symptom exacerbation during VVI pacing compared to DDD or DDI pacing mode in 40 patients. Symptom severity rated by questionnaire on a scale from 0 to 10. Reproduced with permission of author and publisher.

TABLE 2
Symptoms of Pacemaker Syndrome

Symptoms	VVI	VVIR	DDD	Statistics
syncope	96%	95%	100%	NS
dizziness	64%	68%	100%	p < 0.02
dyspnea	56%	57%	78%	p < 0.04
weakness	56%	68%	80%	p < 0.02

Adapted from Dateling F, Obel IWP. PACE 1989;12:1278.[7]

contrast to these studies, older studies using a more "rigid" definition of pacemaker syndrome (e.g., syncope, shock, dizziness, congestive heart failure, cough) and perhaps identifying only patients with more severe symptomology, have generally reported an incidence of pacemaker syndrome of only 5–15%.[9,10]

Pacemaker syndrome occurs in patients of both sexes and all ages and in patients paced for a wide variety of etiologies. Pacemaker syndrome has been reported to occur both immediately after implantation, and in its milder forms may not be noted for months or years. In these patients, symptoms may be milder or intermittent, or patients may assume this level of disability is to be "expected" with a pacemaker.[11] Other potential explanations for the variability of symptoms in some patients include changes in drug treatment, variability of retrograde VA conduction, and changes in myocardial substrate. A variety of clinical factors may predispose patients to the development of pacemaker syndrome, and they are summarized in Table 3.

The diagnosis of pacemaker syndrome requires a high degree of suspicion and a willingness to evaluate a patient's complaints, even when nonspecific or mild. Diagnosis is best confirmed by exclusion of pacing system malfunction and correlation of the patient's cardiac rhythm before and during his/her symptoms. This can be accomplished with Holter monitoring and/or use of a transtelephonic cardiac monitor. Demonstration or correlation of symptoms with ventricular pacing, echo beats, and the presence of retrograde VA conduction are all helpful findings (Fig. 2).[12] The absence or relief of symptoms with the resumption of sinus bradycardia (or an underlying rhythm with AV synchrony) is also consistent with this diagnosis. On physical examination, the presence of cannon A waves in the neck (or systolic reversal of hepatic flow) may also be helpful. Other tests that are helpful include the measurement of blood pressure in the supine and erect position during ventricular (and atrial) pacing.[5] In general, if there is a significant drop in arterial pressure with ventricular pacing (e.g., greater than 20 mm Hg), pacemaker syndrome is likely to be present. However, the absence of a significant drop in arterial pressure does not eliminate the possibility that pacemaker syndrome is responsible for the patient's symptoms. In some patients, ocular pneumoplethysmography or Doppler measurement of cardiac output can document a significant decrease in cardiac output during shifts from VVI to sinus rhythm, atrial pacing, or dual chamber pacing.[13–15] When changes in cardiac output are measured, they provide important docu-

TABLE 3
Pacemaker Syndrome: Clinical Features

Author	No. of Patients	Predictive of Pacemaker Syndrome	Not Predictive
Pearson et al.[14]	24	VA conduction SV during VVI pacing <50 mL % atrial contribution to LV filling >38%	LV EDD FS LA size
Nishimura et al.[5]	50	VA conduction	CHF present CT ratio on CXR
Sulke et al.[8]	22	greater increase in SV with DDD pacing	LA size FS PA pressure VA conduction Mitral regurgitation during VVI pacing
Erlebacher et al.[44]	20	cannon A waves VA conduction	Baseline SV, Baseline PCW presssure
Rediker et al.[16]	19	sinus bradycardia VA conduction	FS LA size LV EDD Exercise duration Increase in CO with DDD pacing
Heldman et al.[6]	40	None	LV function VA conduction SSS vs. AV block as indication for implant
Stewart et al.[15]	29	VA conduction % increase in CO with DDD pacing	LV function

CHF = congestive heart failure; CO = cardiac output; CT = cardiothoracic ratio; CXR = chest radiograph; FS = fractional shortening; LA = left atrial size; LV EDD = left ventricular end-diastrolic dimension; PA = pulmonary artery pressure; PCW = pulmonary capillary wedge pressure; SSS = sick sinus syndrome; SV = stroke volume; VA = ventriculoatrial conduction.

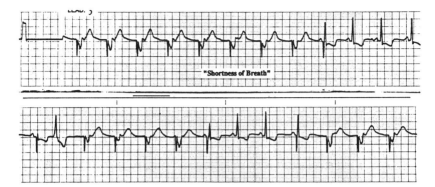

Figure 2. Continuous rhythm strips recorded with a transtelephonic cardiac monitor in a 65-year-old farmer with pacemaker syndrome. This patient's underlying rhythm disorder was sick sinus syndrome with sinus bradycardia and one episode of atrial fibrillation 1 year earlier. His sinus bradycardia was exacerbated by treatment with quinidine, verapamil, and digoxin. He had a VVI(R) device implanted and returned to his physician complaining of fatigue, weakness, dizziness, malaise, and shortness of breath 1 month later. Following documentation of this rhythm by a cardiac event monitor, he underwent further testing. During VVI pacing, there was VA dissociation. During VVI pacing at 90 beats/min, his blood pressure dropped to 90/68 mm Hg; during AAI pacing it was 160/90 mm Hg (at 90 beats/min). During sinus rhythm at 58–64 beats/min, the blood pressure measured 136/70 mm Hg. A DDDR pacemaker was implanted and within 48 hours the patient's symptoms were abolished. He has returned to his active, vigorous lifestyle.

mentation of the physiologic benefit of DDD pacing and will serve as adequate documentation or justification that a generator upgrade is necessary for treatment of "pacemaker syndrome," especially when appropriate symptoms are present. The presence of VA conduction is thought by most to be a factor that increases the chances that a patient will experience pacemaker syndrome.[16] Retrograde conduction may be intermittent in some patients, dependent on position, autonomic tone, and antiarrhythmic drugs.[17] Thus, it seems likely that even if intact VA conduction is not present, pacemaker syndrome may still occur.

In summary, pacemaker syndrome is a diffuse clinical entity which includes many symptoms that are poorly defined and nonspecific. In the elderly population, these symptoms may be attributed to coexisting conditions. Historically, the incidence of pacemaker syndrome was estimated to be about 7%. However, if the diagnosis of pacemaker syndrome is based on objective signs (hypotension), decreased cardiac output (measured by Doppler echocardiography), or patient symptoms (patient questionnaires); the "true" incidence of pacemaker syndrome varies from 20% to 65%. Nonspecific complaints in patients who have VVI pacemakers should not be readily attributed to other etiologies, until an evaluation for possible pacemaker syndrome is undertaken.

Multiple factors may contribute to pacemaker syndrome. These factors include hemodynamic considerations, humoral factors, and neural reflexes. In the following pages we will review each of the above factors and the potential role they play in producing pacemaker syndrome.

Hemodynamic Considerations

A number of physiologists have acknowledged the importance of atrial contraction to ventricular filling.[18-20] The atrium provides a booster pumplike function, and in a broad-based population contributes 15–25% to cardiac output.[19,20] In patients with heart failure or aortic stenosis, the contribution of the atrial "kick" may vary even further, between 5% and 35%.[21] The contribution of atrial systole to cardiac output depends on heart rate, myocardial function (both systolic and diastolic), presence of valvular heart disease, and left atrial size, contractility, and compliance.

Initial studies showing a benefit to AV sequential pacing relied primarily on measurements of cardiac output or intracardiac pressures. Comparing atrial to ventricular pacing in patients, ventricular pacing is associated with higher right atrial, pulmonary artery, pulmonary capillary wedge, and left ventricular end-diastolic pressures. These findings have been further extended by Doppler ultrasound measurement of cardiac output. In one study of 29 patients with DDD pacemakers, the mean cardiac output dropped from 5.0 ± 0.3 L/min to 4.3 ± 0.3 L/min during shifts from DDD to VVI pacing.[15] Patients with retrograde VA conduction and symptoms of pacemaker syndrome showed the greatest improvement in cardiac output during DDD pacing (Fig. 3). These patients showed a mean increase in cardiac output of about 30% compared to a mean increase in cardiac output of 14% in patients without VA conduction or symptoms of pacemaker syndrome. The change in cardiac output was not related to the baseline left ventricular ejection fraction.

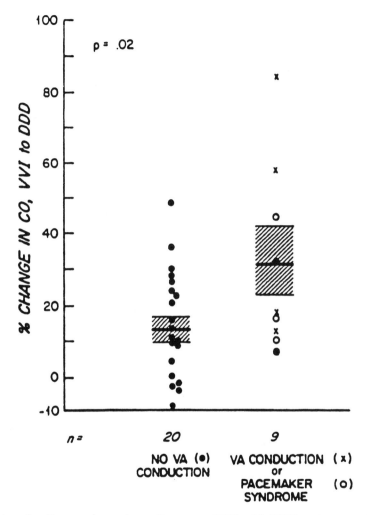

Figure 3. Percent change in cardiac output (CO) with DDD pacing according to the presence (x) or absence (●) of ventriculoatrial (VA) conduction or pacemaker syndrome (○). VA conduction is assessed at time of pacemaker implant. Reproduced with permission of author and publisher.

In patients without VA conduction, there was a wide range of changes in cardiac output during shifts from DDD to VVI pacing. The study of Rediker et al. also showed that cardiac output was significantly greater during DDD pacing than during VVI pacing (6.3±2.6 L/min vs. 4.4±2.2 L/min). In this study, a subgroup of eight out of the 19 patients demanded early crossover from VVI to DDD pacing because of intolerable symptoms after 1.8±1.4 weeks. There were no characteristics of LV function, LA size, or LV size that identified this patient subgroup; however, seven of the eight patients had VA conduction or a sinus rate <60 beats/min. In another study of 24 patients with DDD pacemakers, a stroke volume <50 mL in the VVI mode and the presence of VA conduction predicted maximal benefit from DDD pacing.[14] In addition, five of the 15 patients with a VVI stroke volume <50 mL but none of the nine patient with a stroke volume >50 mL had VA conduction, suggesting that VA conduction predicts hemodynamic benefit from DDD pacing.

While changes in cardiac output and blood pressure are often the primary focus of most discussions about the importance of AV synchrony, it is likely that significant changes in these hemodynamic variables are responsible for only the most severe cases of pacemaker syndrome. It is likely that in the majority of cases, increases in atrial pressure during ventricular pacing are the most common mechanism by which symptoms are produced.[11,12] During ventricular pacing, mean and phasic right and left atrial pressures are elevated (Fig. 4). This elevation of atrial pressures, specifically the giant or cannon A wave occurs because of left (or right) atrial contraction against a closed mitral (or tricuspid) valve, with the increased pressure wave transmitted from the atria into the pulmonary veins and across a closed tricuspid valve to the jugular and hepatic veins. Symptoms such as headaches, fullness in the head or neck, cough, and jaw pain probably arise from this phenomenon.

The importance of AV dyssynchrony as a potential factor in the production of pacemaker syndrome is underscored by reports of patients with DDD(R) or AAI(R) pacemakers who develop pacemaker syndrome (Table 4). During AAI or AAIR pacing, a long stimulus to QRS interval or A-R interval may result, especially during faster sensor-driven rates or after the addition of AV nodal blocking agents. Prolongation of the A-R interval results in simultaneous atrial and ventricular systole and symptoms of pacemaker syndrome due to AV dyssynchrony.[23]

Pacemaker syndrome may also occur during dual chamber pacing.

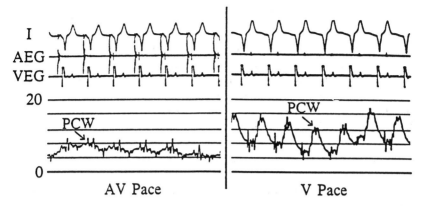

Figure 4. Surface electrocardiographic lead I, atrial electrogram (AEG), ventricular electrogram (VEG), and pulmonary capillary wedge (PCW) pressure recordings from a single patient during AV pacing (AV Pace) on the left and ventricular pacing (V Pace) on the right at 80 beats per minute with AV interval = 150 ms. The cannon A wave is noted on the PCW tracing. Reproduced with permission of author and publisher.

In one report of a patient with a pacemaker programmed to the VDD mode, when the patient's sinus rate dropped below his lower rate, VVI pacing ensued and symptoms consistent with the pacemaker syndrome occurred.[24] Pacemaker syndrome due to programming of the VDD mode became obsolete after the introduction of other DDD pacing modes. The increased popularity of single pass leads for VDD pacing may make this problem more common again.

TABLE *4*

Pacemaker Syndrome with Atrial or Dual Chamber Pacing

- Long programmed AV delay (A—R or P—R >200 ms)
- Pacemaker-mediated or endless loop tachycardia
- DDI or DDIR pacing mode (variable P—V intervals)
- Sinus bradycardia below lower rate limit in VDD pacing mode
- Pacing mode switching (DDDR → VVIR) with Telectronics Meta DDDR
- Rate smoothing or fallback during DDD pacing (CPI Vista DDD)

Utilization of the DDI and DDIR pacing modes may lead to pacemaker syndrome because in this mode P waves are not tracked above the lower rate.[25,26] During DDI or DDIR pacing, the P-V relationship varies and leads to AV dissociation. Pacemaker syndrome may occur during DDI pacing when the sinus rate exceeds the programmed rate; leading to periods of AV dyssynchrony. Likewise, in the DDIR pacing mode, if the sinus rate exceeds the sensor-driven ventricular pacing rate, the atria will be dissociated from the paced QRS leading to AV dyssynchrony. Pacemaker-mediated or endless loop tachycardia occurs when a retrograde P wave occurs after the PVARP and is sensed. This can occur after a loss of atrial sensing, failure to capture the atrium, or after a PVC with retrograde conduction to the atrium when a short PVARP is programmed. Pacemaker-mediated tachycardia is an uncommon cause of pacemaker syndrome today because of widely programmable values for the AV interval and PVARP, and algorithms that prolong the PVARP following a PVC.

The recently approved Meta DDDR (Telectronics, Englewood, Co.) uses an algorithm that provides for mode switching from DDDR to the VVIR mode when an atrial sensed event falls within the PVARP (Fig. 5). VVIR pacing is temporary and reversion to DDDR pacing may occur later. AV dissociation leading to AV dyssynchrony may occur during fallback or rate smoothing, features provided by some dual chamber pacemakers (e.g., CPI's Vista DDD and Precept DDDR). When these features are programmed on, at the upper rate limit or with changes in atrial cycle length exceeding the rate smoothing factor, variable PV intervals will occur leading to transient AV dyssnchrony.

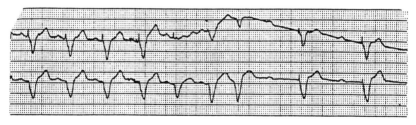

Figure 5.   Rhythm strip from Holter monitor in a patient with a Meta DDDR. In the initial portion of the tracing there is tracking of the atrial rhythm. The P wave following a PVC occurs during the extended PVARP, leading to mode switching, from DDDR to VVIR.

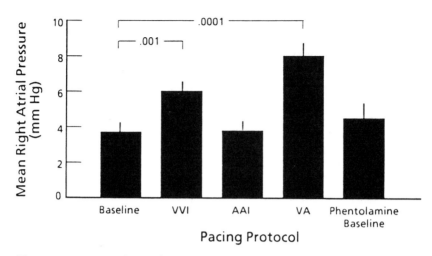

Figure 6. Mean right atrial pressure (mm Hg) measured during VVI pacing, AAI pacing and ventriculoatrial pacing (VA interval = 100–150 ms). Pacing in each mode was performed for 5 minutes at a rate of 100 beats per minute in 16 men without significant heart failure.

The specific hemodynamic consequences of VA conduction have also been studied. In those patients with intact VA conduction, there is a greater decrease in blood pressure and cardiac output during VVI pacing with 1:1 retrograde VA conduction than during ventricular pacing without VA conduction. These findings were reported by Reynolds and Ellenbogen et al.[7,27,28] They reported measurements of intracardiac pressures, arterial pressure, cardiac output, and systemic and pulmonic vascular resistance during both pacing modes. Ellenbogen et al. also compared VA pacing with a fixed VA interval of 100–150 ms, to ventricular pacing.[28] There was a slightly greater decrease in mean arterial pressure and cardiac output, but a greater increase in right atrial and pulmonary capillary wedge pressure during VA pacing than during ventricular pacing in patients without VA conduction (Fig. 6).

Exercise Studies

Prominent symptoms in patients with pacemaker syndrome include fatigue, tiredness, dyspnea, and dyspnea on exertion. In one study, two patients presenting with pacemaker syndrome manifesting as dyspnea on exertion only underwent cardiopulmonary exercise testing. A heightened ventilatory response to exercise manifested as decreased peak $\dot{V}O_2$, shortened exercise duration, higher respiratory rate, and an increased VE/VCO_2 ratio during ventricular pacing.[29] These abnormal ventilatory parameters were improved when the pacing mode was switched from VVI or VVIR to AAIR. Several recent double-blind crossover studies have shown that the mean symptom-limited maximal exercise tolerance time increased by variable amounts (10–15%) during AV synchronous pacing.[8] However, most patients do not perform their daily routine at maximal effort. At lower levels of exercise, which occur more commonly during daily life, the atrial contribution to cardiac output and exercise tolerance is more important than at maximal workload.[30] The importance of the atrial contribution to ventricular filling on exercise performance is probably an additional factor contributing to exercise-induced pacemaker syndrome.

Valvular Regurgitation

Mitral and/or tricuspid regurgitation occur during ventricular pacing, but are not typically as severe or as frequently seen as during AV sequential pacing.[8,11,31–33] The mechanism for the production of cannon or giant A waves is the contraction of the atria against the closed AV valves. Some have speculated, based on animal studies, that an increase in AV valvular regurgitation is responsible for the increase in atrial pressure measured with ventricular pacing.[31,32] However, utilizing left ventricular cineangiography in patients during AV and VA pacing for assessment of mitral regurgitation, only about 30% of patients had slight or mild worsening of mitral regurgitation.[33] Of the five patients in this study experiencing worsening mitral regurgitation, two patients developed trace mitral regurgitation and three patients developed mild mitral regurgitation. There are, however, occasional patients with a marked increase in valvular regurgitation during VVI pacing.

In another study of patients with DDDR pacemakers, the presence and severity of mitral and/or tricuspid regurgitation was assessed by Doppler echocardiography.[8] The presence of tricuspid and mitral regurgitation was greater during VVI pacing than in any dual chamber mode (e.g., VVI, 73% [TR]; DDD, 57% [TR]; and VVI, 75% [MR];

DDD, 34% [MR]). These changes did *not* reach statistical significance (p value not given by authors). The extent of mitral regurgitation assessed by color flow imaging was similar during VVI and DDD pacing; however, the extent of tricuspid regurgitation was greater during VVI than DDD pacing. Importantly, the presence of tricuspid regurgitation did not correlate with the development of pacemaker syndrome, subjective improvement during DDD pacing, or exercise treadmill time. Based on these results, the mechanism for atrial pressure increases during VVI pacing in most patients is likely related to pressure changes from atrial contraction against a closed AV valve and not increased valvular regurgitation.

Humoral Changes

Many investigators have studied the humoral changes during ventricular and atrial pacing. We and others have shown that plasma norepinephrine and epinephrine levels increase acutely in patients during shifts from normal sinus rhythm to ventricular pacing.[34,35] In one report, acute increases in coronary sinus norepinephrine levels were higher in the VVI pacing mode at rest and during exercise than during the VAT pacing mode.[35] Arterial concentrations of catecholamines also increased more during exercise in the VVI mode, but the differences are less striking than those measured from the coronary sinus. In this study, cardiac norepinephrine overflow (calculated as the difference between plasma concentrations of norepinephrine in the coronary sinus and arterial plasma multipled by coronary sinus blood flow) were well correlated with pulmonary capillary wedge pressure ($R = 0.79$). Since coronary sinus norepinephrine overflow is a reasonable measure of cardiac sympathetic nerve activity, this study demonstrates that VVI pacing caused a greater increase in cardiac sympathetic activation than AV synchronous VAT pacing. In our study, the increase in plasma norepinephrine levels appeared to correlate best with the decline in systolic pressure during ventricular pacing. In our earlier study, we showed that plasma norepinephrine, but not epinephrine or dopamine, was significantly elevated during ventricular pacing with VA conduction.[28] In another study of 10 patients with complete AV block, VVIR and DDD pacing produced similar increases in plasma norepinephrine and epinephrine during exercise. There was, however, a large degree of variation in individual patient responses during each pacing mode.[36] These studies suffer from several limitations. In some studies, plasma catecholamine levels, instead of coronary sinus catecholamine levels, are measured. Plasma catecholamines are only a rough approximation of overall sympathetic activity because they are influenced by the rate of release and clearance of catecholamines from different vascular beds. Plasma catecholamine levels may poorly reflect cardiac sympathetic activation during non-steady-state conditions (e.g., changes in pacing modes). The increase in both plasma and coronary sinus catecholamines during VVI pacing probably reflects the compensatory response of the sympathetic nervous system to the decrease in cardiac output and blood pressure with AV dyssynchrony.

ANP (atrial natriuretic peptide) is a 28 amino acid polypeptide produced in granules located within the atrium. ANP is an arterial and venous vasodilator, and in rats results in a vagally mediated inhibition of regional sympathetic nervous activity. Plasma ANP levels are increased when atrial pressure or atrial distension is increased.[37] In patients with DDD pacemakers, because of total AV block, lower ANP levels during rest and exercise were seen with DDD pacing. Peak ANP levels were reached 5 minutes after termination of exercise with DDD pacing and 17 minutes after exercise with VVI pacing.[38] We have also shown that VA pacing increases ANP levels more than ventricular pacing does with VA dissociation (Fig. 7).[34] In this study, the changes in vascular tone measured by venous occlusion plethysmography did not correlate with the changes in ANP levels during ventricular or VA pacing in our study.

Two other studies have also shown that ANP levels were higher during VVI than DDD pacing.[40,41] In one study, ANP release was higher during rate-matched VVI pacing with exercise than DDD pacing. Both of these studies emphasize that AV synchrony reduces ANP release during exercise-induced sinus tachycardia as well as at rest. A preliminary report of five patients with pacemaker syndrome showed they had higher plasma concentrations of ANP during shifts from sinus rhythm to VVI pacing (from 79 pmol/L to 298–341 pmol/L during VVI pacing) than during shifts from sinus rhythm to DDD pacing (79 pmol/L to 131–188 pmol/L during DDD pacing).[36,42] These studies show that ANP is elevated far more during VVI pacing than during AV synchronous pacing modes.[40–42] Whether ANP plays a role in producing the symptoms associated with pacemaker syndrome is still unclear. The observation that ANP levels are raised significantly during VA pacing is intriguing. A

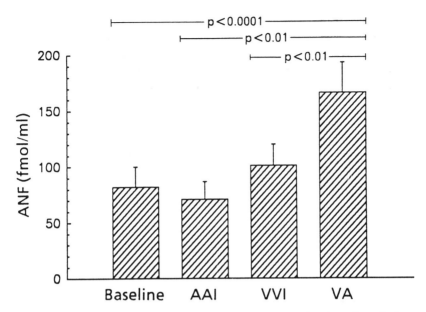

Figure 7. ANF levels measured during VVI, AAI, and VA pacing. Patient population studied are same patients as described in Figure 6.

critical issue remaining to be solved is whether changes in ANP are the cause or the result of pacemaker syndrome. Until there is a specific inhibitor of ANP, it will be difficult to be certain whether ANP plays a primary or secondary role in the pacemaker syndrome.

Role of Atrial and Cardiovascular Reflexes

Alicandri and colleagues at the Cleveland Clinic carefully investigated three patients with hypotension and near-syncope during ventricular pacing due to severe pacemaker syndrome.[43] They measured arterial pressure, cardiac output, total peripheral vascular resistance, and right atrial pressure in these patients. There was a small but variable decrease in cardiac output (ranging from 0% to 15%) during shifts from ventricular pacing to normal sinus rhythm in these three patients. Four patients with stable blood pressure during ventricular pacing were studied as controls. These patients also demonstrated a small but variable decrease in cardiac output during shifts from sinus rhythm to ventricular pacing. The striking difference between the controls and patients with pacemaker syndrome was the approximately 20% increase in peripheral resistance in the control patients and the failure of peripheral vascular resistance to increase in patients with pacemaker syndrome (Fig. 8). In fact, the control patients showed a greater decrease in cardiac output during ventricular pacing than the three patients with pacemaker syndrome, but were well compensated by a mean increase in total peripheral resistance of 22%, compared to pacemaker syndrome patients who had a 1.5% decrease in total peripheral resistance. The investigators concluded that ventricular

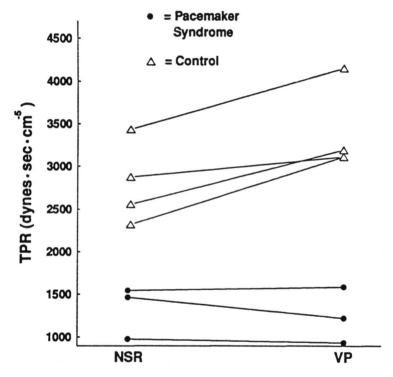

Figure 8.   Changes in total peripheral vascular resistance (dynes·sec·cm^{-5}) during normal sinus rhythm and ventricular pacing in four control patients and three patients with pacemaker syndrome. Data derived from reference 41.

pacing gives rise to a decrease in cardiac output that elicits a vasoconstrictor reflex. With a decrease in cardiac output of 15–30% (e.g., as during assuming the upright position), a normal compensatory response of sympathetic peripheral vasoconstriction to maintain arterial pressure is seen in most patients. In addition, the authors hypothesized that the abnormally timed atrial contraction during VVI pacing gives rise to an atrial vasodilator reflex (possibly due to release of ANP) resulting from stimulation of inhibitory vagal receptors on the atrial wall that are elicited by atrial distension. These two opposing reflexes lead to a wide range and severity of physiologic responses to AV dyssynchrony, resulting in widely variable clinical manifestations during VVI pacing.

In another study, Erlebacher et al. studied 20 patients post cardiac surgery with indwelling Swan-Ganz catheters to detect cannon A waves in the pulmonary capillary wedge tracing during ventricular pacing.[44] They noted a greater decrease in stroke volume index during ventricular pacing in those patients with cannon A waves (cannon A waves = new waves on the pulmonary capillary wedge tracing >4 mm Hg when pacing is switched from AV synchronous to the ventricular pacing mode). Mean systemic blood pressure decreased only in patients with cannon A waves. Ten of 13 patients with cannon A waves had 1:1 retrograde VA conduction. Those patients without cannon A waves had a significant increase (22.8%) in total peripheral vascular resistance during ventricular pacing, while those with cannon A waves had a much smaller increase (4.9%, p<0.002) in total peripheral vascular resistance. Therefore, the response to ventricular pacing in patients with cannon A waves was less than 25% the response seen in patients without cannon A waves. These authors caution that although pacing-induced hypotension is most often attributed to a decrease in stroke volume due to loss of atrial transport, the available data do not show a close correlation between the decrease in stroke volume and the decrease in blood pressure. In fact, the blood pressure (and vasoconstrictor) response to a decrease in cardiac output is variable. In some reports, a decrease in stroke volume or cardiac output during ventricular pacing has been associated in symptomatic patients with a minimal increase, no change, or a *decrease* in peripheral vascular resistance.[43,45,46] These authors suggested that the principal mechanism involved in the failure to elicit significant peripheral vasoconstriction may be due to an "atrial vasodepressor reflex."

Atrial receptors and reflexes are the subject of a recent review.[47] Atrial receptors with myelinated afferents are attached to venoatrial junctions primarily and respond to changes in atrial pressure and volume. Unmyelinated vagal nerve endings increase discharge frequency directly related to atrial pressure or atrial volume and may play a role in pacemaker syndrome. Other inhibitory receptors are located in the atria and cardiopulmonary region and are subserved by nonmyelinated afferent vagal fibers. Activation of these endings causes vagal stimulation and sympathoinhibition leading to vasodilation and bradycardia.

Further insight into the potential mechanism of pacemaker syndrome is provided by Ellenbogen et al.[28] Our group measured the changes in forearm blood flow and forearm vascular resistance during atrial, ventricular, and VA pacing. Forearm blood flow was measured by venous occlusion plethysmography, which provides accurate measurement of changes in regional blood flow and thereby reflects changes in regional vasomotor tone. During VA pacing, but *not* ventricular pacing, striking increases in forearm vascular resistance occur within 30 seconds (Fig. 9). These changes were correlated with changes in systolic arterial pressure, suggesting that these vascular responses (e.g., forearm vasoconstriction) are largely mediated by arterial baroreceptors (Fig. 10). This increase in vascular resistance is mediated by alpha sympathetic vasoconstriction, as it is blocked by intraarterial phentolamine (alpha-sympathetic antagonist).

Further documentation of these reflex changes and their almost immediate time course is provided with peroneal microneurography, a technique that allows recording of postganglionic muscle sympathetic efferent nerve activity.[48] This technique utilizes a tungsten microelectrode advanced through the skin to record muscle sympathetic nerve activity from the peroneal nerve after being amplified (total gain, 70,000) and filtered (bandwidth 700–2000 Hz). Recordings were considered acceptable when spontaneous, pulse-synchronous bursts with signal-to-noise ratios >3:1 were obtained. Muscle sympathetic nerve activity was identified by its relation to cardiac and respiratory activity, its tendency to increase during held expiration and Valsalva straining, and its lack of response to arousal stimuli or skin stroking. In addition, muscle sympathetic nerve activity is characterized by fairly regular pulse synchronous bursts of impulses sometimes occurring in short sequences separated by periods of nerve silence. Nerve activity was then quantified by an off-line custom program for signal processing designed to integrate the nerve traffic signal above the baseline noise level over 2-second time periods.[49] Several lines of evidence confirm the sympathetic nature of these im-

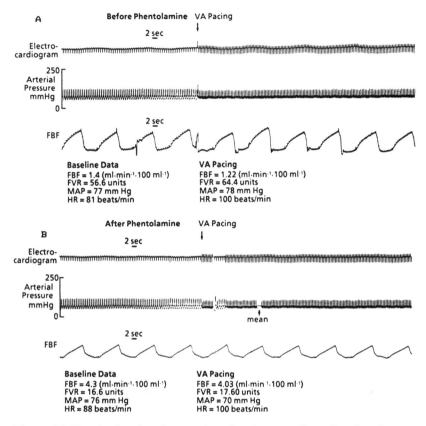

Figure 9A,B. Analog data from patient showing recording of surface electro-cardiogram, phasic arterial pressure (mm Hg), and forearm blood flow during ventriculoatrial (VA) pacing before and after phentolamine infusion. Reproduced with permission of author and publisher.

pulses, such as increases in nerve activity preceding sympathetic responses in effector organs by several seconds. Muscle sympathetic nerve activity is also greatly influenced by fluctuations of blood pressure, especially diastolic blood pressure. It appears that sympathetic outflow to the vascular bed of skeletal muscle may play an important role in buffering acute changes in blood pressure.

Using this technique, we have also recently been able to demonstrate

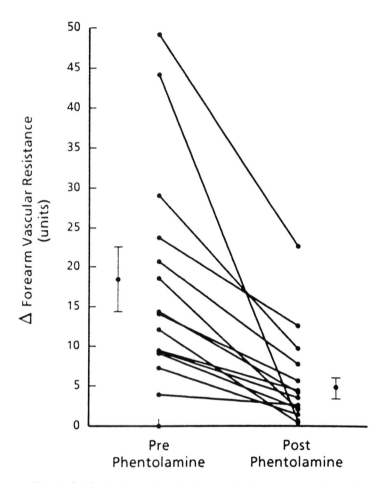

Figure 10. Individual values for the change in forearm vascular resistance (FVR) in 16 male patients during ventriculoatrial pacing before and after phentolamine infusion. During the shift from sinus rhythm to ventriculoatrial pacing, there was a significant increase in FVR to 18 ± 4.1 U (units) before phentolamine and to 5.8 ± 1.5 U after phentolamine. There was a 67% decrease in FVR during shift to VA pacing after phentolamine. Reproduced with permission of author and publisher.

that in patients undergoing electrophysiology study, there is an increase in sympathetic efferent activity to the leg during ventricular, but not atrial pacing (Fig. 11). These observations suggest that sympathetic activation and vasoconstriction of regional (muscle) beds is the "normal response" to ventricular pacing.

We hypothesize that during ventricular pacing, especially with retrograde VA conduction, regional vasomotor tone and humoral sympathetic activation occurs in most people. The changes in sympathetic tone are correlated with the change in systolic arterial pressure and are probably mediated by arterial baroreceptors (Fig. 12). In the upright position, blood is pooled in the extremities and arterial baroreceptors are further activated to compensate for the decreased cardiac output and systolic arterial pressure. In *some* patients, pacemaker syndrome may result due to the inability to compensate by further augmenting sympathetic tone in the face of both of these stimuli. Further, these vascular responses may be additionally altered by the effect of drugs, underlying organic heart disease, volume status, and autonomic defects. The role of atrial and cardiopulmonary reflexes (e.g., inhibitory reflexes) and humoral substances (ANP) will await the results of further investigation. It is unclear whether pacemaker syndrome results from inadequate sympathoexcitation or to a predominance of inhibitory vagal reflexes from the atria and cardiopulmonary region.

Treatment

The treatment of pacemaker syndrome is straightforward. Once the diagnosis is made, symptoms can be eliminated by changing to atrial pacing (AAI or AAIR) if AV conduction is relatively intact or upgrading to a dual chamber pacemaker. In an occasional patient with sinus node dysfunction, the ventricular pacing rate can be lowered or hysteresis can be programmed so that the frequency and/or duration of ventricular pacing is decreased. Certainly, it is preferable to identify patients at high risk of pacemaker syndrome prior to implantation by assessing for retrograde VA conduction or measuring blood pressure changes during ventricular pacing. Patients at risk of pacemaker syndrome should be paced in a mode that allows for AV synchrony.

Pacemaker syndrome produces a wide variety of symptoms, some secondary to the decrease in cardiac output from VVI pacing, some sec-

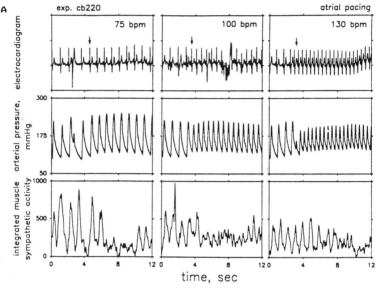

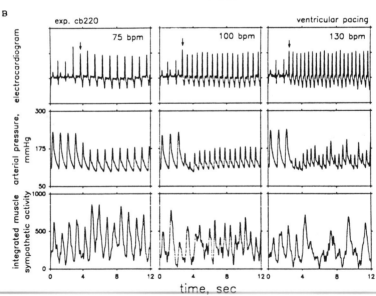

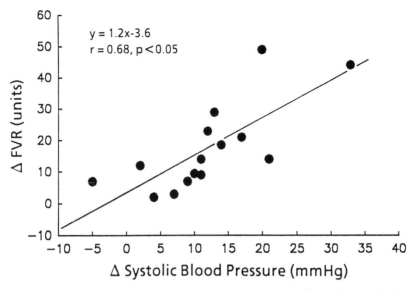

Figure 12. Change in forearm vascular resistance was well correlated with the decrease in systolic blood pressure during VA pacing, suggesting that arterial baroreceptors mediate vasoconstriction during ventricular pacing.

ondary to decreased arterial pressure, and others from the increased venous and atrial pressure occurring during ventricular pacing. An understanding of the hemodynamic, vascular, and humoral effects of ventricular pacing and AV dyssynchrony will lead to a better appreciation of the importance of choosing the appropriate pacing mode in an individual patient.

←————————————————————————————————

Figure 11A,B. Tracings of surface ECG, arterial pressure, and integrated muscle sympathetic nerve activity during transition from sinus rhythm to atrial pacing (arrows) at rates of 75, 100, and 130 beats per minute (bpm) and ventricular pacing (arrows) at rates of 75, 100, and 130 bpm in a 76-year-old man with sick sinus syndrome and hypertension. Note the progressive decrease in integrated muscle sympathetic nerve activity during atrial pacing, but the increase in burst amplitude and width during ventricular pacing. Ventricular pacing is a stimulus to sympathetic activation.

Acknowledgments: We thank Michael Smith, Ph.D., Larry Beightol, M.S., Regina Rogers, R.N., Carolyn McNamara, R.N., and Dave Brands for their help in undertaking and performing these investigations.

References

1. Mitsui T, Hori M, Suma K, Wanibuchi Y, Saigusa M. The "pacemaking syndrome." In: Jacobs JE (ed): Proceedings of the Eighth Annual International Conference on Medical and Biological Engineering, Association for the Advancement of Medical Instrumentation, Chicago, 1969, pp 29–33.
2. Haas JM, Strait GB. Pacemaker-induced cardiovascular failure. Am J Cardiol 1974;33:295–299.
3. Patel AK, Yap VU, Thomsen JH. Adverse effects of right ventricular pacing in a patient with aortic stenosis: hemodynamic documentation and management. Chest 1977;72:103–105.
4. Edhag O, Fagrell B, Lagergren H. Deleterious effects of cardiac pacing in a paient with mitral insufficiency. Acta Med Scand 1977;202:331–334.
5. Nishimura RA, Gersh BJ, Vliestra RE, Osborn MJ, Ilstrup DM, Holmes DR. Hemodynamic and symptomatic consequences of ventricular pacing. PACE 1982;5:903–910.
6. Heldman D, Mulvihill D, Nguyen H, Messenger JC, Rylaarsdam A, Evans K, Castellanet MJ. True incidence of pacemaker syndrome. PACE 1990;13:1742–1750.
7. Dateling F, Obel IWP. Clinical comparison of VVI, VVIR and DDD pacemakers in symptomatic relief of bradyarrhythmias. PACE 1989;12:1278.
8. Sulke N, Chambers J, Dritsas A, Sowton E. A randomized double-blind crossover comparison of four rate-responsive pacing modes. J Am Coll Cardiol 1991;17:696–706.
9. Cohen SI, Frank HA. Preservation of active atrial transport: an important clinical consideration in cardiac pacing. Chest 1982;81:51–54.
10. Ausubel K, Furman S. The pacemaker syndrome. Ann Intern Med 1985;103:420–429.
11. Reynolds DW. Hemodynamics of cardic pacing. In: Ellenbogen KA (ed): Cardiac Pacing, Blackwell Scientific Publications, Boston, MA (in press).
12. Levine PA, Mace RC. Pacing Therapy: A Guide to Cardiac Pacing for Optimum Hemodynamic Benefit, Futura Publishing Co, Mount Kisco, New York, 1983, pp 3–18.
13. Miller M, Fox S, Jenkins R, Schwartz J, Toonder FG. Pacemaker syndrome: a non-invasive means to its diagnosis and treatment. PACE 1981;4:503–506.
14. Pearson AC, Janosik DL, Redd RM, Buckingham TA, Labovitz AJ. Hemodynamic benefit of atrioventricular synchrony: prediction from baseline Doppler echocardiographic variables. J Am Coll Cardiol 1989;13:1613–1621.
15. Stewart WJ, Dicola VC, Harthorne JW, Gillam LD, Weyman AE. Doppler ultrasound measurement of cardiac output in patients with physiologic pacemakers. Am J Cardiol 1984;54:308–312.

16. Rediker DE, Eagle KA, Homma S, Gillam LD, Harthorne JW. Clinical and hemodynamic comparison of VVI versus DDD pacing in patients with DDD pacemakers. Am J Cardiol 1988;61:323–329.
17. Akhtar M. Retrograde conduction in man. PACE 1981;4:548–562.
18. Baig MW, Perrins EJ. The hemodynamics of cardiac pacing: clinical and physiological aspects. Prog Cardiovasc Dis 1991;33:283–298.
19. Mitchell JH, Gilmore JP, Sarnoff SJ. The transport function of the atrium. Factors influencing the relation between mean left atrial pressures and left ventricular end-diastolic pressure. Am J Cardiol 1962;9:237–247.
20. Samet P, Castillo C, Bernstein WH. Hemodynamic consequences of sequential atrioventricular pacing. Subjects with normal hearts. Am J Cardiol 1968;21:207–212.
21. Greenberg B, Chatterjee K, Parmley WW, Werner JA, Holly AN. The influence of left ventricular filling pressure on atrial contribution to cardiac output. Am Heart J 1979;98:742–751.
22. Reynolds DW, Wilson MF, Burow RD, Schaefer CF, Lazzara R, Thadani U. Hemodynamic evaluation of atrioventricular sequential vs. ventricular pacing in patients with noral and poor ventricular function at variable heart rates and posture. J Am Coll Cardiol 1983;1:636–636.
23. Den Dulk K, Lindemands FW, Brugada P, Smeets JLRM, Wellens HJJ. Pacemaker syndrome with AAI rate variable pacing: importance of atrioventricular conduction properties, medication, and pacemaker programmability. PACE 1988;11:1226–1233.
24. Levine PA, Seltzer JP, Pirzada FA. The "pacemaker syndrome" in a properly functioning physiologic pacing system. PACE 1983;6:279–282.
25. Cunningham TM. Pacemaker syndrome due to retrograde conduction in a DDI pacemaker. Am Heart J 1988;115:478–479.
26. Torresan J, Ebagosti A, Allard-Latour G. Pacemaker syndrome with DDD pacing. PACE 1984;7:1148–1151.
27. Reynolds DW, Olson EG, Burow RD, Thadani U, Lazzara R. Hemodynaic evaluation of atrioventricular and ventriculoatrial pacing (abstr). PACE 1984;7:476.
28. Ellenbogen KA, Thames MD, Mohanty PK. New insights into pacemaker syndrome gained rom hemodynamic, humoral and vascular responses during ventriculoatrial pacing. Am J Cardiol 1990;65:53–59.
29. Fujik A, Tani M, Mizumaki K, Asanoi H, Sasayama S. Pacemaker syndrome evaluated by cardiopulmonary exercise testing. PACE 1990;13:1236–1241.
30. Duncan JL, Eisinger G, Florio J, Hayes D, Juszy R. Characterization of rate response during normal daily activities with a dual chamber pacemaker (abstr). PACE 1989;12:1189).
31. Ogawa S, Dreifus LS, Shenoy PN, Brockman SK, Berkovitz BV. Hemodynamic consequences of atrioventricular and ventriculoatrial pacing. PACE 1978;1:8–15.
32. Morgan DE, Norman R, West RO, Burgaff G. Echocardiographic assessment of tricuspid regurgitation during ventricular demand pacing. Am J Cardiol 1986;58:1025–1029.

33. Reynolds DW, Olson EG, Burow RD, Thadani U, Lazzara R. Mitral regurgitation during atrioventricular and ventriculoatrial pacing (abstr). PACE 1984;7:463.
34. Hull RW, Snow F, Herre J, Ellenbogen KA. The plasma catecholamine responses to ventricular pacing: implications for rate responsive pacing. PACE 1990;13:1408–1415.
35. Pehrrson SK, Hjemdahl P, Nordlander R, Astrom H. A comparison of sympathoadrenal activity and cardiac performance at rest and during exercise in patients with ventricular demand or atrial synchronous pacing. Br Heart J 1988;60:212–220.
36. Oldroyd RG, Rae AP, Carter R, Wingate C, Cobbe SM. Double blind crossover comparison of the effects of dual chamber pacing (DDD) and ventricular rate adaptive (VVIR) pacing on neuroendocrine variables, exercise performance, and symptoms in complete heart block. Br Heart J 1991;65:188–193.
37. Bishop VS, Haywood JR. Hormonal control of cardiovascular reflexes. In: Zucker IH, Gilmore JP (ed): Reflex Control of the Circulation, CRC Press, Boca Raton, 1991, pp 253–271.
38. Stagl K, Weil J, Seitz K, Laule M, Gerzer R. Influence of AV synchrony on the plasma level of atrial natriuretic peptide (ANP) in patients with total AV block. PACE 1988;11:1176–1181.
39. Ellenbogen KA, Kapadia K, Walsh M, Mohanty PK. Increase in plasma atrial natriuretic factor during ventriculoatrial pacing. Am J Cardiol 1989;64:236–237.
40. Blanc JJ, Mansourati J, Ritter P, Nitzsche R, Pages Y, Genet L, Morin JF. Atrial natriuretic factor release during exercise in patients successively paced in DDD and VVIR mode. PACE (in press).
41. Vardas PE, Travill CM, Williams TDM, Ingram AM, Lightman SL, Sutton R. Effect of dual chamber pacing on raised plasma atrial natriuretic peptide concentrations in complete atrioventricular block. Br Med J 1988;296:94.
42. Travail CM, Williams TDW, Vardas P, Ingram A, Chalmers J, Lightman S, Sutton R. Pacemaker syndrome is associated with very high plasma concentrations of atrial natriuretic peptide (ANF). J Am Coll Cardiol 1989;13:111.
43. Alicandri C, Fonad F, Farazi RC, Castle L, Morant V. Three cases of hypotension and syncope with ventricular pacing: possible role of atrial reflexes. Am J Cardiol 1978;42:137–142.
44. Erlebacher JA, Danner RL, Stelzer PE. Hypotension with ventricular pacing: an atrial vasodepressor reflex in human beings. J Am Coll Cardiol 1984;4:550–555.
45. Erbel R. Pacemaker syndrome (letter). Am J Cardiol 1979;47:771–772.
46. Lewis ME, Sung RJ, Alter BR, Myerburg RJ. Pacemaker-induced hypotension. Chest 1981;79:354–356.
47. Hainsworth R. In: Zucker IH, Gilmore JP (eds): Atrial Receptors in Reflex Control of the Circulation, CRC Press, Boca Raton, 1991.
48. Vallbo AB, Hagbarth KE, Torebjork HE, Wallin BG. Somatosensory, proprioceptive and sympathetic activity in human peripheral nerves. Physiol Res 1979;59:919–957.

Chapter 6

Noninvasive Hemodynamic Evaluation of Pacing

SVEIN FAERESTRAND

Introduction

Pacemakers should be implanted not only to improve life expectancy of the patients but also to treat heart failure, to improve working capacity, and to improve the patients' feeling of general well-being. VVI pacemakers are unable to normalize or optimize circulatory performance, and the patients' exercise capacity often remains markedly reduced during VVI pacing. In addition, in many patients, VVI pacing can have deleterious effects on long-term hemodynamics compared to DDD pacing.

Since improvement of exercise hemodynamics is strongly related to increment of heart rate, a physiologic pacemaker should incorporate both restoration of normal AV synchrony and provide normal chronotropic response.

Previously, assessment of hemodynamics during cardiac pacing was performed mostly by invasive methods, and many of the studies elucidated only the acute hemodynamic effects of pacing. Noninvasive Doppler echocardiography has proved to be able to distinguish even small hemodynamic changes between different modern pacing modes. The gated blood pool equilibrium radionuclide ventriculography, which is not a completely noninvasive method, has also been used in the assessment of hemodynamics during pacing. However, this method is often unable to distinguish small but nevertheless important hemodynamic effects provided by modern pacing systems.[1]

New Perspectives in Cardiac Pacing, Vol. 3, edited by S. Serge Barold and Jacques Mugica, Mount Kisco, NY, Futura Publishing Co., © 1993.

In this chapter, the focus will be on the use of the noninvasive Doppler, M-mode, and two-dimensional echocardiographic methods, and relevant data on hemodynamic evaluation of different acute and long-term pacing modes will be presented.

Noninvasive Ultrasonic Methods

Improvement of the apparatus as well as thorough research using the noninvasive Doppler, M-mode, and two-dimensional echocardiographic methods in experimental and human studies have resulted in establishment of reliable, reproducible, and sensitive methods for noninvasive measurement of cardiac output (CO), cardiac dimensions, and valvular functions. A great advantage with the ultrasonic methods compared to invasive methods is that the stroke volume (SV) can be measured on a beat-to-beat basis. In this way, hemodynamic measurements can easily be timed to the electrocardiographic events, which is important during arrhythmias as well as during different pacing modes. Furthermore, the noninvasive nature of these techniques make it possible to repeat the measurements with minimal discomfort to the patient in time-related studies of cardiac diseases and therapeutic interventions, including pacemaker treatment.

Several studies have demonstrated a good correlation between the measurement of CO by combining Doppler, two-dimensional, and M-mode echocardiography when compared to invasive methods both in patients with and patients without aortic valve disease. Furthermore, Doppler aortic and mitral flow velocity measurements can be performed with acceptable intraobserver, interobserver, and day-to-day variability.[2-30]

The aortic orifice area is almost constant during the systole, and therefore changes in the SV will affect the aortic flow velocity measured by Doppler echocardiography.[3,31] The aortic flow profile is relatively flat during systole, and hence, the systolic flow distance multiplied by the aortic area is equal to the SV.[32]

Instrumentation

A combined echocardiographic machine with a two-dimensional sector scanner and M-mode echo, in which a Doppler instrument is incorporated, is used for simultaneous sector scanning and Doppler examination. The direction of the Doppler ultrasound beam and the depth of the sample volume, which can be changed, are indicated by a line and a rectangle on the two-dimensional picture. Thus, the sample volume can be located in the region of interest guided by the two-dimensional picture. The Doppler instrument has an audio amplifier and a loudspeaker where the Doppler frequency shift is heard. The highest frequency of the Doppler shift produces a whistling sound, indicating sampling from the blood-jet in the center of the vessel and at a small angle to the blood-jet. The Doppler instrument estimates velocities by converting the Doppler shift frequencies into analog voltages proportional to the frequency shifts (Fig. 1).[2] The spectral analyzer of the Doppler instrument displays all Doppler shift frequencies, using a gray scale to indicate the amount of scatterers (red blood cells) at the various velocities (Fig. 1). In the spectrum, recording echoes from the valves produce strong reflections and thus tall, sharp spikes on display and clicks in the loudspeaker. Valve movements towards the transducer yield taller spikes than movements away from the transducer. Consequently, these amplitudes of the Doppler signal can be used to locate the sample volume in relation to the valves and to time the valve motion in relation to the electrocardiogram. The sound of the Doppler shift frequencies and the direction of the Doppler beam, as well as the location of the sample volume in relation to the region of interest visualized on the sector scanner, are used to achieve a small angle between the blood-jet direction and the Doppler beam direction, which is necessary in order to estimate the true velocity of blood flow.[2]

The location of the Doppler sample volume in the blood-jet in the aortic root does not significantly influence the measured flow velocity.[7] However, in patients with aortic valve diseases leading to a turbulent flow pattern and increased velocity distal to the valves because of valve obstruction, the aortic flow profile is not flat distal to the aortic valves. In the typically old patient population treated with pacemakers, calcification and/or stenosis of the aortic valves is often seen. Therefore, when SV is measured by Doppler echocardiography, the transducer should routinely be located at the apex of the heart and the Doppler sample volume in the left ventricular outflow tract just below the aortic valves. In patients with normal aortic flow profile, the Doppler transducer can be placed in the suprasternal notch, and the Doppler sampling can be performed from the aortic root without guidance from the two-dimen-

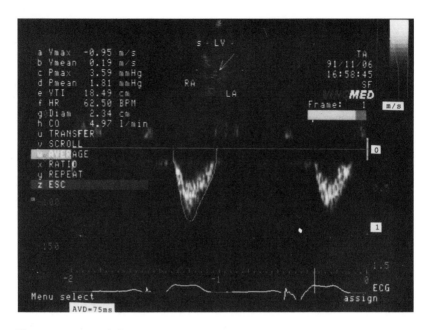

Figure 1.   Recorded parameters during measurement of aortic flow velocity by pulsed wave Doppler echocardiography. The Doppler transducer is located at the apex of the left ventricle with the sample volume located in the left ventricular outflow tract. In the spectrum of velocities, the more commonly occurring velocities are assigned a darker gray scale representation than those occurring less frequently. In this way, sampling from the blood-jet results in the darkest gray scale representation at the highest velocities. The electrocardiogram shows AV synchronous pacing pacing. The velocity-time integral (VTI, cm) of maximum aortic velocity is measured by envelope tracing of the aortic velocity profile demonstrated on the left-hand side velocity profile. HR = heart rate; LV = left ventricle; RV = right ventricle; LA = left atrium; Vmax = maximum velocity; Vmean = mean velocity; Pmax = maximum pressure gradient; Pmean = mean pressure gradient: Diam = measured diameter in the left ventricular outflow tract.

sional picture. The two transducer positions are equally good in the supine patient, but to the less trained investigator there is a great advantage in using the apical position because the sample volume then can be visualized on the sector scanner, thus making it easier to place the sample volume correctly in the region of interest.

The suprasternal location of the Doppler transducer is best during measurement of CO in patients performing exercise tests. It is difficult to maintain a constant sample volume site during the progressive stages of exercise because of excessive chest wall motion. Therefore, often smaller dedicated continuous wave Doppler tranducers are used to measure CO during exercise, but the technique is the same as that applied at rest. The Doppler method for measurement of CO is reliable compared to the thermodilution technique at low levels of exercise, but tend to underestimate the CO during moderate to heavy exercise. However, the thermodilution method may overestimate the CO during exercise.[33–37]

By using the calculation program incorporated in the echo machine, the velocity profile of aortic flow is traced from the beginning to the end of flow. Based on this envelope around the spectrum tracing, the maximum and mean velocities, the maximum and mean pressure gradients, and the velocity-time integral (VTI, cm) are calculated (Fig. 1). The aortic VTI is proportional to the volumetric blood flow so that the integral reflects changes in SV. The integral of maximum aortic velocity has been used because it is less affected by errors caused by small changes in the transducer position than the mean velocity.[2] The VTI includes both the velocity and the ejection time, and this is probably the best Doppler estimate of changes in blood velocity and hence in the SV.[4] A difference of 10% in aortic VTI suggests a significant hemodynamic change.[26,27]

Measurement of Left Ventricular Outflow Area

Guided by a parasternal long-axis picture of the heart, the aortic orifice diameter can be measured by locating the cursor line perpendicular to an imaginary central longitudinal axis of the left ventricular outflow tract just below the aortic valves (Fig. 2). If the aortic area measured in the aortic root distal to the aortic valves is used as the flow area and not the aortic orifice area, the SV will be significantly overestimated.[3]

Calculations

The left ventricular outflow tract diameter (D; Fig. 2) and aortic VTI (Fig. 1) have been calculated as the mean of 10 beats. In this way, variations of the aortic VTI caused by respiration, variable atrial contribution to the ventricular filling during VVI pacing, and minor changes

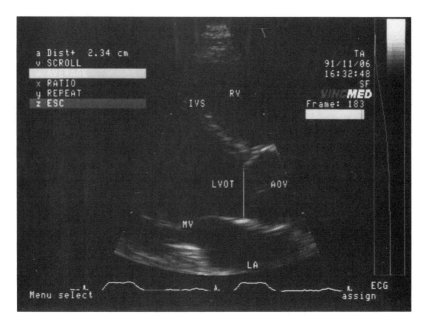

Figure 2. Measurement of aortic orifice diameter (Dist +) from a parasternal long-axis sector scan picture of the heart. LVOT = left ventricular outflow tract; AOV = aortic valves; MV = mitral valves; LA = left atrium; IVS = interventricular septum; RV = right ventricle.

in transducer position during the measurements are compensated for. The SV is calculated as:

$$SV(mL) = (\tfrac{1}{2}D[cm])^2 \times 3.14 \times VTI(cm)$$

Mitral Flow Pattern and Diastolic Dynamics

With the ultrasonic transducer located at the apex or just medial to the apex of the left ventricle, the mitral flow profile can be recorded by locating the Doppler sample volume in the mitral ostium guided by the four-chamber sector scan echocardiographic picture (Fig. 3).[2] The two-dimensional picture and the spectrum of Doppler shift frequencies are recorded simultaneously. The mitral flow profile demonstrates an early

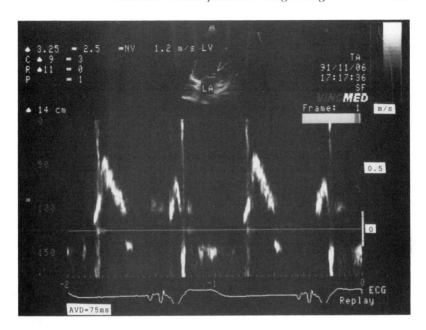

Figure 3. Recorded parameters during measurement of mitral flow velocity by pulsed wave Doppler echocardiography. The transducer is located at the apex of the left ventricle and the sample volume is located in the mitral ostium guided by the four-chamber sector scan picture. The early diastolic peak flow velocity (E) is normally higher than the late peak velocity (A) after atrial contraction, and the E:A >1. The tall A wave indicates a mechanically effective atrial contraction. The high amplitudes of echoes at the opening and closure of mitral valves are clearly demonstrated. Arrow indicates mital valves. For abbreviations, see Figures 1 and 2.

peak flow velocity (E) indicating the peak of early rapid filling, followed by a reduction of the flow velocity in the mid-diastole, and finally an increase of flow velocity to a late atrial peak flow velocity (A) corresponding to the peak flow velocity caused by atrial contraction. In normal hearts, the E wave velocity is higher than the A wave velocity with an E:A ratio >1 also in elderly people.[37,39] Doppler studies have revealed that several factors can influence the left ventricular filling pattern assessed by transmitral flow velocity profile. These factors include the sampling site in the mitral ostium, age, AV delay, heart rate, loading conditions, left ventricular systolic function, and left ventricular compliance and relaxation.[28,40-52] It has also been shown that similar mitral inflow velocity patterns can be produced by different conditions causing similar changes in time course of transmitral pressure difference.[53]

In patients with reduced compliance of the left ventricle, as seen in arterial hypertension and aortic stenosis with left ventricular hypertrophy, and in hypertrophic cardiomyopathy, the A wave velocity usually increases and E:A ratio usually decreases below 1 (Fig. 4).[54-56] The contribution to the left ventricular filling by the early rapid filling phase, and that caused by atrial contraction can be estimated by calculating the velocity-time integral of the mitral flow velocity profile for the E and A wave contribution, respectively.[57] In this way, the contribution of a synchronized atrial systole to the diastolic filling of the left ventricle can be measured. A P wave in the electrocardiogram does not in itself prove

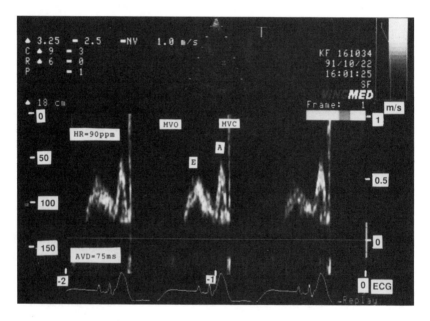

Figure 4.   Measurement of mitral flow velocity by pulsed wave Doppler echocardiography in a patient with hypertrophic obstructive cardiomyopathy during AV synchronous pacing. A pathological E:A <1 is demonstrated. MVO = mitral valve opening; MVC = mitral valve closure. For other abbreviations, see Figure 3.

that atrial contraction is taking place, but the increment of mitral flow velocity after the P wave in the ECG indicates that atrial contraction is actually taking place (Figs. 3 and 4). Patients with a large atrial contribution to left ventricular filling will have the largest increase in CO during DVI versus VVI pacing.[58]

Some recent human Doppler studies of mitral flow profiles have indicated that an increment of heart rate of 10 beats/min can decrease the E:A ratio by approximately 30%.[59] Rate increase during DDD pacing also results in an increment of A velocity and atrial velocity-time integral.[60,61] Animal experiments using atrial pacing, infusion of isoproterenol, or atropine to increase the heart rate from an average of 97 to 146 beats/min resulted in similar increase of the transmitral A velocity with a significant decrease of E:A ratio, and an increase of mitral velocity at the onset of atrial contraction. In these experiments, the E velocity and total mitral flow velocity-time integral either did not change or changed nonsignificantly.[42] Blood flow velocity across the mitral valve is related to the transmitral pressure gradient,[62] and thus, the cited studies indicate that increasing heart rate result in a higher pressure gradient at the onset of atrial contraction. Furthermore, data from a recent animal study seem to suggest that atrial pacing in itself may increase the atrial phase of left ventricular filling.[63] In conclusion, DVI pacing at a fixed AV delay seems to result in increasing atrial contribution with increasing pacing rate at rest, and this change in left ventricular diastolic filling pattern mimics changes seen in patients with abnormal left ventricular diastolic function. When the mitral flow velocity profile and hence the diastolic filling are evaluated in paced patients, the heart rate must therefore be taken into account.

At high pacing rates and with AV delays of 150–250 ms, it is often impossible to differentiate between E and A waves, and even more difficult to calculate the VTI for the two filling phases (Fig. 5). Thus, it is difficult to calculate the atrial contribution to left ventricular filling from the mitral flow velocity profile at high heart rates.

During DVI pacing, the time delay between the atrial pacing spike and the onset of left atrial contraction and hence to the A wave of mitral flow velocity can be measured by using the mitral flow velocity profile and the ECG, which is recorded simultaneously. With the same programmed AV delay, large differences are seen in the time delay from atrial contraction to the onset of left ventricular contraction during DVI pacing. Measurement of mitral flow velocity profile by Doppler echo-

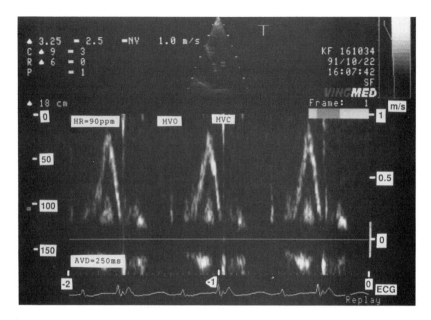

Figure 5. Measurement of mitral flow velocity by pulsed wave Doppler echocardiography during AV sequential pacing at a rate of 90 ppm, and a long AV delay. It is very difficult to identify the E and A waves of mitral flow velocity profile. For abbreviations, see Figures 3 and 4.

cardiography is valuable in deciding whether atrial stimulation results in mechanical contraction, to measure the time delay from right atrial stimulation to left atrial contraction and also the duration of the diastole. Furthermore, left ventricular filling dynamics have been studied from the mitral flow velocity profile during different pacing modes, during different AV delays, and during different pacing rates.

AV Valvular Regurgitation

Noninvasive Doppler echocardiography is a sensitive method for detecting mitral regurgitation[64] and is a suitable method to study acute and time-related effects of different pacing modes on AV valvular function. By combining the Doppler and two-dimensional echocardiographic techniques, the Doppler ultrasonic beam and sample volume can be located in the tricuspid or mitral orifice guided by the apical four-chamber sector scan picture.[65–68] Mitral and tricuspid regurgitation are diagnosed when reverse systolic flow from the left or right ventricle to the corresponding atrium occur (Figs. 6 and 7). If this reverse systolic blood flow can be followed from the AV valves and back into the atrium by pulsed wave Doppler, it represents a true AV valvular regurgitation. During ventricular pacing or arrhythmias, contraction of the atrium can occur during the ventricular systole, resulting in reversal of blood flow from the atrium to the systemic and pulmonary veins. This can be misinterpreted as AV valvular regurgitation when the Doppler sampling of flow velocity is performed only from the atrial side. Thus, it is important

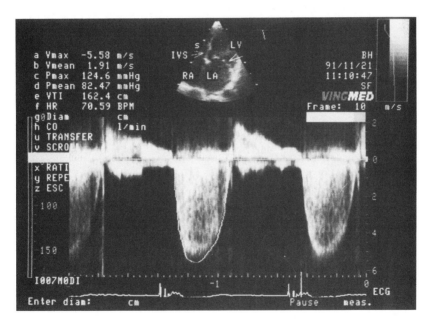

Figure 6. Simultaneous recording of apical four-chamber two-dimensional echocardiography of the heart and continuous wave Doppler recording of mitral flow velocity during VVI pacing. Negative deflections in the spectrum of mitral flow velocities indicate flow away from the Doppler transducer, and hence, flow from the left ventricle to the left atrium. This systolic reversed mitral flow represents valvular regurgitation. RA = right atrium; for other abbreviations, see Figure 1.

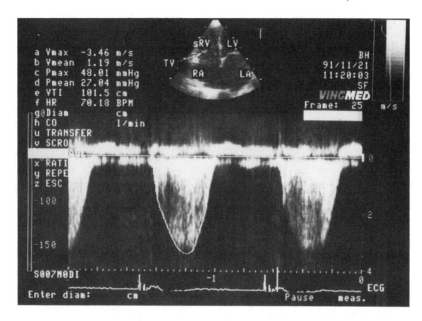

Figure 7. Simultaneous recording of apical four-chamber two-dimensional echocardiography of the heart and continuous wave Doppler recording of tricuspid flow velocity during VVI pacing. Negative deflections in the spectrum of tricuspid flow velocities indicate flow away from the Doppler transducer, and hence, flow from the right ventricle to the right atrium. This systolic reversed tricuspid flow represents valvular regurgitation. TV = tricuspid valves; IVS = interventricular septum; for other abbreviations, see Figures 1 and 6.

also to sample from the orifice of the AV valves in order not to diagnose the reversed blood flow caused by asynchronous atrial and ventricular contraction as AV valvular regurgitation. When AV valvular regurgitation has been diagnosed by pulsed Doppler, the true velocity of the high velocity regurgitant flow can be measured by continuous wave Doppler. By using the Bernoulli equation, the pressure gradient can be calculated (Figs. 6 and 7)[68]

$$\text{pressure gradient} = 4 \times (\text{peak velocity})^2$$

In pacemaker patients and in patients with AV block, even diastolic mitral regurgitation can be found by Doppler echocardiography.[69-71] In this case, the mitral flow is reversed during the late diastole, resulting in blood flow from the left ventricle to the left atrium causing reduced filling of the left ventricle.

Several criteria for estimation of the severity of mitral regurgitation using pulsed Doppler two-dimensional echocardiography, two-dimensional color-coded Doppler, and transesophageal echocardiography have been proposed. The intensity of the regurgitant Doppler signal, its extension into the left atrium, and the increase of forward flow velocity across the mitral valve were initially used to assess the severity of mitral regurgitation. Two-dimensional color-coded Doppler echocardiography has extended these methods further. Another Doppler technique was used to quantify mitral regurgitation as the difference between the total SV measured from mitral flow velocity profile and forward SV measured from aortic velocity profile. However, several studies using two-dimensional color-coded Doppler flow mapping have greatly enhanced the appreciation of the complexity of the regurgitant blood-jet and provided new insight into the dynamics of regurgitant flow. By using color flow mapping, it was initially proposed that the spatial distribution of mitral regurgitant jets within the left atrium is closely related to the severity of regurgitation. However, this mode of quantification has not proved to be accurate, and can at best provide a rough estimate of the severity of mitral regurgitation. Both hemodynamic and instrument-related factors can affect the spatial distribution of the mitral regurgitant jet visualized by Doppler echocardiography. The spatial distribution of mitral regurgitant jet is dependent on the regurgitant pressure drop and, hence, on the velocity of the regurgitant blood jet and also on the compliance of the left atrium. Furthermore, a wide range of velocity values of varying directions in the turbulent regurgitant jet within the left atrium make accurate velocity measurements for assessment of the severity of regurgitation very difficult.[71–83] In spite of thorough research in this field, it is still difficult to reliably quantify the degree of mitral regurgitation by the available echocardiographic methods.

Cardiac Dimensions

The M-mode echocardiographic methods that have been used to measure cardiac dimensions are well established and have proved to be accurate and reproducible (Fig. 8).[84,85] It is important to insure that the

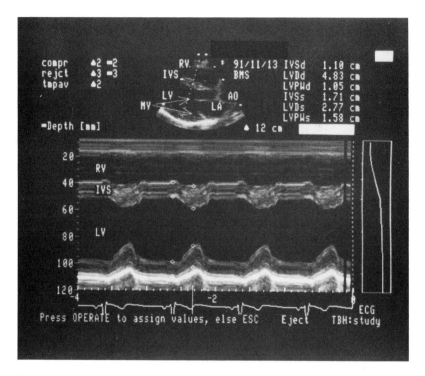

Figure 8. Simultaneous recording of parasternal long-axis two-dimensional echocardiography of the heart and M-mode measurement of left ventricular dimensions. The M-mode ultrasonic beam direction is perpendicular on the interventricular septum and on the left ventricular posterior wall. IVSd = interventricular septum dimension in diastole; LVDd = left ventricular end-diastolic dimension; LVPWd = left ventricular posterior wall dimension in diastole; IVSs = interventricular septum dimension in systole; LVDs = left ventricular end-systolic dimension; LVPWs = left ventricular posterior wall dimension in systole; AO = aortic root; MV = mitral valves; for other abbreviations, see Figure 1.

M-mode cursor line is located perpendicular to the interventricular septum and left ventricular posterior wall in order not to overestimate the dimensions. Based on these M-mode measurements, left ventricular fractional shortening is calculated as the difference between end-diastolic and end-systolic dimension divided by the end-diastolic dimension. M-mode echocardiography has been used to demonstrate that acute changing of pacing mode from DVI to VVI resulted in a significant reduction of both left ventricular end-diastolic and end-systolic dimensions and an increase in left atrial size, indicating a reduction of left ventricular filling during VVI compared to DVI pacing.[86]

Left ventricular end-diastolic and end-systolic volumes can also be measued from two-dimensional echocardiographic apical orthogonal views of the left ventricle by using Simpson's biplane rule.[87] Left ventricular ejection fraction can be calculated from the two-dimensional echocardiographic picture by the method of Quinones et al.[88]

The degree of dysfunction of the left ventricle can play a key role for the hemodynamic improvement effected by DDD pacing versus VVI and rate-adaptive VVIR pacing. However, it is important to realize that chronic bradycardia may result in a dilatation of the heart and may even result in development of mitral regurgitation. DDD pacing with restoration of a normal chronotropic response in such patients may reduce the left ventricular dimension and the mitral regurgitation and result in a time-related increase of the hemodynamic benefit of DDD pacing compared to VVIR pacing.

Measurement of left ventricular dimensions and volumes can be used in long-term studies to measure the hemodynamic differences caused by different pacing modes in the individual patient who serves as his/her own control.

Left Atrial Size

The mechanical activity of the left atrium can be significantly reduced in patients with left ventricular dysfunction. The atrial contribution to left ventricular filling does not only depend on the left ventricular filling pressure, but also on the contractility of the left atrium. Labovitz et al.[89] found that the SV was reduced on average 30% in patients with normal left atrial size versus approximately 10% in patients with left atrial enlargement when the pacing mode was changed from DVI to VVI pacing.

Selection Pacing Mode

The noninvasive echocardiographic methods have been used to quantify the hemodynamic response to temporary DVI pacing, to VVI pacing, and VVI pacing with ventriculoatrial (VA) conduction.[90] A temporary pacing lead system can be introduced to the right atrial appendage and to the right ventricular apex.[91] Recording of the electrogram from the right atrium during VVI pacing is used to verify the presence of VA conduction. A negative AV delay mimicking spontaneous VA conduction can be achieved by connecting the atrial lead to the ventricular channel, and the ventricular lead to the atrial channel of a temporary dual chamber pacemaker. By measuring the SV continuously during spontaneous rhythm and during the different temporary pacing modes, the instantaneous effects of different pacing modes on hemodynamics can be evaluated (Fig. 9). It is also important to verify that atrial pacing actually results in atrial contraction by measuring the mitral flow velocities (Fig. 3).

Although VVI resulted in a significant increase in the CO both in patients without (42% increase) and with (31% increase) valvular heart disease, DVI was the best temporary pacing mode, and the corresponding increases in CO during DVI compared to that during spontaneous bradycardia were 83% and 53%, respectively. Temporary DVI proved to be hemodynamically superior, especially in patients with no valvular heart disease, and resulted in average 29% higher CO than that during VVI, in agreement with other published data.[92-94] Patients with valvular heart disease achieved an average 17% increment in CO during DVI compared to VVI (Fig. 10).

Restoration of AV synchrony will have a variable effect on CO, depending on the mechanical efficiency of atrial contraction, the passive filling pressure, the ventricular compliance, and AV conduction time.[95-102] The hemodynamic benefit from DVI compared to spontaneous bradycardia seems to decrease when the left ventricular end-diastolic dimension increases (Fig. 11). Furthermore, patients with a large end-systolic dimension will have a slighter hemodynamic benefit from AV synchrony than patients with a small end-systolic dimension (Fig. 12). An explanation of this may be that the end-systolic dimension increases when the left ventricular filling pressure increases, and a high filling pressure often results in a slighter benefit of DVI versus VVI.[90,99] It has been demonstrated by Doppler echocardiography that the influence of fortuitous atrial synchrony on SV during VVI pacing is strongly predictive of the improvement in CO achieved with chronic DVI versus VVI pacing (Fig. 13).[103] This observation can be used clinically in patients with complete AV block as a means of identifying, prior to permanent pacemaker im-

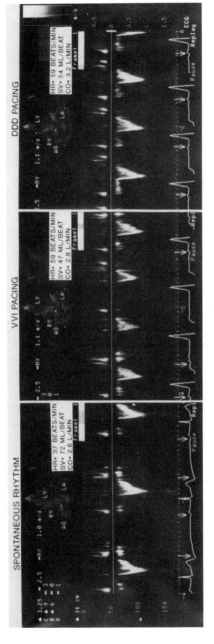

Figure 9. Measurement of aortic flow velocity by pulsed wave Doppler echocardiography and calculation of stroke volume (SV) and cardiac output (CO) during spontaneous rhythm (left), ventricular pacing (center, VVI), and AV synchronous pacing (right, DDD) in a patient with implanted DDD pacemaker; arrows indicate P waves.

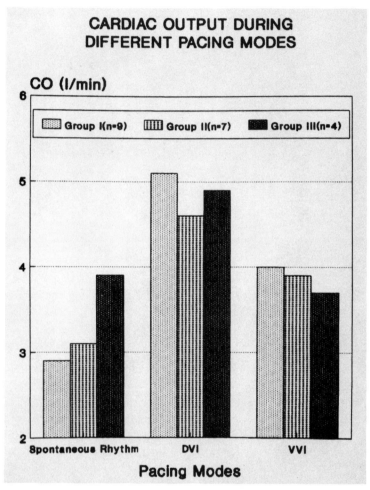

Figure 10.   Continuous measurement of cardiac output (CO) by pulsed Doppler echocardiography during spontaneous rhythm, during temporary AV sequential pacing (DVI), and ventricular pacing (VVI). Group I = patients with no valvular heart disease and no ventriculoatrial conduction; group II = patients with valvular heart disease and no ventriculoatrial conduction; group III = patients with ventriculoatrial conduction.[90]

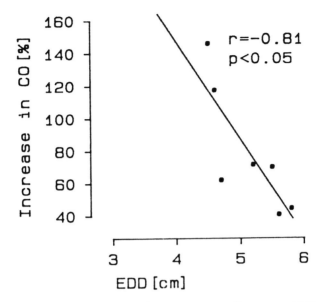

Figure 11. Correlation between the increase in cardiac output (CO) measured by pulsed wave Doppler echocardiography during temporary AV sequential pacing compared to spontaneous rhythm and left ventricular end-diastolic dimension (EDD).[90]

plantation, those who will derive the greatest benefit from AV synchrony.

Temporary VA pacing resulted in average 20% reduction of CO compared to that during VVI without VA conduction (Fig. 14). In patients with spontaneous VA conduction, DVI resulted in 35% increase in CO compared to that during VVI pacing. Other studies using noninvasive Doppler echocardiography have also confirmed that patients with VA conduction have a significantly higher increase in CO during DVI pacing compared to VVI pacing than patients with no VA conduction.[104]

Spontaneous retrograde atrial activation during ventricular pacing has been found in 40–90% of patients with sinus node disease and in 50–60% of patients paced for high degree AV block.[105] This undesirable situation has a significant effect on cardiac performance and may produce quite disabling symptoms, the so-called "pacemaker syndrome" char-

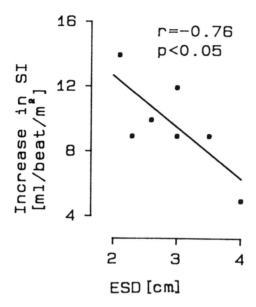

Figure 12. Correlation between increase of stroke index (SI) measured by pulsed wave Doppler echocardiography during temporary AV sequential pacing compared to ventricular pacing and left ventricular end-systolic dimension (ESD).[90]

acterized by a fall in blood pressure leading to weakness, light-headedness, low output symptomatology, and syncopal episodes.[106] The profound fall in blood pressure seen in some patients with retrograde atrial activation during VVI pacing can only partly be explained by an acute drop in CO, and it was suggested that the sudden atrial distension produced by atrial contraction against closed AV valves activates an atrial reflex that abruptly reduces systemic vascular resistance.[107]

In a recent study it was demonstrated that VA conduction during VVI pacing resulted in an elevated level of plasma norepinephrine, indicating an increase of sympathetic neural activity that was absent during atrial pacing. It was postulated that during VA conduction, the decrease in systolic pressure is sensed by arterial baroreceptors, resulting in heightened sympathetic neural tone and increased norepinephrine level. These changes result in increased alpha-mediated vasoconstriction.[108] During VVI pacing and VA conduction, retrograde blood flow into the pul-

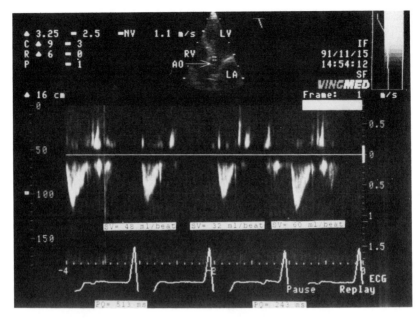

Figure 13. Measurement of beat-to-beat stroke volume (SV) by pulsed wave Doppler eehocardiography during ventricular pacing. The AV delay (PQ) and measured SV are indicated. The recording clearly demonstrates the instantaneous variations in the SV dependent on the synchronization between P and QRS complexes. The lowest SV was measured when no P wave was seen preceding the QRS complex (velocity profile number 3 from the left-hand side). AO = aortic root; for other abbreviations, see Figure 1.

monary venous system and elevation of pulmonary capillary wedge pressure have been demonstrated.[109] This can lead to a deterioration of pulmonary gas exchange because of a ventilation-perfusion mismatching. Recently it was demonstrated that during exercise in VVIR pacing in patients with VA conduction, high pulmonary wedge pressures and heightened ventilation were induced.[110]

In cases with the "pacemaker syndrome," the CO can be measured noninvasively by Doppler echocardiography both during VVI pacing and during spontaneous bradycardia achieved by inhibition of the pacemaker. If the CO is unaltered or reduced during VVI pacing compared to the CO during spontaneous bradycardia, the reason can be VA conduction

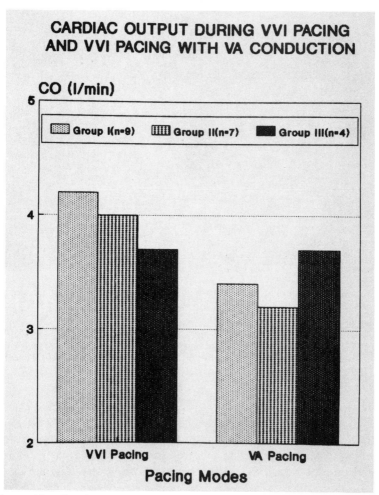

Figure 14.   Continuous measurement of cardiac output (CO) by pulsed wave Doppler echocardiography during temporary ventricular pacing (VVI) and during AV sequential pacing at an AV delay of −175 ms mimicking ventriculoatrial conduction (VA pacing) in the same patient as in Figure 10.[90]

resulting in atrial contraction against closed AV valves. VVI and VVIR pacing should generally be avoided in patients with VA conduction.

Evaluation of Hemodynamics in Physiologic Pacing

From rest to peak exercise, the SV can increase an average of 1.5-fold and the heart rate an average of threefold in a trained healthy person. However, if heart rate cannot be increased during exercise, the SV may increase some more in an attempt to maintain CO during exercise, but this will not be sufficient to provide normal hemodynamics during exercise. On the other hand, heart rate alone will often be the only determinant of CO during exercise in patients with left ventricular dysfunction, resulting in inability to increase the SV during exercise.

Several studies have demonstrated that in patients with complete heart block but normal sinus node function, the CO increases 15–50% during exercise in DDD pacing compared to VVI pacing, and exercise capacity increases 20–45% during DDD pacing compared to VVI pacing also in children.[111–119] Randomized controlled trials have demonstrated a significant improvement in the patient's subjective status as symptoms such as shortness of breath, dizziness, fatigue, angina pectoris, and palpitations were markedly reduced and the sensation of well-being was much improved during DDD pacing compared to VVI and VVIR pacing. Furthermore, the hemodynamic improvement with DDD pacing is long-lasting and may even improve with passage of time.[121–124]

During long-term DDD pacing, the mean increase in aortic velocity-time integral at rest at four follow-up periods was on average 21% during DVI pacing compared to VVI pacing in patients with normal contractility of the left ventricle (Fig. 15).[125] Further, the mean aortic velocity-time integrals fell on average 16% over a follow-up period from 1 to 6 months, and remained constant from 6 to 12 months (Fig. 16).[125] This reduction of SV at rest was seen both during DDD and after reprogramming to VVI pacing. Neither occurrence nor disappearance of mitral regurgitation can explain the differences in SV during DVI versus VVI pacing, and in all cases DVI pacing did actually lead to atrial contraction. A possible explanation for the time-related reduction of SV during long-term DDD pacing may be that the patients have the ability to increase the heart rate significantly during DDD pacing. They can therefore keep the SV lower and still have a significant increase of CO during exercise.

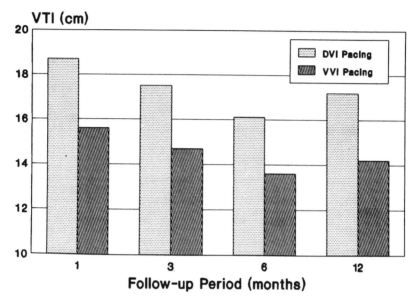

Figure 15. Measurement of aortic flow velocity-time integral (VTI) by pulsed wave Doppler echocardiography during AV sequential pacing (DVI) and during ventricular pacing (VVI) at different follow-up periods during long-term DDD pacing (n = 13).[125]

The patients who received the DDD pacemakers as their first pacemaker suffered from bradycardia before the implantation. This may have resulted in compensatory higher SV achieved by increasing the diastolic dimension and contractility of the left ventricle. Therefore, one can expect reduction in SV after implantation of a DDD pacemaker, leading to reduction of the heart size.

In supine patients, Karlöf et al. found, by using invasive measurements, an average difference of 18% in CO between AV synchronous pacing and rate-matched VVI pacing at rest, while during exercise AV synchronous pacing provided only 8% more CO than rate-matched VVI pacing.[126] Ausubel et al. demonstrated by using gated blood pool equilibrium radionuclide ventriculography that at rest in the upright position

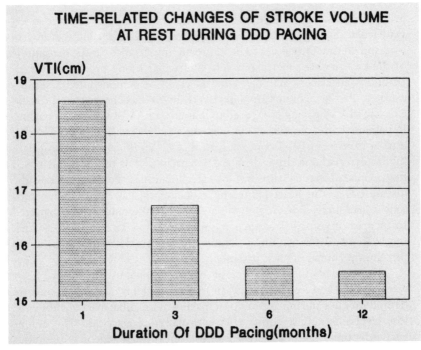

Figure 16. Measurement of aortic flow velocity-time integral (VTI) by pulsed wave Doppler echocardiography at different follow-up periods during long-term DDD pacing (n = 56).[125]

the CO was the same in AV synchronous pacing and in rate-matched VVI pacing, and during exercise AV synchrony provided only 4% more CO than rate-matched VVI pacing.[127] Although these studies demonstrated that CO was similar during AV synchronous pacing and rate-matched VVI pacing during exercise, preload and contractility differ significantly in the two modes. During rate-matched VVI pacing, the reduced end-diastolic filling compared to that during AV synchronous pacing is compensated for by an increase in ejection fraction, thus achieving almost the same CO in the two pacing modes. Studies have also demonstrated that rate-matched VVI pacing can provide the same symptom-limited maximal exercise capacity as AV synchronous pacing, and the same maximum oxygen uptake and maximum CO.[112,128,129]

During exercise and rate increase, the catecholamine drive on the heart increases contractility and peak rates of increase and decrease in left ventricular dimensions. Thus, during heavy exercise, the increase in preload and contractility seem to be of greater importance for the magnitude of the CO than the increase in left ventricular filling provided by synchronous atrial contraction. Pehrsson et al.[130] demonstrated a significantly higher level of noradrenalin overflow to the coronary sinus during exercise in VVI pacing compared to that during AV synchronous pacing. In patients with complete AV block, the atrial rate is significantly higher during exercise in VVI compared to that in VVIR pacing, indicating a higher sympathetic drive during VVI pacing.[131] It has been proposed that increased cardiac turnover of catecholamines would accelerate the disease process in heart failure by reducing cardiac beta adrenoceptor sensitivity. Increased sympathetic nerve activity would also be expected to increase myocardial oxygen requirements and cardiac work, which might lead to deterioration of already compromised hearts, and influence the clinical course of such patients.

During daily life, the typical pacemaker patient usually needs a heart rate variation between 60 and 110 beats/min, and it is relevant to compare hemodynamics during physiologic pacing with other pacing modes at low levels of exercise compatible with daily life activities. The noninvasive Doppler methods have been used in the assessment of hemodynamic response during low level exercise tests in different permanent pacing modes in the same patient by reprogramming of the pacing mode and repeating the hemodynamic measurements. Lau et al. used Doppler echocardiography to compare the relative hemodynamic profile between physiologic pacing and activity sensing VVIR pacing during randomized treadmill exercise tests.[132] At peak exercise, the heart rate in DDD was 108 and in VVIR 106 ppm. The CO was significantly higher at rest, during exercise, and in the first minute of recovery in DDD mode compared with those in VVIR mode. A decrease in SV occurred during VVIR pacing whereas SV was comparable to VVI pacing in DDD mode during exercise. This study demonstrated that during low-level exercise, AV synchrony enhanced the left ventricular filling substantially compared to VVIR pacing at the same rate, and resulted in 15–20% improvement of CO compared to VVIR pacing. Higano et al. measured the changes in hemodynamics during exercise tests by using the acetylene rebreathing technique for measurement of cardiac index as demonstrated in Figure 17. The cardiac index was significantly higher during exercise at all exercise levels in DDD and DDDR pacing compared to VVIR pacing

Hemodynamic Importance of AV
Synchrony During Low Levels of Exercise

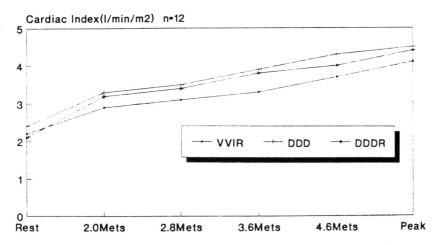

Figure 17. Measurement of cardiac index by acetylene rebreathing technique during treadmill exercise testing in activity-sensing rate-responsive ventricular pacing (VVIR), in AV synchronous pacing (DDD), and in dual chamber rate-responsive pacing (DDDR) in the same patients.[133]

mode. The difference in cardiac index ranged between 0.4 and 0.6 L/min/m^2. At 4.6 mets, the pacing rate in VVIR was 114 ppm, in DDD 105 ppm, and in DDDR 115 ppm. At peak exercise, the heart rate in VVIR was 127 ppm, in DDD 119 ppm, and in DDDR 125 ppm.[133] These data indicate that during exercise at a workload compatible with daily life activities of the average pacemaker patient, physiologic pacing gives added hemodynamic benefit to VVIR pacing. There are also data indicating that physiologic pacing is probably not so energy-consuming as VVIR pacing,[134] and can preserve a higher contractile reserve during exercise than VVIR pacing.[127]

When seeking the mechanism behind the diminishing importance of the atrial contribution to CO at high levels of exercise, one must recall that the contribution of atrial systole to ventricular filling is dependent on the atrial pressure and the left ventricular pressure just at the start of atrial systole. During heavy exercise, the atrial pressure increases substantially because of increased venous return to the heart, and most of the left ventricular filling is taking place in the early rapid filling phase. Thus, the contribution to left ventricular filling effected by atrial contraction is not so significant during heavy exercise as at rest and during low level exercise. When the left ventricular filling pressure increases, the contribution to ventricular filling provided by atrial contraction diminishes.[135] At high passive filling pressures, the ventricle is maximally dilated prior to the onset of atrial kick, and thus the kick makes relatively little contribution to ventricular filling. A negative correlation was found between improvement of CO during DVI pacing and the left ventricular end-diastolic dimension (Fig. 11), and even in a long-term study of DDD pacing, no significant improvement of SV was found during DVI pacing compared to VVI pacing in patients with permanently severe dilatation of the left ventricle.[125] Others have claimed that DVI pacing improved CO on average 20% compared to VVI pacing at different pacing rates in patients with congestive heart failure. Results were similar, but even more dramatic in patients with hypertrophic cardiomyopathy.[136] However, wide variations in the benefit of physiologic pacing in patients with left ventricular dysfunction have been reported.

In patients with left ventricular diastolic dysfunction and reduced compliance of the left ventricle more of the filling comes during atrial systole and less during early passive filling, indicated as a reduced E:A ratio of the mitral flow velocity profile (Fig. 4).[41] Usually these patients will demonstrate a significant improvement of SV during DVI pacing compared to VVI pacing.

AV synchronous pacing at a short AV delay (50–100 ms) can reduce the subaortic pressure gradient significantly compared to spontaneous rhythm in patients with hypertrophic obstructive cardiomyopathy without changing arterial pressure or CO. In these patients, significant improvement of angina pectoris and dyspnea have also been seen during AV synchronous pacing. It is suggested that the altered ventricular activation pattern during pacing with delayed contraction of the subaortic hypertrophic myocardium is the mechanism for this beneficial effect of pacing, which has been shown by Doppler echocardiography to also persist on a long-term basis.[137]

To predict the hemodynamic improvement of physiologic pacing compared to VVIR pacing is obviously very difficult in patients with pre-pacing left ventricular dysfunction, and more reseach is needed in this field. The best approach is probably to regard AV synchrony as worth considering also for patients with left ventricular dysfunction, especially in cases with diastolic dysfunction, and to use physiologic pace-makers in these patients.

Hemodynamic Evaluation of Long-Term Rate-Responsive Ventricular Pacing

Measurement of CO by Doppler echocardiography has recently demonstrated that the increase of CO during symptom-limited exercise in VVIR compared to VVI is in the same range as that observed during physiologic pacing and published previously.[111–119,138] A significant positive correlation between the increase of pacing rate during VVIR pacing and the symptom-limited maximum exercise time on treadmill (r = 0.83; p<0.001) has been demonstrated.[131] Further, a significant positive correlation has been found between the improvement of symptom-limited exercise time on treadmill during VVIR compared to VVI pacing and the time-related reduction of left ventricular end-diastolic dimension measured by combined two-dimensional and M-mode echocardiography during long-term VVIR (Fig. 18).[139] Thus, those patients who can improve their exercise capacity most during VVIR versus VVI will also demonstrate the greatest reduction in heart size during long-term VVIR pacing.

By using noninvasive echocardiography, it has been demonstrated that during VVIR pacing, the resting CO was reduced an average of 17% from 1 to 6 months of pacing (Fig. 19), left ventricular end-diastolic dimension was reduced an average of 13% (Fig. 20), and left ventricular fractional shortening was reduced an average of 16% during the first 6 months of pacing (Fig. 21).[140] The reduction in CO and left ventricular fractional shortening was most significant in the patients not paced previously. This study and others seem to demonstrate that the initial beneficial effect on resting hemodynamics achieved by VVIR pacing is not maintained on a long-term basis.[141,142] However, the time-related reduction of the resting SV during long-term VVIR and DDD pacing (Fig. 16) does not necessarily indicate a deterioration of hemodynamics. During bradycardia, the SV can be increased by the normal compensatory mechanisms consisting of increment of left ventricular end-diastolic dimension and of left ventricular contractility to obtain a sufficient resting CO.[143–145] When the heart rate is increased by pacing, the SV can be adjusted to a lower level and still yield a sufficient CO at rest. After 6

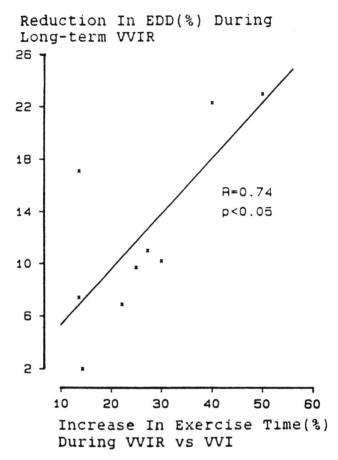

Figure 18. Correlation between increase in symptom-limited treadmill exercise time during activity-sensing rate-responsive ventricular pacing (VVIR) versus ventricular pacing (VVI), and the time-related reduction of left ventricular end-diastolic dimension (EDD) measured by combined M-mode and two-dimensional echocardiography during long-term VVIR pacing.[139]

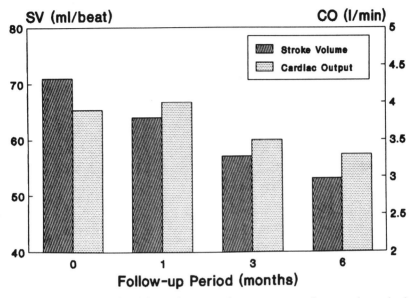

**TIME-RELATED CHANGES IN STROKE VOLUME
AND CARDIAC OUTPUT DURING LONG-TERM VVIR**

Figure 19. Time-related hemodynamic changes measured at rest by pulsed wave Doppler echocardiography at different follow-up periods during long-term activity-sensing rate-responsive ventricular pacing (VVIR; n = 13).[140]

months of VVIR pacing, the CO was almost exactly the same in the patients paced previously in VVI mode and in those who were not, suggesting that this CO probably was high enough to meet the circulatory need at rest.[140] A higher cardiac sympathetic activity has been found during exercise in VVI than in AV synchronous pacing,[130] and a reduction of sympathetic activity may explain the time-related decrease of SV at rest during long-term VVIR pacing. During VVI pacing at a steady heart rate, the SV is increased 30–60% during exercise, and the increase in SV is higher than that during AV synchronous pacing.[115,146–148] During VVIR pacing, it is not necessary to have as high SV as in the VVI mode at a steady pacing rate to achieve a high CO, and this may also explain the reduction of SV during long-term VVIR. The reduction of left ventricular fractional shortening at rest during long-term VVIR pac-

TIME-RELATED CHANGES IN LEFT VENTRICULAR DIMENSIONS DURING LONG-TERM VVIR

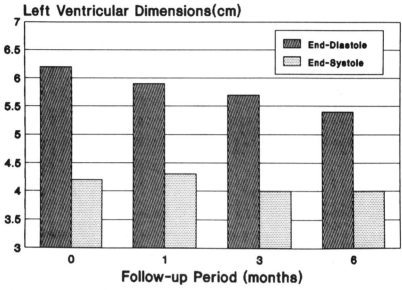

Figure 20.   Time-related changes of heart size measured by combined M-mode and two-dimensional echocardiography at different follow-up periods during long-term activity-sensing rate-responsive ventricular pacing (VVIR; n = 13).[140]

ing is valuable because it indicates that the contractile reserve is increased during VVIR when compared to VVI pacing (Fig. 21).[127] The ability to increase the CO independently of the Frank-Starling mechanism by increasing the heart rate during exercise in VVIR pacing may explain the observed reduction in left ventricular end-diastolic dimension during long-term VVIR. According to the LaPlace formula, a decrease in left ventricular end-diastolic dimension is associated with less wall tension at any given pressure, and may thus be associated with a reduction of the oxygen consumption of the heart which is important in coronary artery disease.[112,149] The effect of rate adaptation on left ventricular dilatation may also have direct prognostic implications, since ventricular dimensions seem to be a critical determinant of survival in patients with heart failure.[150]

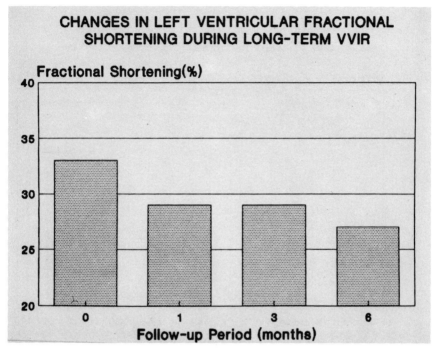

Figure 21.   Time-related changes of left ventricular fractional shortening measured at rest by combined M-mode and two-dimensional echocardiography at different follow-up periods during long-term activity-sensing rate-responsive ventricular pacing (VVIR; n = 13).[140]

Evaluation of the Hemodynamic Importance of the AV Delay

Since preservation of AV synchrony is considered hemodynamically beneficial for the patients, it is important to examine factors that might optimize that benefit for paced patients. One of these factors which has drawn increasing attention is the role of the duration of the AV delay. Noninvasive Doppler echocardiographic examination during routine follow-up can reveal whether atrial pacing is leading to atrial contraction (Fig. 3), which AV delay produces the highest SV (Fig. 13), and whether any particular AV delay leads to mitral regurgitation.[125,151]

No particular average AV delay was found that resulted in a statis-

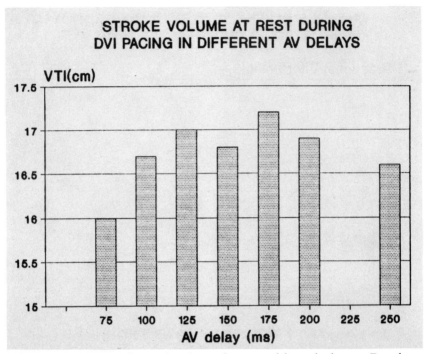

Figure 22. Aortic velocity-time integral measured by pulsed wave Doppler echocardiography at seven different AV delays (75 to 250 ms) in patients with DDD pacemakers implanted (n = 29).[125]

tically significant higher mean SV, but there was a tendency for AV delays of 150–200 ms to yield the highest SV (Fig. 22).[125] For the individual patient, there is an optimal AV delay for the SV (Fig. 23), and this AV delay can vary from 100 to 250 ms among different patients.[125]

The time delay between the right atrial depolarization and the peak velocity of the A wave in the mitral flow velocity profile is significant and independent of the programmed AV delay in the individual patient. By using a bipolar esophageal lead, Wish et al.[152] demonstrated that the conduction time from the atrial pacing artifact to left atrial depolarization ranged from 70 to 380 ms (mean 144 ± 82 ms) among different patients. Thus, DVI pacing at a programmed AV delay of 150 ms resulted in an average time from onset of left atrial depolarization to ventricular pacing spike of 6 ± 81 ms. Furthermore, left atrial depolarization started after

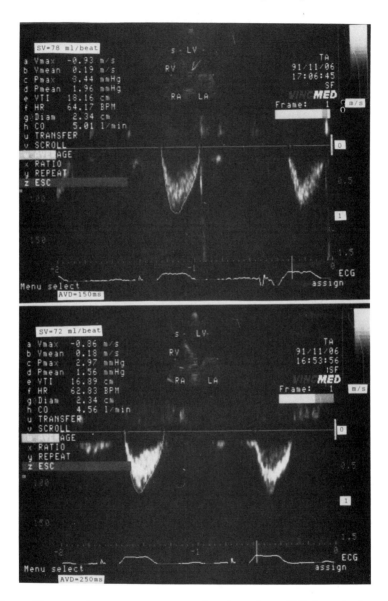

Figure 23. Continuous measurement of stroke volume (SV) by pulsed wave Doppler echocardiography during AV synchronous pacing at two AV delays (AVD) in a patient with normal left ventricular function and implanted DDD pacemaker. For abbreviations, see Figure 1.

ventricular activation in three out of 16 patients, with a programmed AV delay of 150 ms. When the pacing mode changed from DVI to AV synchronous pacing, the left atrial to ventricular sequence increased to an average of 137 ± 50 ms at a programmed AV delay of 150 ms. Shorter interatrial delays were associated with shorter hemodynamically optimal programmed AV delays, and longer interatrial conduction delays were associated with longer optimal programmed AV delays.

Ritter et al.[153] found that during DVI pacing at a programmed AV delay of 150 ms, the mechanical AV delay ranged from 90 to 170 ms, and during AV synchronous pacing from 115 to 175 ms among patients. Janosik et al.[154] found by using Doppler echocardiography that the optimal AV delay during AV synchronous pacing was 164 ± 53 ms compared to 202 ± 40 ms during DVI pacing, with a mean difference of 39 ms (range 0–100 ms). Other studies have also pointed out the benefit of adaptive and differential AV delay during physiologic pacing.[155,156]

The prolongation of conduction time from atrial spike to mitral valve closure during DVI pacing compared to the conduction time from the P wave to the mitral valve closure during AV synchronous pacing may be due to a delay in the time from right atrial stimulus to right atrial activation, prolonged interatrial conduction time, delayed sensing of the intrinsic P wave during AV synchronous pacing, or a combination of these three factors.

Figure 24 demonstrates measurement of the diastolic filling time from the mitral valve opening to the mitral valve closure during AV synchronous pacing. When the programmed AV delay was increased from 75 ms to 150 ms, and further to 250 ms, the corresponding diastolic filling time was reduced from 492 ms to 424 ms and 315 ms, respectively. This is in accordance with other studies using Doppler echoeardiography to demonstrate on average 49% reduction of diastolic filling time when the AV delay was increased from 50 ms to 300 ms.[157] The reason for the reduction of diastolic filling time when the AV delay is increased is that the time delay from mitral valve opening to the onset of atrial contraction, and hence to the A wave in the mitral flow velocity profile, is decreased, and this is clearly demonstrated in Figure 24. As demonstrated in Figure 23 from the same patient as in Figure 24, the SV was 78 mL/beat at an AV delay of 150 ms and 72 mL/beat at an AV delay of 250 ms. A long AV delay might shorten the time delay from early diastolic peak velocity to late diastolic peak velocity so much that the left atrium is underfilled by the pulmonary venous return, leading to failure to main-

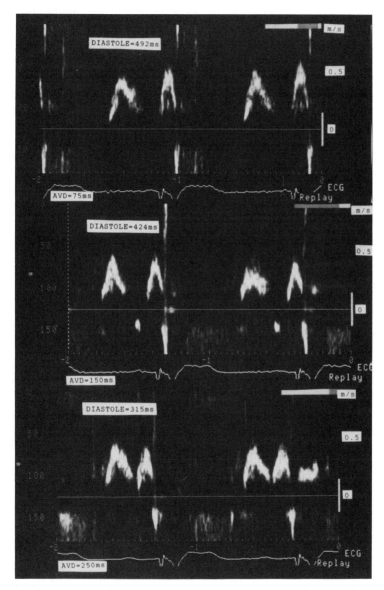

Figure 24. Measurement of the diastolic filling time (DIASTOLE) from recordings of mitral flow velocity by pulsed wave Doppler echocadiography during AV synchronous pacing at three different AV delays (AVD). Same patient as in Figure 23.

tain the left atrial pressure at the onset of atrial contraction. This can result in a reduction of the atrial contribution to left ventricular filling, resulting in a reduction of the SV compared to that at a shorter AV delay.

In patients with advanced interatrial conduction delay, pacing in the right atrium will increase the delay in left atrial activation, resulting in reduction of the mechanical AV delay during DVI pacing, and reduction of the left atrial contribution to left ventricular filling when a conventional AV delay of 150–200 ms is used. This can be avoided by increasing the programmed AV delay, but then the upper rate limit would be significantly reduced. Pacing simultaneously the right atrium and left atrium via coronary sinus during DVI pacing has been shown to improve the CO significantly in these cases compared to stimulation only in the right atrium.[158]

Comparison between patients in DDD pacing at an average AV delay of 150 ms and healthy controls of the same age and at the same heart rate have demonstrated 30–50% longer diastolic filling time in the healthy people with AV delay of average 172 ms. The difference in diastolic filling time seemed to be caused by an earlier opening of mitral valves in the healthy persons compared to the DDD paced patients.[157]

Figure 25 shows Doppler echocardiographic measurement of mitral flow velocities during DVI pacing at different AV delays in a patient with hypertrophic cardiomyopathy. It is clearly demonstrated that when the AV delay is shortened from 250 ms to 150 ms, and further to 75 ms, the duration of diastole is increased because the closing of the mitral valve is progressively delayed. Accordingly, the period of slow ventricular filling between rapid filling and atrial contraction lengthens when the AV delay decreases. At this heart rate of 90 ppm, the E wave and the A wave are superimposed on one another at the longest AV delay. The time interval from the mitral valve opening to the subsequent Q wave is not affected by changes of the AV delay, but progressive increase of the AV delay causes a progressive earlier closing of the mitral valve. With longer AV delay, the peak mitral flow velocity caused by atrial contraction (A wave) increases, indicating a higher pressure gradient between left atrium and the left ventricle at end-diastole, which indicates lower diastolic filling of the left ventricle. At an AV delay of 250 ms, atrial systole often coincides with and prolongs the early diastolic rapid filling phase, which is then followed by an extensive phase of slow ventricular filling.[159] A long AV delay can also cause a premature closure of the mitral valves as demonstrated in Figure 26 from a patient with

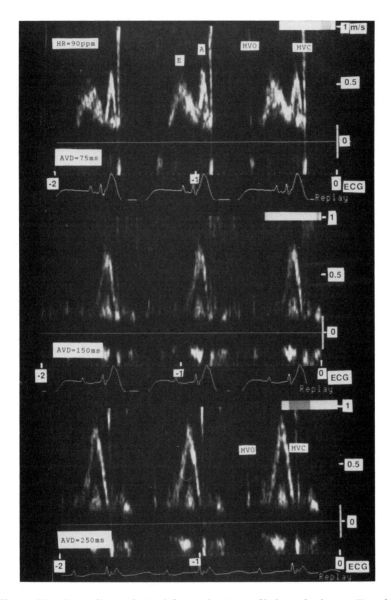

Figure 25. Recordings of mitral flow velocity profile by pulsed wave Doppler echocardiography during AV synchronous pacing at three different AV delays (AVD) in a patient with hypertrophic cardiomyopathy. For abbreviations, see Figures 3 and 4.

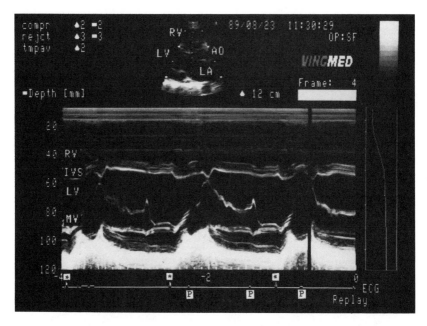

Figure 26.   Two-dimensional and M-mode echocardiography of mitral valves in a patient with complete AV block (atrial rate = 83 beats/min; ventricular rate = 43 beats/min). Premature coaptation and almost complete closure of the mitral valves long before the QRS complex (★) and early reopening of the mitral valves in the late ventricular systole, just after the P wave is demonstrated. For abbreviations, see Figures 1 and 8.

complete AV block. The mitral valve demonstrates a tall E wave and a smaller A wave occurring long before the QRS complex. The atrial contraction causes a premature coaptation and almost complete closure of the mitral valves, and later at the onset of ventricular contraction, the mitral valve closes completely. The P wave occurring just in the latter part of the left ventricular systole causes a premature opening of the mitral valves. Premature mitral valve closure and diastolic mitral regurgitation were demonstrated by pulsed Doppler echocardiography in nine (56%) of 16 patients with first degree AV block, but in none with normal PR intervals. In a study of 41 patients with DDD pacemakers, Doppler echocardiography revealed a critical AV delay averaging 230 ± 30 ms (range 140–260 ms) for appearance of diastolic mitral regurgitation.[69,71] Thus, a long AV delay can cause premature closing of the AV valves and reduce the left ventricular filling time significantly and can also result in diastolic AV valvular regurgitation. These findings provide support for the concept of an "atriogenic" mechanism for initiation of mitral valve closure. However, the hemodynamic significance of diastolic mitral regurgitation has yet to be established.

In an early study from 1983 using Doppler echocardiography, systolic mitral regurgiation was found during DVI pacing at certain AV delays but not at others.[151] Two-dimensional color-coded echocardiography and pulsed Doppler echocardiography have indicated an increased extent of both systolic tricuspid and mitral regurgitation at an AV delay of 250 ms compared to an AV delay of 175 ms, and 125 ms during DDDR pacing. However, this increase was significant only at pacing rates of 100 ppm and not at rates of 80 and 90 ppm.[160]

It has been known for a long time that the AV delay is shortened by sympathetic nervous activity, for example during exercise and emotions with increased heart rate, but only recently has this relationship been fully examined. Luceri et al.[161] demonstrated in 631 patients an average reduction in AV delay from at rest 170 ms to 154 ms at mid-exercise when the heart rate was 110 beat/min, and further to 143 ms at a heart rate of 126 beats/min. In another study, a linear relationship was found between the decrease of the AV delay during increasing heart rates with an average reduction of 4 ± 2 ms for every increase of 10 beats/min in heart rate.[162] This adaptation of AV delay to heart rate occurs not only in healthy hearts, but also in failing hearts and in the presence of beta blockade or antiarrhythmic treatment.[161] A reduction of the AV delay actually results in an increase of the left ventricular filling time, which must be considered beneficial when the heart rate and venous return to the heart are increased during exercise, and the filling of the left ventricle should be augmented to increase the SV.

Doppler echocardiography was used to demonstrate a significant improvement of SV at a pacing rate of 100 ppm when the AV delay was reduced from 175 or 250 ms to 125 ms. Further, those patients who demonstrated these improvements of SV also preferred an AV delay of 125 ms in a double-blind crossover study. Subjectively, an AV delay of 175 ms with rate-adaptive reduction to 100 ms at a rate of 130 ppm or a fixed AV delay of 125 ms were preferred in 90% compared to a fixed AV delay of 175 or 250 ms, while 70% found a fixed AV delay of 250 ms least acceptable during DDDR pacing.[160]

By using the thermodilution method for measurement of CO, Ritter et al. demonstrated that an AV delay of 200 ms produced the highest cardiac index during AV synchronous pacing at a pacing rate of 100 beats/min, and at a pacing rate of 120 beats/min an AV delay of 150 ms yielded the highest cardiac index. Further, at pacing rates higher than 120 beats/min, a rate-adaptive AV delay with a decrease of 20 ms for every 10-beat increase of pacing rate produced better cardiac indexes than fixed AV delay.[153] A limitation of this study and others[163] is that the measurements were carried out with the patients resting supine.

Mehta et al.[164] used Doppler echocardiography to demonstrate that in the standing position the CO was 31% lower than in the supine position on four different AV delays. Even in the standing position, the AV delay of 150 ms resulted in a significantly higher CO versus an AV delay of 75 ms at rest before exercise. During treadmill exercise at a pacing rate averaging 101 beats/min, an AV delay of 75 ms resulted in 11%, on average, higher CO than an AV delay of 150 ms.

A recent multicenter study of 22 chronotropically competent patients with DDD pacemakers demonstrated a significant improvement of oxygen consumption during exercise testing both at the anaerobic threshold and at peak exercise with adaptive AV delay which decreased linearly from 156 to 63 ms, compared to a fixed AV delay of 156 ms.[165]

The duration of the AV delay may be of even more significance in selected patients such as patients with different types of cardiomyopathies. In patients with E:A <0.5 calculated from the mitral flow velocity profile, the effect of changing the AV delay on left ventricular diastolic filling pattern and on SV are augmented compared to those with E:A >1.[52] It has been shown that short AV delays of 75 to 125 ms may improve myocardial function both in hypertrophic cardiomyopathy and in patients with terminal phase dilated cardiomyopathy.[166] In the latter category of patients, Hochleitner et al.[167] demonstrated an improvement of left ventricular function, reduction of left ventricular end-diastolic dimension, increase of systemic blood pressure, and significant improvement of symptoms during AV synchronous pacing at an AV delay of 100 ms.

In studies elucidating the hemodynamic effect of different AV delays, CO or oxygen consumption has been measured during exercise in one AV delay and compared with those in other AV delays, and often no significant differences have been demostrated.[128] The individual large differences in the time delay between left atrial and left ventricular contraction at the same programmed AV delay results in significant differences of the optimal AV delay for the CO among patients.[125] Therefore, in studies elucidating the hemodynamic effect of different AV delays during exercise, the optimal AV delay for the individual patient should be compared with other AV delays. More research on the hemodynamic importance of rate-adaptive AV delay during exercise should be done to elucidate the importance of adaptive AV delay for optimizing the hemodynamics.

Evaluation of Valvular Function During Long-Term Pacing

In a prospective long-term study, the AV valvular function was determined by Doppler echocardiography in 13 patients with DDD pacemakers and in 16 patients with activity-sensing VVIR pacemakers.[168] No patient had systolic AV valvular regurgitation before DDD or VVIR pacing was started. After a mean follow-up period of 33 months in patients treated with DDD pacing, one patient demonstrated systolic mitral regurgitation after a follow-up period of 41 months, and another patient developed systolic tricuspid regurgitation after a follow-up period of 12 months. The other patients with DDD pacemakers had persisting normal AV valvular function. After a mean follow-up period of 20 months of the patients with VVIR pacemakers, two patients demonstrated systolic mitral regurgitation, two patients had systolic tricuspid regurgitation, and four patients had both systolic mitral and tricuspid regurgitation. Thus, systolic AV valvular regurgitation developed in 15% of the patients in long-term DDD pacing and in 50% of the patients in VVIR pacing. In the patients with VVIR pacemakers, no significant difference either in left atrial size or left ventricular end-diastolic dimension were found between those patients with mitral regurgitation and those without mitral regurgitation. In the patients who developed mitral regurgitation after starting VVIR pacing, neither left atrial size nor left ventricular end-diastolic dimension increased significantly during the follow-up period. Furthermore, no clinical evidence of development of heart failure was demonstrated in the latter patients. Thus, the AV valvular regurgitation that developed during VVIR was probably mild. In a recent study, mitral and tricuspid regurgitation was least in DDD compared to VVI pacing mode, but this did not correlate with decreased symptomatology during

DDD versus VVI pacing in a group of 16 patients studied by Doppler echocardiography.[169]

It can be concluded that AV synchrony is important for maintaining normal AV valvular function on a long-term basis. The mechanism behind the difference in the occurrence of systolic AV valvular regurgitation between DDD and VVI pacing is not clarified yet. However, a properly timed atrial and ventricular contraction is important to avoid diastolic AV valvular regurgitation, to initiate AV valvular closure by atrial contraction just before the start of ventricular systole, to avoid a beat-to-beat variation of the filling volume of the left ventricle seen during VVI pacing, and hence avoid a variation of left ventricular end-diastolic pressure, which is important for proper closure of the AV valves. However, the importance of the pacing mode for AV valvular function has to be further investigated.

The high incidence of development of AV valvular regurgitation during VVIR pacing and the recent published data demonstrating increase of CO at low levels of exercise in DDD and DDDR pacing compared to VVIR pacing are good reasons for generally considering DDD pacing a better alternative than VVIR pacing in patients with normal chronotropic response and to implant DDDR pacemakers in patients with combined AV block and chronotropic incompetence.

References

1. Sulke N, Chambers J, Blake G. A comparison of echocardiography and radionuclide angiography in the noninvasive assessment of modern pacemaker hemodynamics (abstr). PACE 1991;14:329.
2. Hatle L, Angelsen B. Doppler Ultrasound in Cardiology. Physical Principles and Clinical Applications, 2nd ed, Lea & Febiger, Philadelphia, 1985, pp 97–188, 306–320.
3. Ihlen H, Amlie JP, Dale J, et al. Determination of cardiac output by Doppler echocardiography. B Heart J 1984;51:54.
4. Ihlen H, Myhre E, Amlie JP, et al. Changes in left ventricular stroke volume measured by Doppler echocardiography. Br Heart J 1985;54:378.
5. Skjaerpe T, Hegrenaes L, Hatle L. Noninvasive estimation of valve area in patients with aortic stenosis by Doppler ultrasound and two-dimensional echocardiography. Circulation 1985;72:810.
6. Mehta N, Iyawe VI, Cummin RC, et al. Validation of a Doppler technique for beat-to-beat measurement of cardiac output. Clin Sci 1985;69:377.
7. Fischer DC, Sahn DJ, Friedman MJ, et al. The effect of variation of pulsed Doppler sampling site on calculation of cardiac output: an experimental study in open-chest dogs. Circulation 1983;67:370.

8. Bennet ED, Barclay S, Mannering, D, et al. The non-invasive assessment of left ventricular performance using Doppler ultrasound (abstr). Clin Sci 1984;66:27.
9. Goldberg SJ, Sahn DJ, Allen HD, et al. Evaluation of pulmonary and systemic blood flow by 2-dimensional Doppler echocardiography using fast Fourier transform spectral analysis. Am J Cardiol 1982;50:1394.
10. Sanders SP, Yeager S, Williams RG. Measurement of systemic and pulmonary blood flow and QP/QS ratio using Doppler and two-dimensional echocardiography. Am J Cardiol 1983;51:952.
11. Stevenson JG, Kawabori I. Noninvasive determination of pulmonic to systemic flow ratio by pulsed Doppler echo (abstr). Circulation 1982;66:232.
12. Meyer RA, Kalavathy A, Korfhagen JC, et al. Comparison of left to right shunt ratios determined by pulsed Doppler/2D-echo (DOP/2D) and Fick method (abstr). Circulation 1982;66:232.
13. Vargas Barron J, Sahn DJ, Valdes-Cruz LM, et al. Quantification of ratio of pulmonary: systemic blood flow (QP:QS) in patients with ventricular septal defect by two-dimensional range-gated Doppler echocardiography (abstr). Circulation 1982;66:318.
14. Valdes-Cruz LM, Mesel E, Horowitz S, et al. Validation of two-dimensional echo Doppler (2DED) for measuring pulmonary and systemic flows (PBF,SBF) in atrial and ventricular septal defects (ASD, VSD): a canine study (abstr). Circulation 1982;66:231.
15. Magnin PA, Stewart JM, Myers S, et al. Combined Doppler and phased-array echocardioghraphic estimation of cardiac output. Circulation 1981;63:388.
16. Huntsman LL, Stewart DK, Barnes SR, et al. Noninvasive Doppler determination of cardiac output in man. Clinical validation. Circulation 1983;67:593.
17. Chandraratna PAN, Nanna M, McKay C, et al. Determination of cardiac output by transcutaneous continuous wave ultrasonic Doppler computer. Am J Cardiol 1984;53:234.
18. Alverson DC, Eldridge M, Dillon T, et al. Noninvasive pulsed Doppler determination of cardiac output in neonates and children. J Pediatr 1982;101:46.
19. Rose JS, Nanna M, Rahimtoola SH, et al. Accuracy of determination of changes in cardiac output by transcutaneous continuous wave Doppler computer. Am J Cardiol 1984;54:1099.
20. Mehta N, Bennett ED. Reduction of ascending aortic blood velocity and acceleration in acute myocardial infarction, using transcutaneous Doppler ultrasound (abstr). Clin Sci 1983;64:6P.
21. Steingart RM, Meller J, Barovick J, et al. Pulsed Doppler echocardiographic measurement of beat-to-beat changes in stroke volume in dogs. Circulation 1980;62:542.
22. Bennett ED, Mannering D, Mehta N. The hemodynamic effects of Domperidone-A dopamine antagonist (abstr). Clin Sci 1983;63:39.
23. Elkayam U, Gardin JM, Berkley R, et al. The use of Doppler flow velocity

measurements to assess the hemodynamic response to vasodilators in patients with heart failure. Circulation 1983;67:377.

24. Distante A, Moscarelli E, Rovai D, et al. Monitoring of changes in cardiac output by transcutaneous aortovelography, a noninvasive Doppler technique: comparison with thermodilution. J Nucl Med Allied Sci 1980;24: 171.

25. Bennet ED, Barclay SA. Davis AL, et al. Ascending aortic blood velocity and acceleration using Doppler ultrasound in assessment of left ventricular function. Cardiovasc Res 1984;18:632.

26. Gardin JM, Dabestani A, Matin K, et al. Reproducibility of Doppler aortic blood flow measurements: studies on intraobserver, interobserver and day-to-day variability in normal subjects. Am J Cardiol 1984;54:1092.

27. Voyles WF, Greene ER, Niranda IP, et al. Observer variability in serial noninvasive measurements of stroke index using pulsed Doppler flowmetry. Biomed Sci Int 1982;18:67.

28. Jaffe WM, Dewhurst TA, Otto CM, et al. Influence of Doppler sample volume location on ventricular filling velocities. Am J Cardiol 1991;68:550.

29. Labovitz AJ, Buckingham TA, Hebermehl K, et al. The effects of sampling site on the two-dimensional echo-Doppler determination of cardiac output. Am Heart J 1985;109:327.

30. Lewis JF, Kuo LC, Nelson JG, et al. Pulsed Doppler echocardiographic determination of stroke volume and cardiac output: clinical validation of two new methods using the apical window. Circulation 1984;3:425.

31. Gussenhoven WJ, Van Leenen BF, Kuis W, et al. Comparison of internal diameter of great arteries in congenital heart disease: a cross-sectional echocardiographic study. Br Heart J 1983;49:45.

32. Seed WA, Wood NB. Velocity patterns in aorta. Cardiovasc Res 1971;5: 319.

33. Loeppky JA, Greene ER, Hoekenga DE, et al. Beat-by-beat stroke volume assessment by pulsed Doppler in upright and supine exercise. J Appl Physiol 1981;50:1173.

34. Ihlen H, Endresen K, Golf S, et al. Cardiac stroke volume during exercise measured by Doppler echocardiography: comparison with the thermodilution technique and evaluation of reproducibility. Br Heart J 1987;58:455.

35. Christie J, Sheldahl LM, Tristani FE, et al. Determination of stroke volume and cardiac output during exercise: comparison of two-dimensional and Doppler echocardiography, Fick oximetry, and thermodilution. Circulation 1987;76:539.

36. Maeda M, Yokota M, Iwase M, et al. Accuracy of cardiac output measured by continous wave Doppler echocardiography during dynamic exercise testing in the supine position in patient with coronary artery disease. J Am Coll Cardiol 1989;13:76.

37. Mackenzie JD, Haites NE, Rawles JM. Method of assessing the reproducibility of blood flow measurement: factors influencing the performance of thermodilution cardiac output computers. Br Heart J 1986;55:14.

38. Spirito P, Maron BJ. Influence of aging on Doppler echocardiographic indices of left ventricular diastolic function. Br Heart J 1988;59:672.

39. Pye MP, Pringle SD, Cobbe SM. Reference values and reproducibility of Doppler echocardiography in the assessment of the tricuspid valve and right ventricular diastolic function in normal subjects. Am J Cardiol 1991;67:269.

40. Appleton CP, Hatle L, Popp RL. Relation of transmitral flow velocity patterns to left ventricular diastolic function: new sights from a combined hemodynamic and Doppler echocardiographic study. J Am Coll Cardiol 1988;12:426.

41. Stoddard MF, Pearson AC, Kern MJ, et al. Left ventricular diastolic function: comparison of pulsed Doppler echocardiographic and hemodynamic indexes in subjects with and without coronary artery disease. J Am Coll Cardiol 1989;13:327.

42. Appleton CP. Influence of incremental changes in heart rate on mitral flow velocity: assessment in lightly sedated, conscious dogs. J Am Coll Cardiol 1991;17:227.

43. Nashimura RA, Abel MD, Hatle L, et al. Assessment of diastolic function of the heart: background and current applications of Doppler echocardiography. Part II. Clinical studies. Mayo Clin Proc 1989;64:181.

44. Gardin JM, Dabestani A, Takenaka K, et al. Effect of imaging view and sample volume location on evaluation of mitral flow velocity by pulsed Doppler echocardiography. Am J Cardiol 1986;57:1335.

45. Harrison MR, Clifton GD, Pennell AT, et al. Effect of heart rate on left ventricular diastolic transmitral flow velocity patterns assessed by Doppler echocardiography in normal subjects. Am J Cardiol 1991;67:622.

46. Miyatake K, Okamoto M, Kinoshita N, et al. Augmentation of atrial contribution to left ventricular inflow with aging as assessed by intracardiac Doppler flowmetry. Am J Cardiol 1984;53:586.

47. Santori MP, Quinones MA, Kuo LC. Relation of Doppler-derived left ventricular filling parameters to age and radius/thickness ratio in normal and pathological states. Am J Cardiol 1987;59:1179.

48. Choong CY, Herrmann HC, Weyman AE, et al. Preload dependence of Doppler-derived indexes of left ventricular diastolic function in humans. J Am Coll Cardiol 1987;10:800.

49. Takenaka K, Dabestani A, Gardin JM, et al. Pulsed Doppler echocardiographic study of left ventricular filling in dilated cardiomyopathy. Am J Cardiol 1986;58:143.

50. deBruyne B, Lerch R, Meier B, et al. Doppler assessment of left ventricular diastolic filling during brief coronary occlusion. Am Heart J 1989;117:629.

51. Bryg RJ, Williams GA, Labovitz AJ. Effect of aging on left ventricular diastolic filling in normal subjects. Am J Cardiol 1987;59:971.

52. Masuyama T, Kodama K, Nakatani S, et al. Effects of atrioventricular interval on left ventricular diastolic filling assessed with pulsed Doppler echocardiography. Cardiovasc Res 1989;23:1034.

53. Levine RA, Thomas JD. Insights into physiologic significance of the mitral inflow velocity pattern. J Am Coll Cardiol 1989;14:1718.

54. Otto CM, Pearlman AS, Amsler LC. Doppler echocardiographic evaluation of left ventricular diastolic filling in isolated valvular aortic stenosis. Am J Cardiol 1989;63:313.

55. Inouye I, Massie B, Loge D, et al. Abnormal left ventricular filling: an early finding in mild to moderate systemic hypertension. Am J Cardiol 1984;53:120.
56. Takenaka K, Dabestani A, Gardin JM, et al. Left ventricular filling in hypertrophic cardiomyopathy: a pulsed Doppler echocardiographic study. J Am Coll Cardiol 1987;7:1236.
57. Pearson A, Janosik DL, Redd RR, et al. Doppler echocardiographic assessment of the effect of varying atrioventricular delay and pacemaker mode on left ventricular filling. Am Heart J 1988;115:611.
58. Pearson A, Janosik D, Redd R, et al. Prediction of hemodynamic benefit of physiologic pacing from baseline Doppler-echocardiographic parameters (abstr). PACE 1987;10:127.
59. Smith SA, Stoner JE, Russell AE, et al. Transmitral velocities measured by pulsed Doppler in healthy volunteers: effects of acute changes in blood pressure and heart rate. Br Heart J 1989;61:344.
60. Herzog CA, Elsperger KJ, Manoles M, et al. Effect of atrial pacing on left ventricular diastolic filling measured by pulsed Doppler echocardiography (abstr). J Am Coll Cardiol 1987;9:197A.
61. Parker TG, Cameron D, Serra J, et al. The effect of heart rate and AV interval on Doppler ultrasound indices of left ventricular diastolic function (abstr). Circulation 1987;76 (Suppl IV):IV-124.
62. Zoghbi WA, Bolli R. The increasing complexity of assessing diastolic function from ventricular filling dynamics. J Am Coll Cardiol 1991;17:237.
63. Lavine SJ, Prcevski P, Held AC, et al. Interrelation of heart rate and preload on diastolic filling in normal and abnormal left ventricle (abstr). J Am Coll Cardiol 1991;17:332A.
64. Blanchard D, Diebold B, Peronneau P, et al. Non-invasive diagnosis of mitral regurgitation by Doppler echocardiography. Br Heart J 1981;45:589.
65. Waggoner AD, Quinones MA, Young JB, et al. Pulsed Doppler echocardiographic detection of right-sided valve regurgitation. Am J Cardiol 1981;47:279.
66. Skjaerpe T, Hatle L. Diagnosis and assessment of tricuspid regurgitation with Doppler ultrasound. In: Rijsterborgh H (ed.). Echocardiography, Martinus Nijhoff, The Hague, 1981, pp 299–304.
67. Melzer RS, Abovich L, Finkelstein M. Doppler disease: Four-valve insufficiency is common though often clinically insignificant (abstr). J Am Coll Cardiol 1986;7:168.
68. Hatle L, Angelsen B: Doppler Ultrasound in Cardiology. Physical Principles and Clinical Applications, 2nd ed, Lea & Febiger, Philadelphia, 1985, pp 22–23, 170–188.
69. Rokey R, Murphy DJ, Nielsen AP, et al. Detection of diastolic atrioventricular valvular regurgitation by pulsed Doppler echocardiography and its association with complete heart block. Am J Cardiol 1986;57:692.
70. Panidis JP, Ross J, Munley B, et al. Diastolic mitral regurgitation in patients with atrioventricular conduction abnormalities: a common finding by Doppler echocardiography. J Am Coll Cardiol 1986;7:768.

71. Ishikawa T, Kimura K, Nihei T, et al. Relationship between diastolic mitral regurgitation and P-Q intervals or cardiac function in patients implanted with DDD pacemakers (abstr). PACE 1991:14:136.
72. Abbasi AS, Allen MW, Decristofaro D, et al. Detection and estimation of the degree of mitral regurgitation by range-gated pulsed Doppler echocardiography. Circulation 1981;61:143.
73. Quinones MA, Young JB, Waggoner AD, et al. Assessment of pulsed Doppler echocardiography in detection and quantification of aortic and and mitral regurgitation. Br Heart J 1980;44:612.
74. Zhang Y, Ihlen H, Myhre E, et al. Measurement of mitral regurgitation by Doppler echocardiography. Br Heart J 1985;54:381.
75. Rockey R, Sterling LL, Zoghbi WA, et al. Determination of regurgitant fraction in isolated mitral or aortic regurgitation by pulsed Doppler two-dimensional echocardiography. J Am Coll Cardiol 1986;7:1273.
76. Blumlein S, Baouchard A, Schiller NB, et al. Quantitation of mitral regurgitation by Doppler echocardiography. Circulation 1986;74:306.
77. Helmcke F, Nanda NC, Hsuin MC, et al. Color Doppler assessment of mitral regurgitation with orthogonal planes. Circulation 1987;75:175.
78. Otsuji Y, Tei C, Kisanuki A, et al. Color Doppler echocardiographic assessment of change in mitral regurgitant volume. Am Heart J 1987;114:349.
79. Miyatake K, Izumi S, Okamoto M, et al. Semiquantitative grading of severity of mitral regurgitation by real-time two-dimensional Doppler flow imaging technique. J Am Coll Cardiol 1986;7:82.
80. Davidoff R, Wilkins GT, Thomas JD, et al. Regurgitant volumes by color flow overestimate injected volumes in an in-vitro model (abstr). J Am Coll Cardiol 1987;9:110A.
81. Sahn DJ. Instrumentation and physical factors related to visualization of stenotic and regurgitant jets by Doppler color flow imaging. J Am Coll Cardiol 1988;12:1354.
82. Bertucci C, Valdes-Cruz LM, Recusani F, et al. Color flow Doppler study of the effects of afterload on spatial distribution of mitral regurgitant jets (abstr). J Am Coll Cardiol 1987;9:67A.
83. Maciel B, Moises V, Shandas R, et al. Effects of receiving chamber compliance on the spatial distribution of regurgitant jets as imaged by color Doppler flow mapping: an in vitro study (abstr). J Am Coll Cardiol 1989;13:23A.
84. Popp RL, Filly K, Brown OR, et al. Effect of transducer placement on echocardiographic measurement of left ventricular dimensions. Am J Cardiol 1975;35:537.
85. Pombo JF, Troy BL, Russell RO Jr. Left ventricular volumes and ejection fraction by echocardiography. Circulation 1971;43:480.
86. Gershony G, Goldman B, Noble E, et al. Mitral valve function and cardiac dimensions during ventricular (VVI) and sequential atrio-ventricular (DVI) pacing. Echocardiographic study. In: Perez Gomez F (ed.). Cardiac Pacing, Futura Media Services, Mount Kisco, NY, 1985, p 205.

87. Feigenbaum H. Echocardiogrphy, 3rd ed. Philadelphia, Lea & Febiger, 1981, pp 149–153.
88. Quinones MA, Waggoner AD, Reduto LA, et al. A new, simplified and accurate method for determining ejection fraction with two-dimensional echocardiography. Circulation 1981;64:744.
89. Labovitz AJ, Williams GA, Redd R, et al. Noninvasive assessment of pacemaker hemodynamics by Doppler echocardiography: importance of left atrial size. J Am Coll Cardiol 1985;6:196.
90. Faerestrand S, Oie B, Ohm O-J. Noninvasive assessment by Doppler echocardiography of hemodynamic response to temporary pacing and to ventriculoatrial conduction. PACE 1987;10:871.
91. Breivik K, Oie B, Faerestrand S, et al. Clinical performance of a new atrioventricular sequential temporary pacing electrode system. In: Perez-Gomez F (ed.). Cardiac Pacing, Futura Media Services, Mount Kisco, NY, 1985, p 390.
92. Leinbach RC, Chamberlein DA, Kastor JA, et al. A comparison of the hemodynamic effects of ventricular and sequential A-V pacing in patients with heart block. Am Heart J 1969;78:502.
93. Chamberlein DA, Leinbach RC, Vassaux CE, et al. Sequential atrioventricular pacing in heart block complicating acute myocardial infarction. N Engl J Med 1970;282:577.
94. Wenke K, Markewitz A. What is the best temporary stimulation mode after open heart surgery? (abstr). PACE 1991;14:619.
95. Greenberg B, Chatterjee K, Parmley WW, et al. The influence of left ventricular filling pressure on atrial contribution to cardiac output. Am Heart J 1979;98:742.
96. Reynolds DW, Wilson MF, Burow RD, et al. Hemodynamic evaluation of atrioventricular sequential versus ventricular pacing in patients with normal and poor ventricular function at variable heart rates and posture (abstr). PACE 1983;6:80.
97. Marco J, Brut A, Gouel Y, et al. Hemodynamic benefits of physiological pacing in patients with severe cardiac insufficiency and complete atrioventricular dissociation (abstr). PACE 1983;6:84.
98. Ruskin J, McHale PA, Harley A, et al. Pressure-flow studies in man. Effect of atrial systole on left ventricular function. J Clin Invest 1970;49:472.
99. Reiter MJ, Hindman MC. Hemodynamic effect of acute atrioventricular sequential pacing in patients with left ventricular dysfunction. Am J Cardiol 1982;49:687.
100. Linderer TV, Leitner ER, Biamino G, et al. Effects of atrial contribution to ventricular filling: the quantitative increase in cardiac output due to AV sequential pacing (abstr). PACE 1983;6:77.
101. Beyer J, Thorban S, Adt M, et al. Physiological vs. VVI pacing: its effect on cardiac output with different left ventricular compliance (abstr). PACE 1983;6:84.
102. Vanovershelde JL, Raphael D, Robert A, et al. Left ventricular filling in dilated cardiomyopathy: relation to functional class and hemodynamics. J Am Coll Cardiol 1990;15:1288.

103. Gillam LD, Homma S, Novick SS, et al. Prediction of the degree of hemodynamic improvement achieved by DDD vs VVI pacing: A Doppler echocardiographic study. PACE 1987;10:123.
104. Stewart WJ, Dicola VC, Harthorne JW, et al. Doppler ultrasound measurement of cardiac output in patients with physiologic pacemakers. Effects of left ventricular function and retrograde ventriculoatrial conduction. Am J Cardiol 1984;54:308.
105. Van Mechelen R, Hagemeijer F, De Boer H, et al. Atrioventricular and ventriculo-atrial conduction in patients with symptomatic sinus node dysfunction. PACE 1983;6:13.
106. Amikam S, Riss E. Untoward hemodynamic concequences of permanent ventricular pacing in patients with ventriculoatrial conduction (abstr). PACE 1979;2:41.
107. Alicandri C, Fouad FM, Tarazi RC, et al. Three cases of hypotension and syncope with ventricular pacing: possible role of atrial reflexes. Am J Cardiol 1978;42:137.
108. Ellenbogen KA, Thames MD, Mohanty PK, et al. New insights into pacemaker syndrome gained from hemodynamic, humoral and vascular responses during ventriculo-atrial pacing. Am J Cardiol 1990;65:53.
109. Naito M, Dreifus LS, David D, et al. Reevaluation of the role of atrial systole to cardiac hemodynamics: evidence of pulmonary venous regurgitation during abnormal atrioventricular sequencing. Am Heart J 1983;105:295.
110. Fujiki A, Tani M, Mizumaki K, et al. Pacemaker syndrome evaluated by cardiopulmonary exercise testing. PACE 1990;13:1236.
111. Yee R, Benditt DG, Kostuk WJ, et al. Comparative functional effects of chronic ventricular demand and atrial synchronous ventricular inhibited pacing. PACE 1984;7:23.
112. Fananapazir L, Srinivas V, Bennett D. Comparison of resting hemodynamic indices and exercise performance during atrial synchronized and asynchronous ventricular pacing. PACE 1983;6:202.
113. Kappenberger L, Gloor HO, Babotai I, et al. Hemodynamic effects of atrial synchronization in acute and long-term ventricular pacing. PACE 1982;5:639.
114. Pehrsson SK, Astrom H. Left ventricular function after long-term treatment with ventricular inhibited pacing compared to atrial triggered ventricular pacing. Acta Med Scand 1983;214:295.
115. Kruse I, Arnman K, Conradson TB, et al. A comparison of the acute and long-term hemodynamic effects of ventricular inhibited and atrial synchronous ventricular pacing. Circulation 1982;65:846.
116. Pehrsson SK. Influence of heart rate and atrioventricular synchronization on maximal work toleranse in patients treated with artificial pacemakers. Acta Med Scand 1983;214:311.
117. Kristensson BE, Arnman K, Ryden L. Atrial synchronous ventricular pacing in ischemic heart disease. Eur Heart J 1983;4:668.
118. Munteanu J, Wirtzfeld A, Stangl K, et al. Is the hemodynamic benefit of

VDD pacing due to AV-synchrony or to rate responsiveness? In: Perez Gomez F (ed.). Cardiac Pacing, Futura Media Services, Mount Kisco, NY, 1985, p 893.

119. Hammill W, Fyfe D, Gillette P, et al. Comparison of cardiac output and exercise performance during atrial synchronized and ventricular pacing (abstr). PACE 1991;14:60.

120. Sutton R, Perrins EJ, Morley C, et al. Sustained improvement in exercise tolerance following physiological cardiac pacing. Eur Heart J 1983;4:781.

121. Perrins EJ, Morley CA, Chan SL, et al. Randomized controlled trial of physiological and ventricular pacing. Br Heart J 1983;50:112.

122. Kenny RA, Ingram A, Mitsuoka T, et al. Optimum pacing mode for patients with angina pectoris. Br Heart J 1986;56:463.

123. Heldman D, Mulvihill D, Nguyen H, et al. True incidence of pacemaker syndrome. PACE 1990;13:1742.

124. Dateline F, Obel IWP. Clinical comparison of VVI, VVIR, and DDDR pacemakers in symptomatic relief of bradyarrhythmias (abstr). PACE 1989;12:1278.

125. Faerestrand S, Ohm O-J. A time-related study of the hemodynamic benefit of atrioventricular synchronous pacing evaluated by Doppler echocardiography. PACE 1985;8:838.

126. Karlöf I. Haemodynamic effect of atrial triggered versus fixed rate pacing at rest and during exercise in complete heart block. Acta Med Scand 1975;197:195.

127. Ausubel K, Steingart G, Shimshi M, et al. Maintenance of exercise stroke volume during ventricular vs. atrial synchronous pacing: role of contractility. Circulation 1985;72(5):1037.

128. Ryden L, Karlsson O, Kristensson B-E. The importance of different atrioventricular intervals for exercise capacity. PACE 1988;11:1051.

129. Wirtzfeld A, Stangl K, Schmidt G. Physiological pacing: AV-synchrony and rate control. In: Perez-Gomez F (ed.). Cardiac Pacing, Futura Media Services, Mount Kisco, NY, 1985, p 875.

130. Pehrsson SK, Hjemdahl P, Nordlander R, et al. A comparison of sympathoadrenal activity and cardiac performance at rest and during exercise in patients with ventricular demand or atrial synchronous pacing. Br Heart J 1988;60:212.

131. Faerestrand S, Breivik K, Ohm O-J. Assessment of work capacity and relationship between rate response and exercise tolerance associated with activity-sensing rate-responsive ventricular pacing. PACE 1987;10:1277.

132. Lau C-P, Wong C-K, Leung W-H, et al. Superior cardiac hemodynamics of atrioventricular synchrony over rate responsive pacing at submaximal exercise: observations in activity sensing DDDR pacemakers. PACE 1990;13:1832.

133. Higano ST, Hayes DL. Hemodynamic importance of atrioventricular synchrony during low levels of exercise (abstr). PACE 1990;13:509.

134. Vogt P, Goy JJ, Kuhn M, et al. Single versus double chamber rate responsive cardiac pacing: comparison by cardiopulmonary noninvasive exercise testing. PACE 1988;11:1896.

135. Myreng Y, Smiseth OA, Risoe C. Left ventricular filling at elevated diastolic pressures: relationship between transmitral Doppler flow velocities and atrial contribution. Am Heart J 1990;119:620.

136. Shefer A, Rozenman Y, Ben David Y, et al. Left ventricular function during physiological cardiac pacing: relation to rate, pacing mode, and underlying myocardial disease. PACE 1987;10:315.

137. Kappenberger L, Jeanrenaud X, Vogt P, et al. Pacemaker treatment of hypertrophic obstructive cardiomyopathy (HOCM): acute and long-term efficacy (abstr). PACE 1991;14:668.

138. Lau C-P, Camm A. Role of left ventricular function and Doppler-derived variables in predicting hemodynamic benefits of rate-responsive pacing. Am J Cardiol 1988;62:906.

139. Faerestrand S, Ohm O-J. Activity-sensing rate-responsive ventricular pacing (RRP) vs. ventricular pacing (VVI): relation between left ventricular dimensions and improvement in work capacity (abstr). J Am Coll Cardiol 1987;11:166A.

140. Faerestrand S, Ohm O-J. A time-related study by Doppler and M-mode echocardiography of hemodynamics. heart size, and AV valvular function during activity-sensing rate-responsive ventricular pacing. PACE 1987;10: 507.

141. Adolph RJ, Holmes JC, Fukusumi H. Hemodynamic studies in patients with chronically implanted pacemakers. Am Heart J 1968;76:829.

142. Nager F, Bühlmann A, Schaub F. Klinische und haemodynamische Befunde beim totalen AV-block nach Implantation elektrischer Schrittmacher. Helv Med Acta 1966;3:240.

143. Sarnoff SJ, Berglund E. Ventricular function. I. Starling's law of the heart studied by means of simultaneous right and left ventricular function curves in the dog. Circulation 1954;9:706.

144. Glower DD, Spratt JA, Snow ND, et al. Linearity of the Frank-Starling relationship in the intact heart: the concept of preload recruitable stroke work. Circulation 1985;71:994.

145. Sarnoff SJ, Mitchell JH. The regulation of the performance of the heart. Am J Med 1961;30:747.

146. Eimer HH, Witte J. Zur Leistungsbreite bei Patienten mit festfrequentem Herzschrittmacher unter Berucksichtigung von Hamodynamik, arteriovenose Sauerstoff differenz und Lungenfunktion. Z Kardiol 1974;63:1099.

147. Koyama T, Nakajima S, Horimoto M. Initial adjustment of cardiac output in response to the onset of exercise in patients with chronic pacemaking as studied by the measurement of pulmonary blood flow. Am Heart J 1976;91: 457.

148. Pehrsson SK, Astrom H, Bone D. Left ventricular volumes with ventricular inhibited and atrial triggered ventricular pacing. Acta Med Scand 1983;214: 305.

149. Kristensson B-E, Ryden L, Arnman K, et al. Atrioventricular synchronous versus ventricular inhibited pacing. A double-blind crossover study (abstr). PACE 1983;6(II):138.

150. Francis G, Kubo S. Prognostic factors affecting diagnosis and treatment of congestive heart failure. Curr Prob Cardiol 1989;11:631.
151. Zugibe FT Jr, Nanda NC, Barold SS, et al. Usefulness of Doppler echo-cardiography in cardiac pacing: assessment of mitral regurgitation, peak aortic flow velocity and atrial capture. PACE 1983;6:1350.
152. Wish M, Fletcher RD, Gottdiener JS, et al. Importance of left atrial timing in the programming of dual-chamber pacemakers. Am J Cardiol 1987;60:566.
153. Ritter P, Daubert C, Mabo P, et al. Haemodynamic benefit of a rate-adapted A-V delay in dual chamber pacing. Eur Heart J 1989;10:637.
154. Janosik DL, Pearson AC, Buckingham TA, et al. The hemodynamic benefit of differential atrioventricular delay intervals for sensed and paced atrial events during physiologic pacing. J Am Coll Cardiol 1989;14:499.
155. Ausubel K, Klementowics P, Furman S. Interatrial conduction during cardiac pacing. PACE 1986;9:1026.
156. Alt EU, Von Bibra H, Blömer H. Different beneficial AV intervals with DDD pacing after sensed or paced atrial events. J Electrophysiol 1987;1:250.
157. Dryander SV, Lemke B, Jaeger D, et al. Diastolic time intervals with different AV-programmings in dual chamber pacemaker carriers compared to a normal population: hemodynamic consequences (abstr). PACE 1991;14:13.
158. Daubert C, Berder V, De Place C, et al. Hemodynamic benefits of permanent atrial resynchronization in patients with advanced interatrial blocks, paced in DDD mode (abstr). PACE 1991;14:130.
159. Freedman RA, Yock PG, Echt DS, et al. Effect of variation in PQ interval on patterns of atrioventricular valve motion and flow in patients with normal ventricular function. J Am Coll Cardiol 1986;7:595.
160. Sulke N, Chambers J, Sowton E. The effects of different AV delay programming in DDDR paced patients during out of hospital activity (abstr). PACE 1991;14:132.
161. Luceri R, Brownstein S, Vardeman L, et al. PR interval behavior during exercise: implications for physiological pacemakers. PACE 1990;13:1719.
162. Daubert JC, Ritter P, Mabo P, et al. Physiological relationship between A-V interval and heart rate in healthy subjects: applications to dual-chamber pacing. PACE 1986;1032.
163. Vogt P, Goy J-J, Fromer M, et al. Hemodynamic benefit of atrio-ventricular delay shortening in DDDR pacing (abstr). PACE 1991;14:14.
164. Mehta D, Gilmour S, Ward DE, et al. Optimal atrioventricular delay at rest and during exercise in patients with dual chamber pacemakers: a non-invasive assessment by continuous wave Doppler. Br Heart J 1989;61:161.
165. Kutalek SP, Harper GR, Ochetta E, et al. Rate adaptive AV delay improves cardiopulmonary performance in patients with complete heart block. PACE 1991;14:108.
166. Ng C-K, Hoertnagel H, Hochleitner M, et al. The effectiveness of physiological pre-exitation pacing to treat terminal phased dilated cardiomyopathy (abstr). PACE 1987;10:371.

167. Hochleitner M, Hoertnagel H, Ng C-K, et al. Usefulness of physiologic dual-chamber pacing in drug-resistant idiopatic dilated cardiomyopathy. Am J Cardiol 1990;66:198.
168. Faerestrand S, Ohm O-J. Dual chamber pacing (DDD) and activity-sensing rate-responsive ventricular pacing (RRP): long-term effect on AV valvular function (abstr). PACE 1988;11:246.
169. Sulke N, Dritsas A, Bostock J. "Subclinical" pacemaker syndrome: A randomized study of asymptomatic patients with VVI pacemakers upgraded to dual chamber devices (abstr). PACE 1991;14:204.

Chapter 7

Natural History of Sick Sinus Syndrome After Pacemaker Implantation

S. SERGE BAROLD, MASSIMO SANTINI

Introduction

Over the last few years, a number of important retrospective but nonrandomized studies have shed light on the natural history of the sick sinus syndrome (SSS) after pacemaker implantation. Important considerations in the SSS include (1) pacemaker syndrome, (2) chronic atrial fibrillation, (3) paroxysmal supraventricular tachyarrhythmias, mostly atrial fibrillation, (4) thromboembolic complications including stroke, (5) congestive heart failure, (6) mortality, and (7) development of second or third degree AV block with AAI pacing. This chapter discusses these issues and the prognosis of SSS patients according to the type of implanted pacemaker.

Pacemaker Syndrome

The adverse hemodynamic consequences of single lead ventricular pacing were first recognized over 20 years ago and called the pacemaker syndrome,[1] recently redefined by Schüller and Brand[2] as follows: "The pacemaker syndrome refers to symptoms and signs present in the pacemaker patient which are caused by inadequate timing of atrial and ventricular contractions." The new definition encompasses the adverse he-

New Perspectives in Cardiac Pacing, Vol. 3, edited by S. Serge Barold and Jacques Mugica, Mount Kisco, NY, Futura Publishing Co., © 1993.

modynamic consequences of (1) single lead ventricular pacing, by far the most common cause of pacemaker syndrome, and (2) other modes of pacing (single lead atrial or dual chamber) due to inappropriate selection of pacing mode or programming.[2]

The pacemaker syndrome consists of a constellation of clinical findings, not all necessarily present in any individual patient, and occurs more commonly with retrograde ventriculoatrial (VA) conduction than with random timing of atrial and ventricular activity.[1,2] About 70–80% of patients with SSS (or carotid sinus syndrome) exhibit VA conduction.[3] Early reports suggested that only 15% of patients with preserved VA conduction would develop symptoms suggestive of the pacemaker syndrome with about half exhibiting its full-blown form.[1,2,4,5] In extreme cases, patients with sick sinus syndrome who develop the pacemaker syndrome may feel worse with a VVI pulse generator than without pacing before implantation.[6] In the past, with only VVI pacing systems and no basis for comparison, only patients with the more severe symptoms were identified as having the pacemaker syndrome.

The true incidence of pacemaker syndrome seems higher than previously realized (as shown in studies where each patient serves as his or her control, comparing various pacing modes) because most patients with dual chamber pulse generators prefer the dual chamber to the VVI mode, with only a small number showing no preference. A number of studies[7–13] have indicated that the majority of patients notice deterioration in their general condition when their pulse generator is programmed from the DDD to the VVI mode (including occasional sleep disturbances that disappeared when the DDD mode was restored). In some cases, patients describe a subjective improvement in their sense of well-being or quality of life and elimination of bothersome nonspecific symptoms in the DDD(R) compared with the VVI(R) mode despite no demonstrable objective improvement of functional exercise capacity.[14,15] Not all patients with demonstrable adverse hemodynamic effects of ventricular pacing are actually symptomatic. However, "asymptomatic" patients often feel better when their VVI pacemakers are upgraded to a DDD system, suggesting the existence of a "subclinical" pacemaker syndrome.[13]

In some patients with intact VA conduction and without a clinical pacemaker syndrome at rest, hemodynamics on exercise may not improve in the VVIR mode because the beneficial effects of an increase in heart rate may be negated by the unfavorable hemodynamic effect of persistent retrograde VA conduction. Implantation of a VVIR pacemaker does not protect the patient against the development of the pacemaker syndrome at rest and/or during exercise.[16-19] The behavior of retrograde VA conduction on exercise has not been studied in detail and it appears that it cannot be predicted individually.[20] The pacemaker syndrome may occur on exercise during VVIR pacing in the following circumstances: (1) Continuous pacing with persistence of VA conduction on exercise.[21,22] (2) Patients with chronotropic atrial incompetence may remain in normal sinus rhythm at rest, but on exercise inadequate increase of the sinus rate gives way to ventricular pacing (at a rate exceeding the sinus rate) associated with retrograde VA conduction.[19] (3) VA conduction is dynamic, and some patients with blocked VA conduction at rest may develop improved and restored VA conduction on exercise during ventricular pacing under the influence of catecholamines or other factors.[20] Alternatively, the pacemaker syndrome at rest may actually disappear on exercise if an increase in the ventricular pacing rate blocks VA conduction.

The pacemaker syndrome is a preventable condition and should be considered a complication of the past. Indeed, Travill and Sutton recently emphasized that the pacemaker syndrome is really an iatrogenic condition.[23] Once established, the pacemaker syndrome can be eliminated simply by restoring AV synchrony.[4,24] Patients with intact retrograde VA conduction represent a high risk group. No single parameter can identify individuals who will develop the pacemaker syndrome. However, at the time of pacemaker implantation, a decrease in the systolic blood pressure of 20 mm Hg or more with ventricular pacing (with or without evidence of VA conduction) suggests a high likelihood for the development of the pacemaker syndrome, and a device that maintains AV synchrony should then be implanted.[4,24,25]

Chronic Atrial Fibrillation

A past history of paroxysmal supraventricular tachyarrhythmias (SVT) appears to be the major determinant of atrial tachyarrhythmias after implantation of VVI, DDD, or DDDR pulse generators.[26-28] Many studies have demonstrated that the development of chronic atrial fibrillation (AF) is higher with VVI than with AAI (DDD, DVI) pacing when all SSS patients are considered as a group regardless of preexistent paroxysmal SVT[26,29-50] (Tables 1A,B and 2). (1) The incidence of chronic

TABLE 1A

Incidence of Chronic Atrial Fibrillation According to Pacing Mode

Diagnosis	Authors	Pacing Mode	No. of Pts.	Mean Follow-up in Months	Incidence of Chronic AF Regardless of Preoperative SVT	Incidence of Chronic AF in Patients Without Preoperative SVT		Incidence of Chronic AF in Patients With Preoperative SVT	
						Number	%	Number	%
SSS	Sutton et Kenny[30]	VVI	651	39	22%*				
		AAI	410	33	4%				
SSS	Markewitz et al.[31]	VVI	87	32	27%				
		AAI/DDD	67/69	51/13	14/3%				
SSS	Rosenqvist et al.[32]	VVI	79	47	47%*	34	18% NS	45	69%*
		AAI	89	44	7%	36	3%	53	9%
SSS	Zanini et al.[34]	VVI	57	40	18%*				
		AAI	53	45	4%				
SSS	Stangl et al.[35]	VVI	112	33	19%	71	0%	41	51%
		AAI	110	40	6%	93	0%	17	41%
SSS	Santini et al.[36]	VVI	125	60	46%*				
		AAI/DDD	135/79	60	4/12%				
SSS	Sethi et al.[37] (No previous SVT)	VVI	47	50	15%*	47	15%*	0	0
		AAI	40	47	0%	40	0%	0	0
SSS	Bianconi et al.[38] (Abstract)	VVI	150	59	39%*				
		AAI/DDD	153	44	18%*				
All	VanErckelens et al.[39] (No previous SVT)	VVI	163	99	M 14%*	163	M 14%*		
		DDD	44	99	M 2%	44	M 2%		
SSS	Nürnberg et al.[40] (Abstract)	VVI	93	41	38%	66	32% NS	27	52%
		AAI/DDD	15/22	41	13/18%	12/20	16/20%	3/2	0/0%
All	Jutila et al.[41] (No previous SVT)	VVI	16	36	M 69%*	16	M 69%*		
		DDD	18	36	M 17%	18	M 17%		
SSS/AVB	Feuer et al.[26]	VVI	110	48	M 18%*				
		DDI/DDD	110	40	M 8%				

172

Indication	Study	Pacing mode	No. of pts.	Follow-up	%	No.	%	No.	%
All	Snoeck et al.[42]	VVI	285	60	M 30%				
		DDD	NR	60	M 10%				
All	Snoeck et al.[48]	VVI/VVIR	230/45	60	M 32%				
		DDD	45	60	M 11%				
SSS	Hesselson et al.[29]	VVI	193	1977–89	26%	140	19%	53	43%
		DVI/DDD	58/308	As above	9/5%	43/204	0/4%	15/104	33/7%
All except SSS	Hesselson et al.[29]	VVI	92	As above	5%				
		DVI/DDD	26/273	As above	8/2%				
SSS	Hesselson et al.[29]	VVI	Act.	84	45%*	Act.	32%*	Act.	63%
		DVI/DDD	Act.	84	12/9%	Act.	0/8%	Act.	47/11%*
All except SSS	Hesselson et al.[29]	VVI	Act.	84	11%				
		DVI/DDD	Act.	84	12/3%				
SSS	Sasaki et al.[43]	VVI	34	62	44%*				
		AAI/DDD	17/24	39	2%				
SSS	Sgarbossa et al.[50] (Abstract)	VVI	112	57	Using UV & MV analyses VVI vs. VVI/dual chamber*				
		AAI/dual chamber	19/375	57					
All	Langerfeld et al.[45]	VVI	203	68	M 31%				
		DDD	43	32	M 2%				
SSS	Kosakai et al.[46] (Abstract)	VVI	51	60	57%*	19	21%	32	78%
		AAI/AV seq.	87/57	60	16/23%	28/29	4/10%	59/58	22/36%
SSS/AVB	Grimm et al.[47] (No previous SVT)	VVI	147	69	M 31%*	147	M 31%*		
		DDD	41	32	M 2%	41	M 2%		
SSS	Grimm et al.[47] (No previous SVT)	VVI	67	69	42%*	67	42%*		
		DDD	14	32	0%	14	0%		
AVB	Grimm et al.[47] (No previous SVT)	VVI	80	69	23%*	80	23%*		
		DDD	27	32	4%	27	4%		
SSS	Ishikawa et al.[49] (Abstract)	VVI	8	71	75%*			8	75%*
		VVI	13	71	8%			13	8%

Act. = Actuarial; CAF = chronic atrial fibrillation; PAF = paroxysmal atrial fibrillation; P = paroxysmal; SVT = supraventricular tachyarrhythmias; AAA = antiarrhythmic agents; pts. = patients; RA = right atrium; AVB = AV block; SSS = sick sinus syndrome; seq. = sequential; NS = not significant; M = mixed patient population, e.g., AVB + SSS. UV = univariate analysis; MV = multivariate analysis (Cox's proportional model). * Statistically significant (P<0.05). For Sgarbossa et al.,[50] See Table 1B for selected comments on the various studies.

TABLE *1B*
Comments on Table 1A

Authors	Comments
Sutton & Kenny[30]	Composite of 18 series.
Markewitz et al.[31]	Presumably CAF.
Santini et al.[36]	Incidence of CAF was not significantly related to age or associated conduction disorders.
Sethi et al.[37]	Additional data: One AAI patient showed intermittent AF controlled with AAA. 3 VVI patients showed PAF (including PAF in data yields 21%* AF with VVI and 2.5% AF with AAI).
Bianconi et al.[38]	Incidence of atrial arrhythmias not specified in terms of chronic vs. paroxysmal.
VanErckelens et al.[39]	Incidence of atrial arrhythmias not specified in terms of chronic or paroxysmal. Authors described "AF was continuously documented." Presumably this means CAF. Authors focused on AF beginning after implantation. 58 pts. with VVIR (F/U 99 months) were also analyzed. AF occurred in 3.4% (statistically less than with VVI), ? mechanism. VVIR may have been preferentially implanted in AV block vs. SSS.
Nürnberg et al.[40]	Incidence of AF not specified in terms of chronic vs. paroxysmal. SSS (98 pts. with code 22–25 and 32 pts. with code 26 BTS European Registry). Number of pts. with PSVT and AAI/DDD too small to be analyzed.
Jutila et al.[41]	AF presumably chronic. Tricuspid regurgitant (TR) jet and RA size were significantly larger in VVI pts. vs. DDD (*) at 24 months F/U. RA size and TR jet in AF > sinus rhythm (*).
Feuer et al.[26]	In the VVI group, PAF before implant vs. no PAF, CAF was 80% vs. 19% (*). Separate analysis of PAF in AV block VVI and PAF in SSS VVI indicated that PAF is a predictor of CAF in each VVI group. PAF is not a predictor of CAF in DDD/DDI mode.
Snoeck et al.[42]	VVI SSS CAF = 39.5%. VVI AVB CAF = 18.5%.
Snoeck et al.[48]	VVI SSS CAF = 49%. VVI AVB CAF = 22%.
Hesselson et al.[29]	By 8 years, all patients >70 treated for SSS with VVI had developed CAF.
Sgarbossa et al.[50]	History of PAF before implantation is an independent predictor of CAF regardless of pacing mode (P≤0.03).
Kosakai et al.[46]	AF presumably CAF.
Grimm et al.[47]	AF presumably chronic. Incidence of AF with VVI after 5 years: SSS 28/67 (42%)* vs. AV block 18/80 (23%) in patients without SVT prior to implantation. Considering all indications (including SSS & AVB) in pts. without SVT prior to implantation, AF occurred in 1/41 (2%) of DDD and 63/203 (32%) of VVI devices.
Ishikawa et al.[49]	Only patients with the bradycardia-tachycardia syndrome were studied. In the VVI mode, one patient not listed developed PAF. In the DDD mode, 4 pts. developed PAF with DDI mode.

See Table 1A for abbreviations.

TABLE 2
VVI Versus Atrial-Based Pacing: Incidence of Complications

Higher Incidence of Complications With VVI Vs. Atrial-Based Pacing	Increased Incidence of Chronic Atrial Fibrillation			Increased Incidence of Stroke and Thromboembolism	Increased Development of CHF After Pacemaker Insertion	Increased Mortality
	Regardless of Preexistent SVT	Preexistent SVT	No Preexistent SVT			
Statistically significant difference P<0.05	29, 30, 32, 34, 36, 37, 38, 43, 44, 46, 47, 49 26M, 39M, 41M	29, 32 26 M	29, 37, 47 39 M, 41 M	30, 32, 36, 40, 43, 46, 50	32	29, 32, 35, 36, 40, 43, 61 (pts. with preexistent CHF—58, 57A, 59A)
Trend and/or no statistical evaluation	31, 35, 40	35, 40, 46, 49	46	34	35	
No statistically significant difference	42 M, 45 M, 48 M		32, 40	37, 38	34, 43	34, 37, 38

Numbers represent references.
A = AV block; M = mixed (sick sinus syndrome, AV block, etc.); SVT = supraventricular tachyarrhythmia; CHF = congestive heart failure.

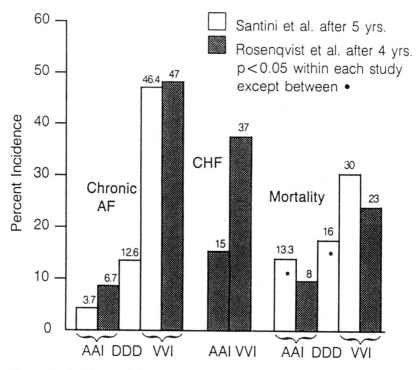

Figure 1: Incidence of chronic atrial fibrillation (AF), development of congestive heart failure (CHF), and mortality in patients with the sick sinus syndrome according to pacing mode. (From Santini et al.[36] and Rosenqvist et al.[32])

AF was higher with VVI than atrial-based pacing in 12 studies involving only SSS patients (all statistically significant with
P<0.05)[29,30,32,34,36–38,43,44,46,47,49] (Figs. 1–3). Three additional studies that included a mixture of patients with either AV block or SSS also demonstrated a statistically significant increase in chronic AF with VVI pacing compared to atrial-based pacing.[26,39,41] (2) VVI pacing possibly increased the incidence of chronic AF during VVI pacing in an additional six studies in which no statistical data were provided (three studies involved SSS patients[31,35,40] and the other three contained a mixed patient population.[42,45,48]

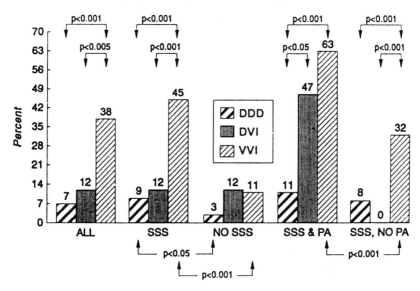

Figure 2: Development of atrial fibrillation 7 years after pacemaker implantation as a function of pacing mode, classified by indication for pacing and history of atrial tachyarrhythmias before pacing. PA = atrial tachycardia before pacemaker implantation; SSS = sick sinus syndrome. (Reproduced with permission from Hesselson et al.[29])

Preexistent Paroxysmal Supraventricular Tachyarrhythmias

Relatively few workers have analyzed the prognostic significance of preexistent paroxysmal SVT in the development of chronic AF[26,29,32,35,40,46,49] (Tables 1 and 2). Two studies in patients with a history of paroxysmal SVT before pacemaker implantation showed a statistically significant increase in chronic AF with VVI compared to atrial-based pacing[29,32] (Fig. 2). An additional study by Feuer et al.[26] also revealed a statistically significant increase in chronic AF with VVI pacing in patients with prior paroxysmal SVT, but these workers, as mentioned above, did not separate patients with AV block from those with SSS. Four studies in patients with preexistent SVT demonstrated a trend towards possible increase in chronic AF with ventricular pacing.[35,40,46,49]

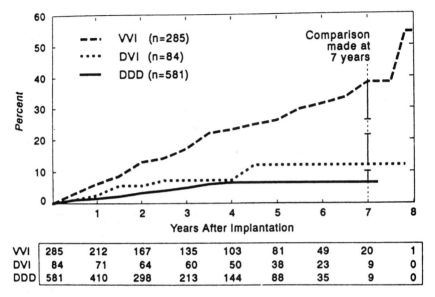

Figure 3: Rate of development of atrial fibrillation after pacemaker implantation as a function of pacing mode determined by actuarial methods. 95% confidence limits at 7 years are inserted for each curve. The numbers in the table at the bottom indicate the number of patients remaining in the study at each time interval. (Reproduced with permission from Hesselson et al.[29])

No Preexistent Paroxysmal Supraventricular Tachyarrhythmias

Some investigators have evaluated the effect of the pacing mode on the incidence of chronic AF specifically in SSS patients without preexistent paroxysmal SVT (Tables 1 and 2). Three studies in patients without preexistent SVT showed a statistically significant increase in chronic AF with VVI compared to atrial-based pacing.[29,37,47] Two other studies showed a statistically significant increase in chronic AF with VVI pacing, but the patient population was mixed and not separated in terms of AV block or SSS.[39,41] One study in SSS patients showed a trend towards an increase in chronic AF.[46] Two studies in SSS patients without preexistent SVT revealed no statistical increase in the incidence of chronic AF with VVI pacing compared to atrial-based pacing.[32,40]

Paroxysmal Atrial Fibrillation

Preliminary evidence suggests that atrial-based pacing pacing also reduces the incidence of paroxysmal atrial fibrillation, but the data are relatively soft compared to the impressive data concerning the beneficial effect of atrial-based pacing in the prevention of chronic AF.[46,51-56] Hayes and Neubauer[53] determined the occurrence of paroxysmal AF in patients who received DDD pacemakers between April 1981 and June 1989 with an average follow-up or 32 months. Forty-nine patients had paroxysmal AF before pacemaker implantation, yet no recurrence of paroxysmal AF was documented in 25 of these 49 patients (51%). However, Hayes and Neubauer[53] failed to indicate the role of pharmacological therapy in producing such a remarkable decrease in paroxysmal AF after dual chamber pacemaker implantation.

Congestive Heart Failure

Alpert et al.[57,58] investigated the influence of pacing mode and congestive heart failure (at the time of pacemaker implantation) on long-term survival (one study concentrated on high degree AV block and the other on SSS[57,58]). In the AV block or the SSS group without congestive heart failure, the mortality did not differ significantly when VVI was compared to dual chamber pacing. On the other hand, in the AV block or the SSS group with congestive heart failure, dual chamber pacing improved survival significantly compared to VVI pacing (Tables 2, 3, Fig. 4). Linde-Edelstam et al.[59] also analyzed the survival of patients with AV block treated with VDD and VVI pacemakers and found a higher mortality in the VVI group compared to the VDD group only in the patients that presented with congestive heart failure at the time of pacemaker implantation (Tables 2 and 3).

Rosenqvist et al.[32] evaluated the development of congestive heart failure *after* pacemaker implantation for sick sinus syndrome and found a statistically higher incidence with VVI than AAI pacing (Fig. 1), while Stangl et al.[35] demonstrated only a trend in the same direction (Table 4). However, two other groups reported no significant difference in sick sinus syndrome patients between VVI vs. AAI pacing with regard to the development of congestive heart failure after pacemaker implantation[34,43] (Table 4).

TABLE *3*

Mortality in Patients With Preexistent Congestive Heart Failure: VVI Versus Atrial-Based Pacing

Diagnosis	Authors	Pacing Mode	Average Follow-up in Months	No. of Pts.	Mortality	Comments
SSS	Alpert et al.[58]	VVI DVI/DDD	12–216 ?12–60	23 16	43%* 25%	Predictive cumulative mortality at 5 years
AVB	Alpert et al.[57]	VVI DVI/DDD	12–216 12–60	53 20	53%* 31%	As above
AVB	Linde-Edelstam et al.[59]	VVI VDD	49 61	24 18	53%* 28%	Estimated mortality at 5 years

* = Statistically significant (P<0.05)
SSS = Sick sinus syndrome; AVB = atrioventricular block; Pts. = patients.

TABLE *4*

Development of Congestive Heart Failure After Pacemaker Implantation: VVI Versus Atrial-Based Pacing

Diagnosis	Authors	Pacing Mode	Average Follow-up in Months	Number of Patients	Incidence of CHF–%
SSS	Sasaki et al.[43]	VVI AAI/DDD	62 39	34 17/24	21% NS 2%
SSS	Rosenqvist et al.[32]	VVI AAI	47 44	79 89	37%* 15%
SSS	Zanini et al.[34]	VVI AAI	40 45	57 53	5% NS 2%
SSS	Stangl et al.[35]	VVI AAI	33 40	112 110	7% 1%

CHF = Congestive heart failure; SSS = sick sinus syndrome; NS = not statistically significant.
* = Statistically significant (P<0.05).

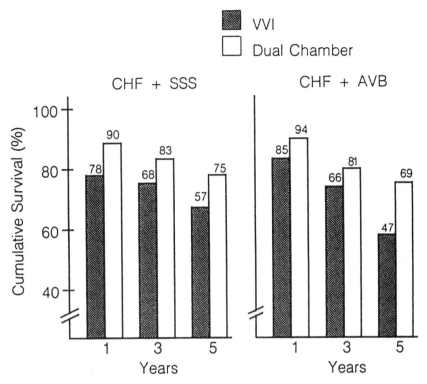

Figure 4: Effect of dual chamber pacing on survival of patients with sick sinus syndrome (SSS) and high degree AV block (AVB) related to the presence of congestive heart failure at the time of pacemaker implantation. (From Alpert et al.[57,58])

Stroke and Thromboembolism

Sutton and Kenny analyzed the incidence of thromboembolic complications in SSS patients with VVI and AAI pacemakers by using data from five previously published reports.[30] In 321 patients with AAI pacemakers, evidence of systemic embolism was found in five patients (1.6%) compared with 69 patients (13%) in 532 patients with VVI pacemakers (P<0.001). No details were given concerning the average duration of follow-up and the site of embolism, though one could rightfully assume that a large number of patients presented with strokes.

TABLE 5
Stroke and Embolism: VVI Versus Atrial-Based Pacing

Diagnosis	S/TE	Authors	Pacing Mode	No. of Pts.	Mean Follow-up in Months	Incidence of Stroke & TE Phenomena	Presence of SVT Before Pacemaker	Absence of SVT Before Pacemaker	Comments
SSS	S	Sutton & Kenny[30]	VVI	532	NR	13%*	M	M	Composite of 5 series
			AAI	321	NR	1.6%	M	M	
SSS	TE	Bianconi et al.[38] (Abstract)	VVI	150	59	10% NS	M	M	
			AAI/DDD	153	44	4%	M	M	
SSS	S	Santini et al.[36]	VVI	125	60	10.4%	M	M	Only VVI vs. AAI attained statistical significance (P<0.05)
			AAI/DDD	135/79	60	2*/3%	M	M	
SSS	S	Sethi et al.[37]	VVI	47	50	10.6% NS	0	All pts.	
			AAI	40	47	2.5%	0	All pts.	
SSS	TE	Sasaki et al.[43]	VVI	34	62	26%*	M	M	
			AAI/DDD	17/24	39	0%	M	M	
SSS	S	Rosenqvist et al.[32]	VVI	79	47	15%	20%*	M	
			AAI	89	44	12%	7.1%	M	
SSS	S/TE	Zanini et al.[34]	VVI	57	52	12%	M	M	
			AAI	53	54	0%			
SSS	TE	Kosakai et al.[46] (Abstract)	VVI	51	60	22%*	M	M	
			AAI/AV seq.	87/57	60	3/0%	M	M	
SSS	S	Nürnberg et al.[40] (Abstract)	VVI	93	41	11%*	M	M	
			AAI/DDD	15/22	41	0/0%	M	M	
SSS	S	Sgarbossa et al.[50] (Abstract)	VVI	112	57	Using univariate (UV) & multivariate (MV) analyses (Cox's proportional model), VVI vs. AAI/dual chamber*	M	M	Ventricular pacing is an independent predictor of CAF. (UV = P<0.003 MV = P<0.01)
			AAI/dual chamber	19/375	57		M	M	

Pts. = patients; SSS = sick sinus syndrome; S = stroke; TE = thromboembolism; SVT = supraventricular tachycardia; seq. = sequential; * = statistically significant (P<0.05) NS = not statistically significant; M = mixed SSS population regardless of SVT before pacemaker implantation.

Including the report of Sutton and Kenny,[30] seven studies (Tables 2 and 5) have demonstrated a statistically significant (P<0.05) higher incidence of stroke/thromboembolism in SSS patients equipped with VVI pacemakers compared to AAI/DDD devices (strokes were analyzed in five studies[30,32,36,40,50] and thromboembolic/stroke complications were grouped together in two studies[43,46]). The study of Rosenqvist et al.[32] comparing VVI to AAI pacing showed a significant increase in the incidence of stroke with VVI pacing only in a group of patients who had paroxysmal SVT before pacemaker implantation. Sgarbossa et al.[50] from the Cleveland Clinic followed 507 patients with SSS who received their initial pacemaker from January 1980 through December 1989 (VVI 112, atrial 19, dual chamber 375) with a mean follow-up of 57 months. Data from Sgarbossa et al.[50] (presented in abstract form) indicated that with univariate and multivariate analysis, single lead ventricular pacing (compared to other modes) was associated with a statistically significant higher incidence of stroke (P = 0.003 and P<0.01, respectively), but no other details were given. In the study of Santini et al.,[36] most patients who developed strokes died, thereby allowing the investigators to analyze stroke mortality according to pacing mode. Santini et al.[36] found a significantly higher stroke mortality in the VVI group (8%) compared to the AAI group (2%). However, stroke mortality showed no difference with VVI pacing compared to atrial-based pacing in patients less than 70 years old.[36] Patients over 70 years showed a statistically significant higher mortality in the VVI group (17%) compared to the AAI group (3%, P<0.001)[36] (Fig. 5). Only one study has shown a trend towards a higher incidence of stroke/thromboembolism with VVI pacing[34] (Tables 2 and 5). Only two studies have shown no statistically significant difference in the incidence of thromboembolic complications (thromboembolism was analyzed in one[38] and strokes in the other[37]) in patients with VVI compared to atrial-based pacing (Tables 2 and 5).

Mortality

In 1980, Shaw et al.[60] suggested that ventricular pacing does not favorably influence mortality in SSS patients. Their study[60] involved 381 patients, 156 with SSS and 225 with sinus bradycardia. Only 61 patients received VVI pacemakers. Shaw et al.[60] found an approximately 80% survival rate at 5 years for the entire group of 381 patients, a figure not

Stroke Mortality
AAI, DDD, and VVI Patients

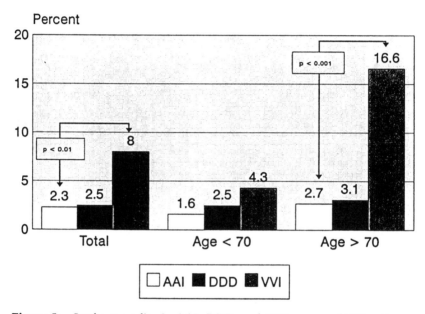

Figure 5: Stroke mortality in AAI, DDD, and VVI groups of SSS patients. Stroke mortality is higher in the VVI group than in the AAI group. Stroke mortality remained higher in the VVI group than in the AAI group only in patients older than 70 years. (Reproduced with permission from Santini et al.[36])

significantly different from the expected survival of a matched population. Patients without pacemakers showed about the same survival as those with pacemakers. We believe that the study is limited because treatment with pacing was not randomized, and pacing was undoubtedly used in the most severe cases, thereby removing from the study patients who were most at risk. Consequently, it is not possible to exclude a favorable effect on the prognosis of SSS patients who received permanent pacemakers. So far there is also no evidence that VVIR (as opposed to VVI) pacing improves survival.

Ten studies have demonstrated a statistically significant reduction in mortality of SSS patients with atrial-based pacemakers compared to those with VVI devices (Tables 2 and 6). These ten studies include (1) the three previously described findings of Alpert et al.[57,58] and Linde-Edelstam et al.[59] of increased mortality with VVI versus atrial-based pacing in patients with congestive heart failure at the time of pacemaker

TABLE *6A*
Mortality: VVI Versus Atrial-Based Pacing

Diagnosis	Authors	Pacing Mode	No. of Pts.	Mean Follow-up in Months	Mortality
SSS	Rosenqvist et al.[32]	VVI	79	47	23%*
		AAI	89	47	8%
SSS	Sasaki et al.[43]	VVI	34	62	24%* (CD) (See Comment 1)
		AAI/DDD	17/24	39	0% (CD)
SSS	Santini et al.[36]	VVI	125	60	30%* (CD) (See Comment 2)
		AAI/DDD	135/79	60	13/16% (CD)
SSS	Zanini et al.[34]	VVI	57	40	18% NS
		AAI	53	45	9%
SSS	Witte et al.[61]	VVI	3440	96	22.3%
		AAI/DDD	1096/156	96	10.5% (See Comment 3)
SSS	Nürnberg et al.[40] (Abstract)	VVI	93	41	47%*
		AAI/DDD	15/22	41	24%
SSS	Stangl et al.[35]	VVI	112	33	27%
		AAI	110	40	17% (See Comment 4)
SSS	Sethi et al.[37]	VVI	47	50	15% NS
		AAI	40	47	10%
SSS	Bianconi et al.[38] (Abstract)	VVI	150	59	31% NS
		AAI/DDD	153	44	14%
SSS	Hesselson et al.[29]	VVI	Actuarial	84	63%*
		DVI/DDD	Actuarial	84	34/40%
SSS	Hesselson et al.[29]	VVI	193	1977–89	47%
		DVI/DDD	58/308	As above	33/20%

SSS = Sick sinus syndrome; CHF = congestive heart failure; CAD = coronary artery disease; Pts. = patients.
* = Statistically significant P<0.05; NS = not statistically significant.

TABLE *6B*
Comments

1. Sasaki et al.[43] Both total mortality and cardiac deaths were statistically higher in the VVI vs. DDD group.

2. Santini et al.[36] Cardiac death (CD) includes CHF in 3 and thrombo-embolism (TE) in 5 patients. CD from TE, VVI = 5, vs. AAI/DDI = 0 (P<0.05).

3. Witte et al.[61] Before the availability of DDD therapy, patients with severe disease and/or a low Wenckebach point were treated with a VVI pacemaker. These patients were excluded for analysis from the VVI group because of their poor prognosis so as to obtain a more accurate statistical evaluation.

4. Stangl et al.[35] When analyzed separately in (1) patients with no underlying disease, mortality was significantly lower in the AAI vs. the VVI group (P<0.02), (2) patients with CAD, mortality was significantly lower in the AAI vs. the VVI group (P<0.05).

implantation. (2) Seven studies all with SSS patients have shown a higher mortality in patients with VVI compared to those with atrial-based pacing[29,32,35,36,40,43,61] (Tables 2 and 6 and Figs. 1, 6, 7). Witte et al.[61] analyzed a large population of SSS patients (4682 patients, VVI 3440, AAI 1096, DDD156). With a follow-up of 8 years, 89.5% of the AAI/DDD patients were alive compared to 77.7% of the VVI patients (P<0.005) Stangl et al.[35] found in the SSS no difference in the overall mortality of the VVI group versus the AAI group, but the mortality was higher in patients with VVI pacemakers who had either coronary artery disease or no underlying heart disease. Three other studies of SSS patients have shown no statistically significant difference in mortality comparing VVI with AAI/DDD pacing[34,37,38] (Tables 2 and 6).

Hesselson et al.[29] (from Parsonnet's group) followed 950 patients (559 with SSS) who received DDD, DVI, or VVI pacemakers from February 1977 to August 1989. All patients were in sinus rhythm at the time of pacemaker implantation. The average duration of follow-up for DDD, DVI, and VVI pacing was 30, 53, and 44 months, respectively. The overall mortality was higher in the VVI group (50%) than in the DDD (22%) or DVI (38%) groups (Figs. 6, 7). At 7 years, survival of all patients (by actuarial analysis) was significantly poorer in the VVI group (36%) than in the DDD (55%, P<0.001) and DVI groups (53%, P<0.025) (Fig. 7). The survival was worse in the VVI group regardless of the indication

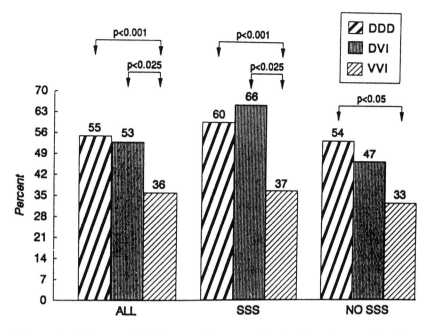

Figure 6: Patient survival 7 years after pacemaker implantation as a function of pacing mode classified by indication for pacing. SSS = sick sinus syndrome. (Reproduced with permission from Hesselson et al.[29])

for pacing. The survival of SSS patients at 7 years was significantly poorer in the VVI group (37%) than in the DDD (60%, P<0.001) and DVI groups (66%, P<0.025) (Fig. 7). Hesselson et al.[29] pointed out that age at the time of pacemaker implantation was important in determining survival. In patients older than 70 years at the time of implantation, at 7 years the survival was significantly poorer (28% versus 56%) in the VVI group than in the DDD group regardless of the indication for pacing. When analyzed in terms of only SSS patients, 7-year survival was 28% in the VVI versus 46% DDD mode (P<0.001) and 55% in the DVI group P<0.025). In patients younger than 70 years of age at the time of implantation, the 7-year survival was 56% with the VVI and 66% with the DDD mode regardless of the indication for pacing (the difference did not reach statistical significance). In SSS patients younger than 70 years, the survival rate in the VVI mode was 56%, DDD mode 66%, and DVI

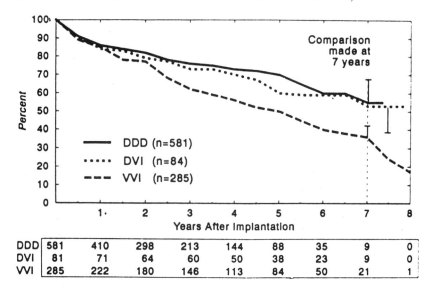

DDD	581	410	298	213	144	88	35	9	0
DVI	81	71	64	60	50	38	23	9	0
VVI	285	222	180	146	113	84	50	21	1

Figure 7: Actuarial survival seven years after pacemaker implantation as a function of pacing mode. 95% confidence limits at 7 years are inserted for each curve. The numbers in the table at the bottom indicate the number of patients remaining in the study at each time interval. (Reproduced with permission from Hesselson et al.[29])

mode 73% (difference did not reach statistical significance) (Fig. 8). The observation by Hesselson et al.[29] that in patients older than 70 years, the survival rate at 7 years is significantly better with DDD than with VVI pacing (including SSS patients) confirms the work of Santini et al.,[36] who suggested that in a more elderly population (older than 70 years), the adverse hemodynamics of VVI pacing in the SSS are less easily tolerated than in younger individuals. Hesselson et al.[29] did not analyze the cause of death in their patients. However, Santini et al.[26] found that cardiac mortality (defined as sudden death or death due to acute myocardial infarction or heart failure) was significantly higher in patients with VVI pacemakers than in patients with AAI pacemakers, but only in patients >70 years old and not in patients <70 years.

Byrd et al.[62] also evaluated the impact of the pacing mode in 666 patients. Thirty percent of the patients received VVI pacemakers, and they had a 62% survival rate at 44 months while 77% of the patients

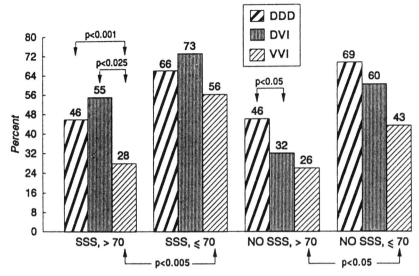

Figure 8: Patient survival at 7 years as a function of pacing mode classified by indication for pacing and age at the time of pacemaker implantation. (Reproduced with permission from Hesselson et al.[29])

with DDD pacemakers had an 82% survival at 44 months. Byrd et al.[62] admitted that their selection criteria precluded drawing conclusions with regard to the merit of either modality, and the data were not analyzed in terms of indications for pacing. However, the survival curve for the DDD group was at least as good or probably better than for the norm of the population.

Critique of Data Favoring Atrial-Based Pacing

All available data favoring atrial-based pacing in the SSS come from retrospective, nonrandomized studies due to the lack of prospective large-scale randomized controlled trials comparing VVI to atrial-based pacing. The limitations[63,64] of the present data base include: (1) selection bias for VVI pacing in older patients at a higher risk of developing atrial fibrillation, (2) selection bias for VVI pacing in the high risk or sicker patients, (3) selection bias for VVI pacing in patients with paroxysmal supraven-

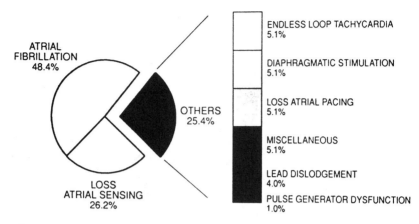

Figure 9: All causes of mode changes out of DDD and their frequency of occurrence. (Reproduced with permission from Gross et al.[28])

tricular tachyarrhythmias. (Note that such arrhythmias were previously considered a contraindication to DDD pacing until recently. However, most studies comparing single lead VVI pacing to atrial-based pacing were performed in Europe with AAI pacing rather than DDD pacing.) (4) Mode selection not at random where a large variety of pacemakers is available in any given institution, (5) unstated criteria for pacemaker selection, (6) unstated left ventricular function. The type of congestive heart failure (diastolic versus systolic) was not analyzed in any of the studies. (7) Different follow-up periods for atrial-based versus VVI pacing without actuarial analysis. (8) Despite many studies comparing AAI to VVI pacing, the fate of the patients rejected for AAI pacing has not been studied. Such patients most probably received VVI rather than dual chamber devices. Patients rejected for AAI pacing because of intraatrial or intraventricular conduction disturbances (even with only right or left bundle branch block) are associated with sicker hearts.

Lamas et al.[63] recently indicated that current data showing a reduced incidence of chronic AF and suggesting improved survival with dual or single lead atrial pacing in SSS patients are inconclusive due to the methodological limitations inherent in the retrospective analyses of incomplete pacemaker data bases.[64] Lamas et al.[63] emphasized that current retrospective data do not allow a definitive recommendation regarding atrial pacing in patients with SSS, but call for a prospective, randomized, controlled trial to determine the benefit of atrial or dual chamber pacing in patients with SSS. Nevertheless, in 1991 the American College of Cardiology/American Heart Association Task Force report concerning the Guidelines for Implantation of Cardiac Pacemakers and Antiarrhythmia Devices stated that "long-term absence of atrioventricular synchrony increases the incidence of atrial fibrillation and stroke and may reduce patient life expectancy. Therefore, the concept that the single chamber pacemaker with rate-adaptive functions is equivalent to the dual chamber pacemaker cannot be supported."[25] Furthermore, also in 1991 the British Pacing and Electrophysiology Group in their working party report on Recommendations for Pacemaker Prescription for Symptomatic Bradycardia stated that "evidence is accumulating of a considerable reduction in the high spontaneous incidence of the development of atrial fibrillation and of systemic emboli in patients with sinus node disease treated by a pacing system that maintains atrioventricular synchrony."[65]

Retrograde Ventriculoatrial Conduction: Risk of Chronic Atrial Fibrillation and Thromboembolic Complications

Irrespective of the pacemaker syndrome, retrograde VA conduction during single lead ventricular pacing appears to constitute an independent prognostic factor for the development of atrial arrhythmias and thromboembolic complications.[48,66,67] For this reason alone, some workers feel that single lead VVI pacing is contraindicated in SSS patients with retrograde VA conduction.[66,67]

Snoeck et al.[48] investigated the importance of retrograde VA conduction during VVI pacing in the genesis of chronic AF. Snoeck et al.[48] evaluated 275 patients with single lead ventricular pacemakers, 230 with VVI and 45 with VVIR devices. At 5 years of follow-up, chronic AF occurred in 32% of the patients (VVI pacing in SSS patients 49%, and VVI in AV block, 22% had chronic AF). Further analysis revealed that retrograde VA conduction increased the risk of chronic AF by a factor of 5 for both the SSS and AV block groups. The patients were divided into two groups according to retrograde VA conduction. *Group I with absent retrograde VA conduction:* The entire group exhibited a 17% incidence of chronic AF at 5 years. The SSS group without retrograde VA conduction exhibited a 23% incidence of chronic AF at 5 years. *Group*

II with retrograde VA conduction: Patients with AV block exhibited an 89% incidence of chronic AF at 5 years. Essentially 100% of the SSS patients developed chronic AF at 5 years. Snoeck et al.[48] also pointed out that in continuously paced patients, the incidence of chronic AF was 46% in contrast to patients with alternating pacing and sinus rhythm (in a balanced fashion) who showed a 17% incidence of chronic AF at 5 years. Thus, it appears that the degree of pacemaker utilization is a very important factor in the genesis of chronic AF in patients with single lead ventricular pacemakers.[39,48] Stangl et al.[35] also demonstrated that VVI pacing in SSS patients at a rate of 50/min was associated with a lower incidence of chronic AF compared to a pacing rate of 70/min, but only in patients with preexistent supraventricular tachyarrhythmias.

Ebagosti et al.,[66] in the follow-up of 45 VVI patients, observed atrial arrhythmias and deaths only in cases with retrograde VA conduction. Curzi et al.[67] compared 110 VVI patients (AV block and SSS) with retrograde VA conduction (group A with a mean follow-up of 85 months) with 120 VVI patients without retrograde VA conduction (group B with a mean follow-up of 124 months). Patients in group A developed 28 thromboembolic episodes (14 in the first year after implantation) in association with atrial fibrillation in only five patients. In group B, four thromboembolic episodes occurred (none within 2 years from implantation) in association with the onset of AF.

In VVI pacing, the incidence of chronic AF is higher in SSS patients than in patients with AV block for several reasons.[45,47,48] (1) VA conduction is more frequent in the SSS. (2) History of SVT (more common in SSS) prior to pacemaker implantation (bradycardia-tachycardia syndrome) represents a predictor for the subsequent development of chronic AF. (3) Atrial disease is more common in the SSS.

Is VVI Pacing Contraindicated in the Sick Sinus Syndrome?

The 1991 ACC/AHA Guidelines for Pacemaker Implantation do not specifically state that single lead atrial (in the presence of normal AV conduction) and dual chamber pacemakers are indicated in patients with retrograde VA conduction. The 1991 ACC/AHA Guidelines[25] recommend VVI pacing as a Class I choice for "any symptomatic bradycardia, but particularly when there is no evidence of pacemaker syndrome due to loss of atrial contribution or negative atrial kick (a replacement pacemaker)." Symptomatic bradycardia in the *absence* of retrograde VA conduction is classified as a Class II choice for VVI pacing. The 1991 ACC/AHA Guidelines make no firm statement that the VVI mode is contraindicated in patients with either the SSS and/or retrograde VA conduction, though they do indicate that "VVIR pacemakers are particularly contraindicated in the presence of retrograde VA conduction." Many workers and the recent report of the British Pacing and Electrophysiology Group have stated categorically that the VVI and VVIR modes are contraindicated in all SSS patients.[65,68-78] The British Pacing and Electrophysiology Group also stated that atrial fibrillation/flutter with AV block or slow ventricular response constitutes the only indication for the VVI or VVIR pacing mode.[65] In contrast, the 1991 ACC/AHA Guidelines are far more liberal with regard to indications for VVI and VVIR pacing.[25]

We generally agree with the recommendations of the British group, but believe that single lead ventricular pacing in the absence of atrial fibrillation still has a place in the occasional patient with rare episodes of bradycardia (providing a safety net or backup pacing). Replacement of a depleted VVI pacemaker with another VVI or VVIR unit is not unreasonable in many asymptomatic patients. Single lead ventricular pacing may also be appropriate in patients who are incapacitated and inactive as well as those with other medical problems associated with a short life expectancy.

Single Chamber Atrial Pacing

Single chamber atrial pacing is popular in Europe, but in the United States perhaps 1% or less of patients requiring pacing receive single chamber atrial pacemakers. AAI and AAIR pacemakers are underutilized and still considered controversial despite the wealth of information showing their superiority over VVI pacing in the SSS.[71,79,80] There is no real scientific justification for underutilizing AAI pacing. Previous problems with atrial pacing such as instability of the leads, poor lead characteristics, and limited device programmability have been solved. Atrial lead dislodgement is relatively rare. Pacing and sensing are reliable on a chronic basis. The only important problem with AAI (AAIR) pacing is the relatively low risk of AV block.

Risk of AV Block

In 1989, Rosenqvist and Obel[80] reviewed 28 different series of SSS patients treated with AAI pacing. There were 1,878 patients with a median follow-up period of 36 months. The total prevalence of second or third degree AV block was 2.1% (median value) with an estimated annual incidence of 0.6%. In 17 studies (60%), the annual rate of second or third degree AV block was 1% and in six studies (22%), the annual incidence was 1–2%. There was no difference in follow-up time between studies showing a low as compared to a high incidence of AV block. Review of a number of series of SSS patients treated with AAI pacing published after the report of Rosenqvist and Obel[80] have confirmed that the development of second and third degree AV block in carefully selected patients with this mode of pacing is quite low[36,37,81–89] (Table 7).

Brandt et al.[88] studied 213 SSS patients with AAI pacemakers for a mean follow-up of 60 months. High grade AV block occurred in 8.5% (1.8%/year). Its incidence was much greater in patients with complete bundle branch block or bifascicular block (6 of 17 patients, 35%) than in patients without such conduction disturbances (12 of 196 patients, 6%, giving an annual incidence of approximately 1.2%). Eight patients exhibited a prolonged P-Q interval of 220–240 ms before pacemaker implantation, but none of the patients developed high grade AV block during follow-up.

Considering the low risk of AV block in the above reports, the question arises as to why Sutton and Kenny[30] found a higher incidence of AV block in their study. Sutton and Kenny[30] reviewed 28 series involving 1,395 SSS patients (with AAI pacing) and reported the development of significant AV block in 8.4% (117 patients) for a mean follow-up of 34 months, giving an annual incidence of 3% per year. Sutton and Kenny[30] therefore concluded that the AAI mode is not safe for SSS patients. The discrepancy appears related to the lack of strict selection of candidates for AAI pacing and therefore overestimation of the incidence of AV block because significant AV block was defined by Sutton and Kenny[30] as (1) PR interval >0.24 second), (2) complete bundle branch block, (3) Wenckebach rate or point (slowest atrial pacing rate where type I second degree AV block develops or the fastest atrial rate associated with 1:1 AV conduction) at the AV node ≤120/min, (4) prolonged HV interval >75 ms, and (5) second or third degree AV block. Furthermore, the deleterious effect of drugs on AV conduction was not specifically analyzed. Only one recent report (not included in Table 7) by Haywood et al.[90] revealed a high incidence of AV block during AAI pacing (in contrast to 1,146 patients in 11 series with longer follow-up shown in Table 7). The study by Haywood et al.[90] consisted of only 24 patients without second or third degree AV block or bundle branch block with a short mean follow-up of 11 months. Four patients developed AV block. The Wenckebach point was tested after pacemaker implantation and not before or during implantation. The four patients that developed AV block all had a Wenckebach point >120/min soon after pacemaker implantation. Drug treatment was not specified and therefore a drug effect on AV conduction cannot be ruled out in the report of Haywood et al.[90]

VanMechelen et al.[91] emphasized that the development of second or third degree AV block during AAI pacing is often due to the effect of drugs on the AV junction. Indeed, in the series of Santini et al.[36] (135 patients, mean follow-up of >61 months), seven patients developed second or third degree AV block, which disappeared in six when drug therapy was discontinued.

Selection of Patients for AAI (AAIR) Pacing

In the 11 studies of AAI pacing[36,37,81–89] since the report of Rosenqvist and Obel[80] in 1989, a variable number of patients were included for AAI pacing despite (1) intraventricular conduction disorder (IVCD) such as bundle branch block, left anterior hemiblock, or left posterior hemiblock, (2) Wenckebach point <120/min, or (3) first degree AV block. In some studies such as the ones by Swiatecka et al.[85] and Brandt et al.,[88] removal of patients more likely to develop second or third degree AV block (low Wenckebach point, first degree AV block, or IVCD) yields an annual incidence of second or third degree block close to 1%. It seems that patients with bundle branch block or bifascicular block are not good candidates for AAI pacing. Although some workers do not recommend dual chamber pacing in patients with isolated left anterior or left posterior hemiblock, patients with this type of IVCD probably have a low risk of developing second or third degree AV block with AAI pacing.

It seems reasonable to conclude on the basis of the published literature that the development of clinically important conduction disturbances in carefully selected patients for AAI (AAIR) pacing is very low

TABLE 7
Sick Sinus Syndrome:
Incidence of Second and Third Degree AV Block in Patients With AAI Pacemakers

Authors	No. of Pts.	Mean Follow-up in Months	Wenckebach Point*	PR Interval in Seconds	Intraventricular Conduction Disorder	Incidence of 2nd & 3rd Degree AV Block	Annual Incidence of 2nd & 3rd Degree AV Block	Comments
Rosenqvist & Obel[8]	1878 (28 Articles)	36 (median)	110–150 & not always stated	NR	NR	2.1%	0.6%	
Santini et al.[36]	135	65	>140	NR	CBBB, LAH, & LPH excluded	5%	<1%	7 pts. developed AVB. In 6, AVB disappeared when drug treatment was discontinued. 2 pts. developed 1st degree AVB.
Sethi et al.[37]	40	47	>130	Normal except for 1 pt.	NR	0%	0%	
Brandt et al.[88]	196	60	>120	≤0.24	Only LAH or LPH included	6%	1.2%	6 (35%) of 17 other pts. with CBBB or BFB developed 2nd or 3rd degree AVB.
Lemke et al.[83]	111	47	>120 (since 1983)	NR	NR	4.5%	1.1%	5 other pts. showed intermittent type 1 2nd degree AVB on Holter recordings. Pacing system not revised because pts. were asymptomatic.

Kallryd et al.[81]	66	32	NR	>0.24 in 3 pts.	5 pts. CBBB, 6 pts. LAH, HV ≤60 ms.	6%	1.5%	No pt. had BFB. Only 1 pt. from group of 14 pts. with IVCD or PR >0.24 sec developed 2nd or third degree AVB.
Kerr et al.[82]	43	27	>130	Normal	No IVCD**. HV normal. No CBBB with AP	1 AVB at rate of 90/min.	0.5%	
Kolettis et al.[84]	91	33	>120	Normal	No BBB	1.1%	0.9%	2 pts. developed 2nd degree AVB at night, asymptomatic, no treatment.
Novak et al.[86]	38	30	>130	≤0.24	NR	0%	0%	
Bernstein et al.[87]	187	30	>120	1st degree AV block included	CBBB included	2.1%	0.9%	
Swiatecka et al.[85]	122	35	30 pts. >120 5 pts. <120	NR	2 pts. CBBB, 1 pt. LAH	5.7% 3.2% (excl. 3 pts.)	1.9% <1% (excl. 3 pts.)	When 3 pts. (2 with W point <120 and 1 with LAH) were excluded, the annual incidence of second or third degree AVB becomes <1%.
Rognoni et al.[89]	117	46	NR	NR	NR	2%		

Whenever possible, patients with 1st degree AVB, CBBB, BFB, LAH, LPH and low W point were excluded from analysis.
NR = Not reported; Pts. = patients; W = Wenckebach; AP = atrial pacing; AVB = AV block (if not specified, AVB refers to 2nd or 3rd degree AV block); CBBB = complete bundle branch block; IVCD = intraventricular conduction disturbance; LAH = left anterior hemiblock; LPH = left posterior hemiblock; BFB = bifascicular block; Excl. = excluding.
* Wenckebach point. Slowest atrial rate at which type I 2nd degree AV block occurs.
** IVCD not defined.

(annual incidence of about 1%), often related to drug therapy and rarely if ever catastrophic at its onset. Consequently, single lead atrial pacing may be considered in the SSS if (1) atrial pacing to rates 120–140 per minute is associated with 1:1 AV conduction with the realization that this is an arbitrary value that may change from day to day. The Wenckebach point may occur at a higher atrial rate when standing during normal life than when lying during testing. The procedure is still recommended, though there is evidence about the poor prognostic value of the Wenckebach point in identifying patients at risk for the subsequent development of AV block.[85,88,92,93] In this regard, Brandt et al.[88] found that in 213 patients treated with AAI pacemakers, a Wenckebach point greater than 130/min was not predictive of the subsequent development of AV block. Eighteen of 213 patients developed high grade AV block, and all had a Wenckebach point $\geq$130/min, and 12 of the 18 had a Wenckebach point >150/min. (2) PR interval <0.24 seconds at rest. (3) Absence of bifascicular or bundle branch block. The presence of isolated left anterior or left posterior hemiblock probably does not constitute an important contraindication to single lead atrial pacing. (4) Absence of a prolonged HV interval.

With careful selection of patients, AAI or AAIR pacing could be used safely in probably half the patients with sick sinus syndrome. Preimplantation stress testing or Holter recordings are useful in determining the presence of atrial chronotropic incompetence. About 40% of patients who are candidates for atrial pulse generators may require rate-adaptive devices (AAIR) because of poor atrial chronotropic response.

Patient Survival

Brandt et al.[88] recently described the natural history of sinus node disease treated with atrial pacing in 213 patients for a mean follow-up period of 60 months. The incidence of permanent AF was 7% (1.4% per year). The 1.4% annual incidence of chronic AF was identical to that reported by Sutton and Kenny[30] in their collective review of patients with AAI pacemakers. The risk of chronic AF increases substantially with age >70 years at the time of AAI pacemaker implantation.[88] In patients >70 years, the incidence of permanent AF was 2.7% per year, whereas it was only 0.2% per year in patients <70 years. The presence of SVT before pacemaker implantation was not a significant predictor of the development of chronic AF. Only two of the 15 patients who developed chronic AF required ventricular pacing. A mode change was performed in 30 patients (lead dislodgement 8, high grade AV block 18, and miscellaneous causes in 4). Eleven leads became displaced and in eight the workers elected to position the displaced lead into the right ventricle for technical reasons. Considering the low displacement rate of modern screw-in leads (assumed to be near 0 if a lead becomes displaced and is successfully repositioned), and excluding patients with bundle branch block or bifascicular block and the 12 patients with AV block, mode change would have been performed in only 12 patients plus 4 for miscellaneous causes, which makes 16 patients (7.5%) or 1.5% per year. For the patients with SSS, the survival rate was 97% at 1 year, 89% at 5 years, and 72% at 10 years. The survival rate in this group did not differ significantly from that of a Swedish age- and gender-matched general population in which the corresponding survival probabilities were 97%, 82%, and 63%, respectively. Only two patients died of strokes. Seven died suddenly, three with dual chamber pacemakers. Brandt et al.[88] felt that the cause of death was due to ventricular arrhythmia rather than AV block.

The data of Brandt et al.[88] concerning survival in the SSS confirm those of Lemke et al.[83] who studied the 5-year survival of 100 patients (followed for a mean of 47 months) with SSS and single lead atrial pacing. The mean age at the start of pacing was 65 years and the survival rate after 5 years was 85%, equivalent to that of a matched population.

AAIR Pacemaker Syndrome

In patients carefully selected for AAIR pacing, the AV interval should shorten like the normal PR interval during exercise (see Chapter 15). During atrial pacing, a marked delay between the pacemaker stimulus and the onset of ventricular systole may produce atrial systole against closed AV valves, producing a hemodynamic situation identical to retrograde VA conduction. This form of pacemaker syndrome is highly unlikely with the pacing rates ordinarily used in the AAI mode, but can occur in the AAIR mode when the atrial pacing rate increases.[94,95]

Mabo et al.[96] reported that with carefully selected patients with single lead atrial pacing, the PR interval does not show a decrease on exercise in about 1/3 of patients (2 of 6 took antiarrhythmic agents). The PR interval was 182 ± 43 ms at rest and on exercise 182 ± 38 ms. The hemodynamic consequences of an unchanged PR interval on exercise are not clear. A fast sensor response in the AAIR mode with a sudden increase in the atrial rate disproportionate to the degree of exercise can lengthen the PR interval before the expected catecholamine surge has the opportunity to improve or shorten AV conduction. The AAIR mode therefore poses the risk of "overstimulation" with rates above exercise requirement that may lead to undesirable paradoxical prolongation of the PR interval. This behavior tends to correct itself as sympathetic tone is progressively increased during the exercise. Paradoxical prolongation of the AV interval is usually seen in patients taking drugs that depress AV conduction.[95–97] The long PR interval places the atrial paced beat too close to the previous QRS complex and atrial contraction occurs against a closed AV valve, producing an exercise-induced AAIR pacemaker syndrome. Drugs that impair AV conduction should therefore be used cautiously in patients with AAIR devices. As a rule, if the clinical situation suggests the patient will require antiarrhythmic therapy at the time of implantation, a dual chamber pacemaker should be used.

Change in Pacing Mode

With contemporary dual chamber devices, the most important cause of change in the pacing mode is the development of chronic atrial fibrillation. Therefore, patients with SSS require a change in the pacing mode more frequently than patients with AV block.

Gross et al.[28] analyzed the causes of change in the pacing mode in 486 patients with DDD pulse generators implanted from December 1981 to December 1988 (a period of almost 8 years) with a mean follow-up of 33 months. Eighty-two percent of pulse generators remained in the DDD mode throughout the follow-up period, i.e., nearly 80% 5-year survival of the DDD mode. The DDD survival rate at 1, 2, 3, 4, and 5 years was 90%, 88%, 84%, 79%, and 78%, respectively. Atrial fibrillation was the most common cause of reprogramming to another mode and it occurred in 10% of all patients. In the study or Gross et al.,[28] loss of atrial pacing was due to (1) chronic AF. About 10% of patients lost DDD pacing because of chronic AF (48 of 486, but in 11, sinus rhythm returned and the DDD mode was restored temporarily; six patients relapsed into AF, five remained in the DDD mode.) (2) Atrial undersensing

(26 of 486 or 5%). Thirteen of the 26 patients (2.7%) required abandonment of the DDD mode because of loss of atrial sensing not attributable to early generation pacemaker technology. Thus, chronic AF and loss of atrial sensing accounted for 73% of all mode changes. About 10% of all mode changes were considered related to early or defective pacemaker technology. The pacing mode was not necessarily downgraded to the VVI mode. For example, with loss of atrial capture or diaphragmatic pacing, the DDD mode was programmed to the VDD mode, and in the presence of atrial undersensing the DVI rather than the VVI mode was used.

Hummel et al.[98] reported an 85% maintenance of dual chamber pacing at 2.5 years with 80% remaining in the DDD mode (5% DDI or VDD). This series involved 122 dual chamber devices and 25 had a permanent mode change (20%). Seven of the 25, however, were left in the DDI or VDD mode so that 85% (18 of 122) remained in the dual chamber mode. Eight patients were programmed out of the DDD mode because of atrial arrhythmias (5%). Sgarbossa et al.[44] from the Cleveland Clinic evaluated 395 DDD pacemakers (implanted in January 1980 through December 1989), with a mean follow-up 57.2 months. Of these, 87.2% were in the DDD mode at 5 years and 74.3% at 10 years. Detollenaere et al.[99] followed 252 DDD pacemakers from October 1982 to December 1990 with a mean follow-up of 30 months. Reprogramming was required in 39 patients (15.5%). In 24 patients, this was due to an atrial arrhythmia (14 for atrial fibrillation and 10 for atrial flutter). These workers were able to convert the atrial arrhythmia to normal sinus rhythm in 33%, giving a survival of 94% at 2 years. Detollenaere et al.[99] indicated the importance of having the option of rapid atrial pacing for conversion of atrial flutter. Other workers have reported basically the same experience with regard to longevity of the DDD mode and the development of chronic AF.[100–103]

In summary, about 85–90% of contemporary DDD pulse generators should remain in the DDD mode at 5 years because of improved pacemaker sensitivity, better leads, and increasing experience. The development of chronic AF in SSS patients constitutes the most common cause of downgrading to the VVI mode.

Special Predictors of Atrial Fibrillation

Hayes et al.[104] showed that the amplitude of the atrial electrogram at the time of pacemaker implantation appears to predict the subsequent development of chronic atrial fibrillation (2.9 mV in patients without chronic atrial fibrillation versus 2.5 mV in patients who subsequently developed chronic atrial fibrillation). Sgarbossa et al.[44,50] also found that an endocardial P wave electrogram <2 mV is predictive of the subsequent development of chronic atrial fibrillation. Both studies failed to state whether the electrogram was unipolar or bipolar. A low atrial electrogram appears to be a marker for fibrosis and fragmented electrical activity of large atria. In this respect, Brandt et al.[105] demonstrated that lower unipolar electrographic atrial voltage is correlated with older age of patients and the presence of SSS.

Other characteristics of the P wave on the surface electrocardiogram that may be useful in predicting the development of chronic atrial fibrillation include: (1) progressive morphologic changes of the P wave in terms of duration (lead 2) and terminal forces in lead V_1,[106] and (2) using signal averaging electrocardiography, Fukunami et al.[107] recently reported that the voltage of the last portion of the filtered P wave (determined by signal averaged electrocardiography) was 95% sensitive in identifying patients with paroxysmal atrial fibrillation. This approach may become valuable in SSS patients.

The ability to predict the development of chronic atrial fibrillation is important because at the time of implantation (or pacemaker replacement), consideration should be given to implanting a pacemaker that will serve the patient should chronic atrial fibrillation develop, i.e., capability of VVIR or automatic mode switching.[104]

Increase in Left Atrial Size

VVI pacing causes left atrial enlargement more than DDD pacing.[56,108,109] Atrial enlargement most probably contributes to the increased incidence of atrial arrhythmias. Chronic elevation of atrial pressure (with impaired atrial motion) causes atrial enlargement that predisposes to atrial fibrillation compared to DDD/AAI pacing. Conversion from VVI to AAI/DDD pacing can reduce atrial enlargement and probably decrease the incidence of atrial arrhythmias.[108]

Is Atrial Rate-Adaptive Pacing Useful in the Prevention of Atrial Arrhythmias?

Preliminary data suggest that rate-adaptive AAIR and DDDR modes may be more efficacious in preventing atrial arrhythmias than their non-rate-adaptive counterparts in the SSS.[110–112] DDDR pacemakers may prevent arrhythmias by eliminating the relative bradycardia during exercise seen in patients with non-rate-adaptive devices where excessive catecholamine release on exercise may increase the propensity to atrial arrhythmias. Thus, the question arises as to whether rate-adaptive pacing provides protection against the development of chronic AF. This question cannot as yet be answered. In this respect, Haywood et al.[113] failed to detect any significant elimination of atrial ectopic activity with AAIR units in the SSS. Feuer et al.[114] warned that DDDR pacing may well be associated with a higher incidence of atrial tachyarrhythmias compared to conventional DDD pacing. There is concern that DDDR pacing may cause atrial arrhythmias whenever an unsensed P wave falling in the postventricular atrial refractory period is closely followed by a sensor-initiated atrial stimulus delivered during the atrial vulnerable period. However, so far preliminary clinical experience suggests that DDDR pacing does not result in a significant increase in atrial arrhythmias.

Progression of Chronotropic Incompetence

Little is known about the progression or even development of chronotropic incompetence in SSS patients (or patients with AV block). Vardas et al.[115] recently indicated that in SSS patients, chronotropic incompetence increases with the passage of time, a finding confirmed by Gwinn et al.,[116] who also emphasized that a substantial number of patients with AV block also developed chronotropic incompetence after pacemaker implantation. Vardas et al.[115] suggested that the presence of syncope and a severely prolonged corrected sinus node recovery time may be predictive of the development of progressive chronotropic incompetence. These findings suggest that rate-adaptive pacemakers should be considered even in chronotropic competent patients at the time of initial implantation because of the possibility of progressive chronotropic incompetence.

Conclusion

Many recent studies suggest that atrial-based pacing as opposed to single lead ventricular pacing improves the natural history of SSS patients after pacemaker implantation. The continuing controversy concerning the basically unimportant contribution of AV synchrony to the cardiac output *on exercise* (as opposed to the increase in heart rate) should not detract from the well-established and significant benefits of maintaining AV synchrony *at rest*. For this reason, we believe that the statement "The atrium should be paced/sensed unless contraindicated" merits being called the golden rule of cardiac pacing for the 1990s, because it focuses on the hemodynamic and electrophysiological advantages of atrial pacing, especially important in patients with SSS. In the 1990s with presently available technology, permanent antibradycardia pacing in the SSS should provide (1) restoration of normal or near-normal hemodynamics at rest and on exercise, remembering that the pacemaker syndrome is basically an iatrogenic condition, (2) a more favorable natural history with reduction or prevention of certain atrial tachyarrhythmias and their thromboembolic complications related to atrial dysfunction. After the institution of atrial pacing, it is mandatory to assess its efficacy in the control of atrial tachyarrhythmias.[117] If atrial arrhythmias recur, increasing the atrial pacing rate to 80/min may help.[117] If not, antiarrhythmic drug therapy is indicated because poor arrhythmia control predisposes to systemic embolism. Atrial arrhythmias seem to respond better to antiarrhythmic agents in patients with atrial and dual chamber pacemakers than in those with single lead ventricular devices.[118] Long-term anticoagulants should be administered in patients with refractory paroxysmal atrial fibrillation, but the efficacy of warfarin versus aspirin is presently unknown in this setting.[117] (3) Protection against rapid ventricular pacing. The presence of paroxysmal atrial tachyarrhythmias in the SSS, previously considered a contraindication to dual chamber pacing, now constitutes an important indication for dual chamber pacing. Patients with paroxysmal supraventricular tachyarrhythmias may benefit from specially designed DDD or DDDR pacemakers that can limit the paced ventricular rate during supraventricular tachyarrhythmias by a variety of mechanisms that include fallback and automatic switching of pacing mode, discussed in other chapters of this book.

References

1. Ausubel K, Furman S. The pacemaker syndrome. Ann Intern Med 1985;103:420.
2. Schüller H, Brandt J. The pacemaker syndrome: Old and new causes. Clin Cardiol 1991;14:336.

3. Furman S. Atrioventricular and ventriculoatrial conduction. In: Furman S, Hayes DL, Holmes DR (eds.). A Practice of Cardiac Pacing, Futura Publishing Co., Mt. Kisco, NY 1986, p 56.
4. Nishimura R, Gersh B, Vliestra R, et al. Hemodynamic and symptomatic consequences of ventricular pacing. PACE 1982; 5:903.
5. Cohen S, Frank H. Preservation of active atrial transport: An important clinical consideration in cardiac pacing. Chest 1982; 81:51.
6. Galvao S. Syndrome du stimulateur monochambre à fréquence asservie. A propos d'un cas. Stimucoeur 1987;15:137.
7. Heldman D, Mulvihill D, Nguyen H, et al. True incidence of pacemaker syndrome. PACE 1990;13:1742.
8. Rediker D, Eagle K, Homma S, et al. Clinical and hemodynamic comparison of VVI versus DDD pacing in patients with DDD pacemakers. Am J Cardiol 1988;61:323.
9. Mitsuoka T, Kenny R, Yeung T, et al. Benefits of dual-chamber pacing in sick sinus syndrome. Br Heart J 1988;60:338.
10. Fromer J, Kappenberger L, Bobotai I. Subjective and objective response to single versus dual-chamber pacing. J Electrophysiol 1987;1:343.
11. Kristensson B, Arnman K, Smedgard P, et al. Physiologic versus fixed rate ventricular pacing. A double-blind crossover study. PACE 1985;8:73.
12. Dateling F, Obel I. Clinical comparison of VVI, VVIR, and DDD pacemakers in the symptomatic relief of bradyarrhythmias. PACE 1989;12: 1278.
13. Sulke N, Dritsas A, Bostock J, et al. "Subclinical" pacemaker syndrome: A randomized study of symptom-free patients with ventricular demand VVI pacemakers upgraded to dual-chamber devices. Br Heart J 1992;67: 57.
14. Sulke N, Dritsas A, Chambers J, et al. A randomized crossover study or four rate-responsive pacing modes. PACE 1990;13:534.
15. Bubien R, Kay G. A randomized comparison of quality of life and exercise capacity with DDD and VVIR pacing modes. PACE 1990;13:524.
16. Wish M, Cohen A, Swartz J, et al. Pacemaker syndrome due to a rate-responsive ventricular pacemaker. J Electrophysiol 1988; 2:504.
17. Liebert H, O'Donoghue S, Tullner W, et al. Pacemaker syndrome in activity-responsive VVI pacing. Am J Cardiol 1989;64:124.
18. Baig M, Perrins E. The hemodynamics of cardiac pacing. Clinical physiological aspects. Prog Cardiovasc Dis 1991;33:283.
19. Wish M, Fletcher R, Cohen A. Hemodynamics of AV synchrony and rate. J Electrophysiol 1989;3:170.
20. Cazeau S, Daubert J, Mabo P, et al. Dynamic electrophysiology of ventriculoatrial conduction: Implications for DDD and DDDR pacing. 1990;13:1646.
21. White M, Gessman L, Morse D, et al. Effects of exercise on retrograde conduction during activity sensing rate-responsive pacing. PACE 1987;10: 424.
22. Fujiki A, Tani M, Mizumake K, et al. Pacemaker syndrome evaluated by cardiopulmonary exercise testing. PACE 1990; 13:1236.

23. Travill CM, Sutton R. Pacemaker syndrome: An iatrogenic condition. Br Heart J 1992;68:163.
24. Nishimura R, Gersh B, Holmes DJ, et al. Outcome of dual-chamber pacing for the pacemaker syndrome. Mayo Clin Proc 1983; 58:452.
25. Dreifus L, Fisch C, Griffin J, et al. Guidelines for implantation of cardiac pacemakers and antiarrhythmia devices. A report of the American College of Cardiology/American Heart Association Task Force on Assessment of Diagnostic and Therapeutic Procedures (Committee on Pacemaker Implantation). J Am Coll Cardiol 1991;18:1.
26. Feuer J, Shandling A, Messenger J, et al. Influence of cardiac pacing mode on the long-term development of atrial fibrillation. Am J Cardiol 1989;54: 1376.
27. Benditt D, Mianulli M, Buetikofer J, et al. Prior arrhythmia history is the major determinant of post-implant atrial tachyarrhythias in DDDR pacemaker patients. RBM 1990;12:95.
28. Gross JN, Moser J, Benedek ZM, et al. DDD pacing mode survival in patients with a dual-chamber pacemaker. J Am Coll Cardiol 1992;19:1536.
29. Hesselson AB, Parsonnet V, Bernstein AD, et al. Deterious effect of long-term single-chamber ventricular pacing in patients with sick sinus syndrome: The hidden benefits of dual chamber pacing. J Am Coll Cardiol 1992;19:1542.
30. Sutton R, Kenny RA. The natural history of sick sinus syndrome. PACE 1986;9:1110.
31. Markewitz A, Schad N, Hemmer W, et al. What is the most appropriate stimulation mode in patients with sinus node dysfunction? PACE 1986;9: 1115.
32. Rosenqvist M, Brandt J, Schüller H. Long-term pacing in sinus node disease: Effects of stimulation mode on cardiovascular morbidity and mortality. Am Heart J 1988;116:16.
33. Rosenqvist M. Atrial pacing for sick sinus syndrome. Clin Cardiol 1990;13: 43.
34. Sanini R, Facchinetti AI, Gallo G, et al. Morbidity and mortality of patients with sinus node disease. Comparative effects of atrial and ventricular pacing. PACE 1990;13:2076.
35. Stangl K, Seitz K, Wirtzfeld A, et al. Differences between atrial single chamber pacing (AAI) and ventricular single chamber pacing (VVI) with respect to prognosis and antiarrhythmic effect in patients with sick sinus syndrome. PACE 1990;13:2080.
36. Santini M, Alexidou G, Ansalone G, et al. Relation of prognosis in sick sinus syndrome to age, conduction defect and modes of permanent cardiac pacing. Am J Cardiol 1990;65:729.
37. Sethi KK, Bajaj V, Mohan JC, et al. Comparison of atrial and VVI pacing modes in symptomatic sinus node dysfunction without associated tachyarrhythmias. Indian Heart J 1990;42:143.
38. Bianconi L, Boccadamo R, DiFlorio A, et al. Atrial versus ventricular stimulation in sick sinus sundrome. Effect on morbidity and mortality. PACE 1989;12:1236.

39. VanErckelens F, Sigmund M, Lambertz, et al. Atrial fibrillation in different pacing modes. J Am Coll Cardiol 1991;17:272A.
40. Nürnberg M, Frohner K, Podczeck A, et al. Is VVI pacing more dangerous than AV sequential pacing in patients with sick sinus syndrome? PACE 1991;14:674.
41. Jutila C, Klein R, Shively B. Deleterius long-term effects of single chamber as compared to dual chamber pacing. Circulation 1990;82(Suppl. III):III-182.
42. Snoeck J, Decoster H, Verherstraeten M, et al. Evolution of P wave characteristics after pacemaker implantation. PACE 1990;13:2091.
43. Sasaki Y, Furihata A, Suyama K, et al. Comparison between ventricular inhibited pacing and physiologic pacing in sick sinus syndrome. Am J Cardiol 1991;67:771.
44. Sgarbossa EB, Pinski SL, Castle LW, et al. Incidence and predictors of loss of pacing in the atrium in patients with sick sinus syndrome. PACE 1992;15:2050.
45. Langenfeld H, Grimm W, Maisch B, et al. Atrial fibrillation and embolic complications in paced patients. PACE 1988;11:1667.
46. Kosakai Y, Ohe T, Kamakura S, et al. Long term follow-up of incidence of embolism in sick sinus syndrome after pacing. PACE 1991;14:680.
47. Grimm W, Langenfeld H, Maisch B, et al. Symptoms, cardiovascular risk prorile, and spontaneous ECG in paced patients: A five-year follow-up study. 1990;13:2086.
48. Snoeck J, Decoster H, Marchand X, et al. Modifications de l'onde P et fibrillation auriculaire après l'implantation d'un pacemaker type VVI. Arch Mal Coeur 1992;85:1419.
49. Ishikawa T, Kimura K, Miyazaki N, et al. Preventive effects of pacemakers on atrial fibrillation in patients with tachycardia-bradycardia syndrome. Eur J Pacing Electrophysiol 1992;22 (Suppl. 1A):A27.
50. Sgarbossa EB, Pinski SL, Castle LW, et al. Determinants of chronic atrial fibrillation and stroke in paced patients with sick sinus syndrome. PACE 1992;15:511.
51. Mabo P, Denjoy I, Leclercq J, et al. Comparative efficacy of permanent atrial pacing in vagal atrial arrhythmias and in bradycardia-tachycardia syndrome. 1989;12:1236.
52. Attuel P, Pellerin D, Mugica J, et al. DDD pacing: An effective treatment modality for recurrent atrial arrhythmias. PACE 1988;11:1647.
53. Hayes DL, Neubauer SA. Incidence of atrial fibrillation after DDD pacing. PACE 1990;13:501.
54. Barr E, Hummel J, Hanich R, et al. VVIR pacing causes more arrhythmias and adverse symptoms than DDDR pacing. RBM 1990;12:57.
55. Galley D, Elharrar C, Ammor M, et al. Is chronic atrial pacing protective against atrial fibrillation? RBM 1990;12:92.
56. Ishikawa T, Taki S, Kimura K, et al. Atrial load and incidence of atrial fibrillation in patients treated by pacemakers. Eur Heart J 1992;13(Abstr. Suppl.):419.

57. Alpert MA, Curtis JJ, Sanfelippo JF, et al. Comparative survival after permanent ventricular and dual chamber pacing for patients with chronic high degree atrioventricular block with and without preexisting congestive heart failure. J Am Coll Cardiol 1986;7:925.

58. Alpert MA, Curtis JJ, Sanfelippo JF, et al. Comparative survival following permanent ventricular and dual chamber pacing for patients with chronic symptomatic sinus node dysruriction with and without heart failure. Am Heart J 1987;113:958.

59. Linde-Edelstram C, Gullberg B, Nordlander R, et al. Longevity in patients with high degree atrioventricular block paced in the atrial synchronous or the fixed-rate ventricular-inhibited mode. PACE 1992;15:304.

60. Shaw DB, Holman RR, Gowers JI. Survival in sinoatrial disorder (sick sinus syndrome). Br Med J 1980;280:139.

61. Witte J, v. Knorre GH, Volkmann HJ, et al. Survival rate in patients with sick sinus syndrome in AAI/DDD vs. VVI pacing. In: Santini M, Pistolese M, Alliegro A (eds.). Progress in Clinical Pacing, Futura Media Services, Mt. Kisco, NY, 1993, p 175.

62. Byrd CL, Schwartz SJ, Gonzales M, et al. DDD pacemakers maximize hemodynamic benefits and minimize complications for most patients. PACE 1988;11:1911.

63. Lamas GA, Estes NM III, Schneller S, et al. Does dual chamber of atrial pacing prevent atrial fibrillation? The need for a randomized controlled trial. PACE 1992;15:1109.

64. Gross JN, Sackstein RD, Furman S. Cardiac pacing and atrial arrhythmias. Cardiol Clin 1992;10:609.

65. Clarke M, Sutton R, Ward D, et al. Recommendations for pacemaker prescription for symptomatic bradycardia. Report of a working party of the British Pacing and Electrophysiology Group. Br Heart J 1991;66:185.

66. Ebagosti A, Gueunoun M, Saadjian A, et al. Long-term follow-up of patients treated with VVI pacing and sequential pacing with special reference to VA retrograde conduction. PACE 1988;11:1929.

67. Curzi G, Mocchegiani R, Ciampani N, et al. Thromboembolism during VVI permanent pacing. In: Perez-Gomez F (ed.). Cardiac Pacing. Electrophysiology Tachyarrhythmias, Editorial Grouz, Madrid, 1985, p 1203.

68. Benditt DG. Atrial-based pacing modes: A review or their important contributions to the care of paced patients. Medtronic News 1991;20:4.

69. Nathan AW, Davies DW. Is VVI pacing outmoded? Br Heart J 1992;67:285.

70. Parsonnet V, Bernstein AD. Adaptive rate pacing. In: Heart Disease Update, Braunwald E (ed.). W.B. Saunders, Philadelphia, PA, 1989, p 97.

71. Santini M, Ansalone G, Cacciatore G, et al. Status of single chamber atrial pacing. In: Barold SS, Mugica J (eds.), New Perspectives in Cardiac Pacing. 2, Futura Publishing Co., Mt. Kisco, NY, 1991, p 273.

72. Sutton R, Bourgeois I. Pacemaker selection. In: Sutton R, Bourgeois I (eds.), The Foundations of Cardiac Pacing: Part I, An Illustrated Practical Guide to Basic Pacing, Futura Publishing Co., Mt. Kisco, NY, 1991, p 149.

73. Bodinot B. Stimulation cardiaque à fréquence asservie. Ann Cardiol Angeiol 1990;39:597.
74. Daubert C, Mabo Ph, Ritter Ph, et al. Quel type de stimulateur pour quel patient? Que Choisir en 1991. Stimucoeur 1991;19:171.
75. Camm AJ, Katritsis D. Ventricular pacing in sick sinus: A risky business? PACE 1990;13:695.
76. Katritsis D, Jones S, Camm AJ. A rational choice of pacemaker mode. Eur J Cardiac Pacing Electrophysiol 1991;1:132.
77. Sulke AN. Which pacemaker? Br J Clin Pract 1991;45:216.
78. deRoy L. Cardiac pacing for bradyarrhythmias. In: Andries E, Brugada P, Stroobandt R (eds.). How to Face "the Faces" of Cardiac Pacing, Kluwer, Boston, 1992, p 29.
79. Rydén L. Atrial inhibited pacing: An underused mode of cardiac stimulation. PACE 1988;11:1375.
80. Rosenqvist M, Obel I. Atrial pacing and the risk for AV block: Is there a time for change in attitude? PACE 1989;12:97.
81. Kallryd A, Kruse I, Ryden L. Atrial inhibited pacing in the sick sinus syndrome: Clinical value and the demand for rate responsiveness. PACE 1989;12:954.
82. Kerr CR, Tyers GFO, Vorderbrugge S. Atrial pacing: Efficacy and safety. PACE 1989;12:1049.
83. Lemke B, Holtmann BJ, Selbach H, et al. Retrospective analysis of complications and life expectancy in patients with sinus node dysfunction. Int J Cardiol 1989;22:185.
84. Kolettis TM, Miller HC, Boon NA. Atrial pacing. Who do we pace and what do we expect? Experiences with 100 atrial pacemakers. PACE 1990;13:625.
85. Swiatecka G, Sielski S, Wilczek R, et al. Atrioventricular conduction disturbances in patients with sinoatrial node disease and atrial pacing. PACE 1992;15:2074.
86. Novak M, Vondracek V, Psenicka M, et al. Atrial pacing: Is it safe in long-term use? Eur J Cardiac Pacing Electrophysiol 1992;2 (Suppl. IA):A17.
87. Bernstein SB, VanNatta BE, Ellestad MH. Experiences with atrial pacing. Am J Cardiol 1988;61:113.
88. Brandt J, Anderson H, Fåhraeus T, et al. Natural history of sinus node disease treated with atrial pacing in 213 patients: Implications for selection of stimulation mode. J Am Coll Cardiol 1992;20:633.
89. Rognoni G, Francalacci G, Occhetta E, et al. Long-term pacing therapy in sick sinus syndrome. Eur Heart J 1991; 12(Abstr. Suppl.):199.
90. Haywood GA, Ward J, Ward DE, et al. Atrioventricular Wenckebach point and progression to atrioventricular block in sinoatrial disease. PACE 1990;13:2054.
91. VanMechelin R, Segers A, et al. Serial electrophysiologic studies after single chamber atrial pacemaker implantation in patients with symptomatic sinus node dysfunction. Eur Heart J 1984;6:628.
92. Barnay C, Joseph IP, Coster A, et al. Use of Wenckebach point to assess AV conduction before AAI pacing. RBM 1990;12:90.

93. Markewitz A, Wenke K, Weinhold C. Predictive value of rapid atrial stim-ulation for occurrence of AV block. PACE 1990; 13:501.
94. Clarke M, Allen A. Rate-responsive atrial pacing resulting in pacemaker syndrome. PACE 1987;10:1209.
95. DenDulk K, Lindemans FW, Brugada P, et al. Pacemaker syndrome with AAI rate variable pacing: Importance of atrioventricular conduction prop-erties, medication and pacemaker programmability. PACE 1988;11:1226.
96. Mabo P, Pouillot C, Kermarrec A, et al. Lack of physiological adaptation of the atrioventricular interval to heart rate in patients chronically paced in the AAIR mode. PACE 1991;14:2133.
97. Ruiter J, Burgersdijk C, Zeeders M, et al. Atrial Activitrax pacing. The atrioventricular interval during exercise. PACE 1987;10:1226.
98. Hummel J, Fazio G, Lawrence J, et al. The natural history of dual chamber pacing. PACE 1991;14:1745.
99. Detollenaere M, VanWassenhove E, Jordaens L. Atrial arrhythmias in dual chamber pacing and their influence on long-term mortality. PACE 1992;15: 1846.
100. Puziak A, Campbell J, Dente C, et al. Frequency of physiologic pacing mode abandonment. PACE 1991;14:732.
101. Chamberlain Weber R, Ingram A, Briers L, et al. Reasons for reprogram-ming dual chamber pacemakers to the VVI mode: a retrospective review using a computer database. J Am Coll Cardiol 1992;19:67A.
102. Oseroff O, Klementowicz P, Andrews C, et al. Indications for permanent mode change during DDD pacing. PACE 1987;10:409.
103. Soler M, Pfisterer M, Cueni T, et al. Long term follow-up of dual chamber pacemakers: Incidence and duration of physiologic pacing. 1987;10:745.
104. Hayes D, VonFeldt L, Neubauer S. Does P-wave amplitude predict oc-currence of atrial fibrillation following DDD implant? PACE 14:675, 1991.
105. Brandt J, Attewell R, Fåhraeus T, et al. Acute atrial endocardial wave am-plitude and chronic pacemaker sensitivity requirements: Relation to patient age and presence of sinus node disease. PACE 1990;13:417.
106. Snoeck J, DeCoster H, Vrints C, et al. Predictive value of the P wave at implantation for atrial fibrillation after VVI pacemaker implantation. PACE 1992;15:2077.
107. Fukunami M, Yamada T, Ohmori M, et al. Detection of patients at risk for paroxysmal atrial fibrillation during sinus rhythm by P wave triggered signal-averaged electrocardiogram. Circulation 1991;83:162.
108. Kubica J, Stolarczyk L, Krzyminska E, et al. Left atrial size and wall motion in patients with permanent ventricular and atrial pacing. PACE 1990;13: 1737.
109. Sakadamis G, Papadopoulos CL, Giannacoulis J, et al. The left atrial size in patients with permanent cardiac pacemakers. Acta Cardiol 1988;43:425.
110. Kato R, Terasawa T, Gotoh T, et al. Antiarrhythmic efficacy of atrial de-mand (AAI) and rate-responsive atrial pacing. In Santini M, Pistolese M, Alliegro A (eds.). Progress in Clinical Pacing, Exerpta Medica, Amsterdam, 1988, p 15.

111. Bellocci F, Nobile A, Spampinato A, et al. Antiarrhythmic effects of DDD rate responsive pacing. PACE 1991;14:622.
112. Marinoni GP, Cundari F, Orlando F, et al. Can the DDDR mode improve the cardiac performance and have an antiarrhythmic effect in patients with a chronotropic failure? Eur J Cardiac Pacing Electrophysiol 1992;2:A51.
113. Haywood G, Katritsis D, Ward J, et al. Rate responsive atrial pacing increases heart rate but fails to increase exercise tolerance in patients with sinoatrial disease. PACE 1991; 14:684.
114. Feuer JM, Shandling AH, Ellestad MH. Sensor-modulated dual chamber cardiac pacing: Too much of a good thing too fast. PACE 1990;13:816.
115. Vardas PE, Fitzpatrick A, Ingram A, et al. Natural history of sinus node chronotropy in paced patients. PACE 1991;14:155.
116. Gwinn N, Leman R, Kratz J, et al. Chronotropic incompetence. A common and progressive finding in pacemaker patients. Am Heart J 1992;123:1216.
117. Sutton R. Pacing in atrial arrhythmias. PACE 1990;13:1823.
118. Barnay C, Coste A, Quittet F, et al. Stimulation auriculaire permanente exclusive. Experience clinique a propos de 65 observations avec un recul de 1 a 5 ans. Arch Mal Coeur 1986; 79:1703.

PART II

Impact of New Technology

Chapter 8

Base Rate Behavior of Dual Chamber Pacing Systems

PAUL A. LEVINE

Introduction

The very first pacemakers were nonprogrammable units that were not capable of sensing. They delivered an output pulse at a rate that was set by the manufacturer, thus mimicking a parasystolic focus in the presence of a native rhythm. Over the past 34 years, there have been dramatic changes in pacing therapy with the artificial devices being able to increasingly approximate normal sinus rhythm. Present generation systems are capable of stimulating and sensing in both the atria and ventricles while some can automatically adjust the base rate of the pacemaker in response to input that is independent of the P wave. In order to achieve this, the timing circuits of the modern pacemaker have increased in complexity in an effort to not only provide for the maintenance of AV synchronization but also to minimize the potential adverse electronic interactions that might result between the two channels of the pacemaker as well as avoid adverse interactions with the native rhythms.[1] This chapter will review base rate timing (also termed lower rate limit behavior) of the currently available dual chamber pacing modes, which includes DDD, DDI, DVI, and VDD. In addition, it will review selected aspects of dual chamber rate-modulated pacing and crosstalk.

The base rate timing intervals of the DDD, DDI, and DVI modes are similar but not identical, although when there is stable AV sequential pacing, the surface appearance of the rhythms appears the same (Fig. 1).

New Perspectives in Cardiac Pacing, Vol. 3, edited by S. Serge Barold and Jacques Mugica, Mount Kisco, NY, Futura Publishing Co., © 1993.

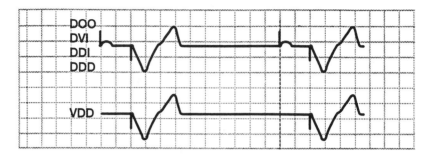

Figure 1. Schematic diagram of base rate pacing in the five dual chamber modes. DOO, DVI, DDI, and DDD all are identical in the absence of native atrial or ventricular activity. Base rate VDD pacing in the same setting looks identical to single chamber ventricular pacing.

The basic interval from a sensed R wave or a paced ventricular event to the next paced ventricular event is termed the ventricular escape interval (VEI). In single chamber pacing systems, this is the primary or basic pacing interval. In dual chamber systems capable of stimulating in both chambers, the VEI is divided into two subintervals. The first is an interval from a sensed or paced ventricular event to the ensuing atrial output pulse. This has been termed the atrial escape interval (AEI). It is followed by a second interval from the atrial output pulse to the ventricular output pulse, which is the atrioventricular interval (AVI). The sum of the AVI and the AEI equals the VEI or basic pacing interval. The base rate has also been called the lower rate limit.

In the DOO mode, there is an absence of sensing and thus an atrial output pulse is released upon completion of the AEI while a ventricular output pulse is issued upon completion of the AVI (Fig. 2). There is no alert period during which sensing might occur and thus one might consider the DOO mode as having a refractory period on both the atrial and ventricular channels which encompass the entire timing period.

When sensing capability is introduced, the refractory period must shorten to something less than the total timing interval in order to allow for an alert period during which sensing can occur. In the DVI mode, sensing is only present on the ventricular channel with the atrial channel remaining refractory at all times (Fig. 3). In the DDI and DDD modes, sensing occurs on both channels but the response is varied slightly between the two modes. The VDD mode is analogous to the DDD mode

DOO

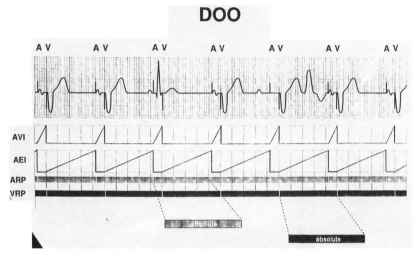

Figure 2. Timing diagram showing DOO pacing. Despite the presence of native atrial and ventricular activity, this mode is not capable of sensing and competes with the intrinsic rhythms. Conceptually, it is as if the refractory periods on both the atrial and the ventricular channels encompassed the entire timing cycle.

but differs in that it is not capable of releasing an atrial stimulus. Thus, at base rate pacing, the VDD mode looks similar to VVI pacing (Fig. 1).

DVI Pacing

DVI pacing was first introduced in the early 1970s with units that were large and uncomfortable, requiring two bipolar leads. It was only with the advent of dual unipolar systems that the hemodynamic benefits associated with the DVI mode were able to be realized due to the increased utilization of dual chamber pacing. In the DVI mode, while atrial pacing followed by ventricular pacing in sequence occurs, sensing is only present on the ventricular channel. As such, only the ventricular channel has a refractory period and an alert period. Depending upon the native rate, atrial competition is extremely common in the DVI mode[2] (Fig. 4) and has been associated with pacemaker-induced atrial tachyarrhythmias[3]

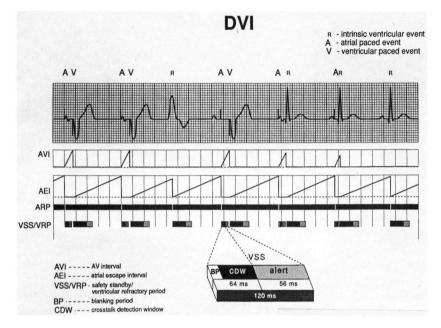

Figure 3. Timing diagram showing DVI pacing. While the atrial channel remains refractory (ARP) precluding any atrial sensing, the ventricular channel can sense. An R wave occurring during the atrial escape interval (AEI) inhibits both atrial and ventricular outputs and resets the AEI. An R wave sensed during the AV interval only inhibits the ventricular output. Depending on the timing design, it may or may not reset the AEI. The subintervals in the safety pacing circuitry are also shown in expanded form. After the blanking period (BP), there is a crosstalk detection window (CDW). If an event is sensed during the CDW, a ventricular output will be triggered upon completion of the safety standby (VSS) interval.

(Fig. 3). Unlike single chamber pacing and unlike the DDI and DDD modes, total inhibition of the pacing system will not occur unless the intrinsic ventricular rate exceeds the rate that is defined by the atrial escape interval.[4]

One of two basic timing systems may be found in the DVI mode. These are ventricular-based timing and atrial-based timing.[5,6] In a ventricular-based timing system, a sensed R wave will always inhibit the ventricular output and reset the atrial escape interval. If the R wave is sensed during the atrial escape interval, it will also inhibit the atrial output

II CONTINUOUS DVI PACING a 70 PPM

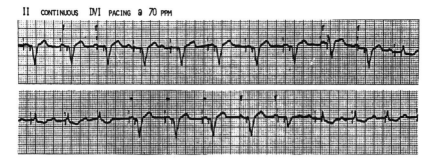

Figure 4. Rhythm strip from a patient with a noncommitted DVI pacing system. There is frequent atrial competition due to the sinus rate being faster than the programmed pacing rate. At times, there is only a single pacing stimulus; this is the atrial stimulus. The pacemaker was programmed to a rate of 70 with an AV delay of 150 ms. Thus, in order to totally inhibit the pacemaker, the native rhythm would have had to exceed a rate of 86 bpm (the cycle length would have had to be shorter than the atrial escape interval of 700 ms).

pulse. In an atrial-based timing system, a sensed R wave will always inhibit the ventricular output pulse; however, its effect on the basic timing of the pulse generator will depend on where the R wave was sensed within the sequence of events. If it is sensed within the atrial escape interval, it also inhibits the atrial output pulse; but rather than resetting the AEI, it resets the base rate which is defined by the AA interval. If sensing occurs within the AV interval, the ventricular output pulse is inhibited but the timing interval is NOT reset.

In the presence of stable functional single chamber atrial pacing due to the intrinsic atrial output to conducted R wave interval being shorter than the programmed AV interval, there will be a slight acceleration of the pacing rate in a ventricular-based timing system.[5,6] The degree of acceleration will be determined by the difference between the AV and the AR intervals, which is subtracted from the basic drive cycle length. In an atrial-based timing system, since the sensed R wave does not reset any timers, there will be stable AR pacing at the programmed base rate. In the presence of 2:1 AV block where only every other atrial paced event is conducted, a ventricular-based timing system will demonstrate an alternation in the pacing interval with one cycle at a faster rate than the programmed base rate with the second being at the programmed base rate in a ventricular-based timing system. In an atrial-based timing system in which 2:1 AV block is encountered, the atrial paced rate will be at the precise programmed rate during both AV and AR pacing; however, the ventricular rate will demonstrate an alternation between a rate that is faster than the programmed base rate and one that is slower than the base rate.

Crosstalk

A unique rhythm was identified with the first generation of the DVI mode. If the atrial lead was in close anatomic proximity to the ventricular lead, the atrial stimulus could be detected by the ventricular sense amplifier, causing inhibition of the ventricular output pulse. This is a form of oversensing termed crosstalk.[7] As the first-generation DVI units utilized ventricular-based timing, when there was concomitant high grade AV block, sequential atrial pacing stimuli would be present at the atrial escape interval but without a visible interceding paced or sensed ventricular event (Fig. 5). More commonly, AV conduction was intact

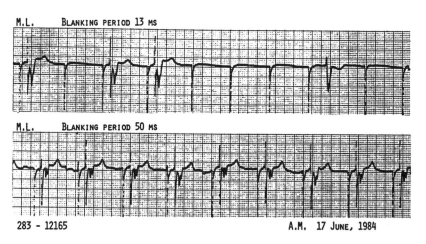

Figure 5. An example of crosstalk-induced ventricular output inhibition induced in a patient with high grade AV block by programming the atrial output amplitude to 10 volts, pulse duration to 1.0 ms, ventricular sensitivity to 1 mV, and a blanking period to 13 ms. Repetitive atrial stimuli are seen at a pacing interval equal to the AEI plus blanking period. Increasing the blanking period, bottom tracing, prevented the ventricular oversensing.

when crosstalk was present, resulting in AR pacing with an AR interval that was longer than the programmed AV interval. This could result in an acceleration of the programmed rate since the AA interval was still equal to the atrial escape interval; the R wave in this setting was not sensed because it coincided with the refractory period initiated by the ventricular oversensing.[8] Another rhythm that could result is AR pacing at a rate that was slower than the programmed base rate of the system. This would occur when the AR interval was very long, allowing the conducted R wave to fall outside the ventricular refractory period that had been initiated by the oversensing; the conducted R wave was then sensed, again resetting the AEI. Atrial bigeminy has also been reported, associated with an interaction between the endogenous AV nodal conduction being more rapid following the longer cycle and thus allowing the R wave to coincide with the first ventricular refractory period. The relative acceleration of the atrial paced rate results in first degree AV block on that next beat, delaying the R wave until it falls outside the ventricular refractory period to again allow it to be sensed.[9]

The advent of dual unipolar DVI pacing systems virtually guaranteed crosstalk if there were not a change in the timing design of the pacemaker. Thus, the ventricular refractory period was triggered by completion of the atrial escape interval. On the surface ECG, one would see the concomitant release of an atrial output pulse which then served as a marker for the initiation of ventricular refractoriness.[10,11] This had two consequences, the first being that a ventricular output pulse was forced to follow an atrial output pulse, leading to this being described as committed DVI pacing. In retrospect, the first generation of DVI systems were called noncommitted. While the first generation of devices had an AV interval that was programmable to 250 ms, this was no longer safe with the committed design since a ventricular output might then be released onto the vulnerable zone of the T wave. As such, AV interval programmability was deleted from this second-generation DVI system with the AV interval limited to 150–155 ms. A normal rhythm in a committed DVI system might show an ineffective atrial stimulus falling within the PR interval followed by an ineffective ventricular stimulus that occurred after the conducted QRS complex (Fig. 6). Both stimuli failed to capture because they occurred during physiologic refractory periods of their respective chambers. Similarly, failure to sense the native R wave occurred as the refractory period of the ventricular sense amplifier began on completion of the AEI. A similar rhythm might be seen in

II

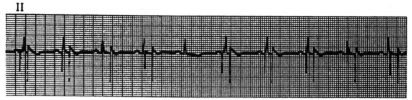

R.M. BUMC 416411 14 JAN, 1982

Figure 6.   An example of committed DVI pacing. The pacing system was functioning normally yet there was atrial and ventricular competition and neither stimulus was effective as it occurred during the physioiogic refractory period of each respective chamber.

either the DDI or DDD modes when there was true atrial undersensing, a state that might appropriately be termed "functional" DVI pacing.

With advancements in technology, the manufacturers were able to modify the ventricular refractory period to allow for a period of sensing during the AV interval. In present generation devices, there is a brief refractory ventricular period termed a blanking period. It is initiated by completion of the atrial escape interval but does not cover the entire AV interval. Depending on the pulse generator, it may be a fixed or programmable parameter varying between a low of 12 ms to a high of 125 ms. The longer the blanking period, the greater the likelihood of failure to sense a native R wave, whether it is a conducted QRS complex or an ectopic beat. When a blanking period is present, one might encounter either noncommitted DVI pacing (an atrial stimulus followed by appropriate inhibition of the ventricular output pulse) or committed pacing, depending on the relationship of the native R wave to the blanking period. Thus, the current design has been called modified committed, reflecting that both behaviors may be present.[4,11]

The only DVI (and some first-generation DDD) design that absolutely prevented crosstalk was the committed mode. Crosstalk did occur in the noncommitted systems and can occur in the modified committed design, particularly at high atrial outputs, high ventricular sensitivities, and short blanking periods. Thus, a separate timing circuit was introduced which had a special detection window following the ventricular blanking period. If a ventricular event was sensed during this crosstalk detection window, the presumption was that it was crosstalk (Fig. 3). Rather than inhibiting an output pulse, one was triggered at the end of an abbreviated AV interval.[1,4] The reason for choosing a shortened AV delay to trigger a ventricular stimulus rather than at the programmed AV delay was that AV intervals are programmable in the new units to as much as 350 ms. If the sensed event were actually a ventricular ectopic beat rather than true crosstalk, a long AV delay would predispose to potentially dangerous competition. Triggering a ventricular output after a short AV delay would be analogous to the fixed AV delay of the committed design, effectively keeping the output pulse away from the vulnerable zone of the native complex. It would also serve as a marker that this feature was enabled. Although a number of terms have been used (Safety Pacing™ introduced by Medtronic, Nonphysiologic AV Delay™ used by Intermedics, and Safety Standby Option™ by Pacesetter), this feature has generically been called safety pacing. Safety pacing does not prevent crosstalk, it simply prevents crosstalk-mediated ventricular output inhibition.

In many current generation devices, safety pacing can be either enabled or disabled. When disabled, one can take advantage of the intentional induction of crosstalk to achieve accelerated atrial paced rates but only in pacing systems that utilized a ventricular-based timing system.[8] This is safe only in patients who have intact AV nodal conduction. In those systems that utilize an atrial-based timing design, crosstalk with safety pacing disabled will be associated with atrial pacing stimuli at the programmed base rate.

When one encounters AA pacing (Fig. 5) in a system that utilizes a ventricular-based timing design and in which safety pacing has been disabled, one can readily differentiate crosstalk from a ventricular open circuit. If the failure to release a ventricular output pulse is due to crosstalk, the AA interval will equal the sum of the atrial escape interval and the blanking period. If it is due to an open circuit, the AA interval will equal the basic pacing interval. This differentiation is not feasible when atrial-based timing is utilized since the AA interval will equal the programmed base rate interval in each case. Crosstalk-mediated ventricular output inhibition and a ventricular open circuit will have an identical appearance.

DDD Pacing

With respect to DDD pacing, the base rate behavior is identical to the DVI mode in its appearance on the surface ECG. Internal to the

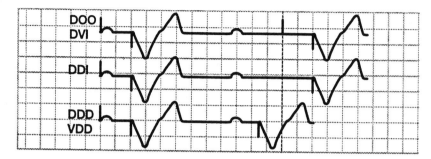

Figure 7.   Schematic diagram showing the behavior of the DOO, DVI, DDI, DDD, and VDD modes when a P wave occurs during the atrial escape interval. The DOO and DVI modes ignore the P wave. The DDI mode senses the atrial activity and inhibits the atrial output, but does not track the P wave. Thus, in the presence of AV block, the DDI mode will provide backup ventricular pacing at the programmed rate. Both the DDD and VDD mode sense the P wave, terminate the atrial escape interval, and initiate and AV interval to track the P wave. The vertical dashed line identifies the end of the atrial escape interval.

pacemaker, there are additional circuits that allow for atrial sensing. Thus, while the DVI mode will ignore a native P wave, the DDD mode will sense it, terminate the atrial escape interval, and initiate an AV interval as it tracks the P wave (Fig. 7). This, however, then takes the system out of lower rate limit behavior.

DDI Pacing

DDI pacing is AV sequential pacing with intact atrial sensing but without the ability to track a sensed P wave.[12,13] Again, at base rate pacing, the rhythm will look identical to that seen with the DVI mode. A sensed P wave that occurs during the AEI will cause inhibition of the atrial output pulse, but unlike the DDD mode, it will not terminate the atrial escape interval timer. The AEI is allowed to complete, at which time the AV interval is initiated. If a native R wave is not sensed before the AV interval completes, then a ventricular output is released at the programmed base rate.

The DDI mode has been described as being the DDD mode but with the upper rate limit interval set to equal the lower rate limit interval.[12] While this might be an effective way to conceptualize the behavior of this mode, it is not correct. A sensed P wave terminates the atrial escape interval in the DDD mode and initiates an AV interval. In the DDI mode, the sensed P wave does not terminate the AEI, which is allowed to complete before an AVI is started (Fig. 8). This is dramatically demonstrated by the first-generation DDI mode. Since the ventricular blanking period was triggered by completion of the atrial escape interval, an oversight in this first iteration of the DDI mode resulted in

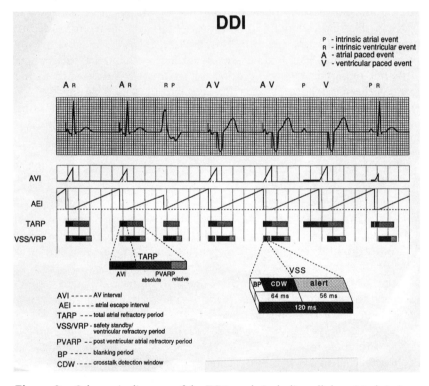

Figure 8. Schematic diagram of the DDI mode including all the critical timing cycles. The timing intervals have been previously described. Note that a sensed P wave as shown in the next to last complex on this rhythm inhibits the atrial output but does not affect the atrial escape interval which continues to time-out. The sensed P wave does, however, begin the atrial refractory period, which is primarily involved with sensing and not timing.

persistence of a blanking period even in the absence of an atrial stimulus. This resulted in blanking period undersensing, which caused some degree of confusion.[14,15] Although many of these pulse generators are still functioning, the present generation DDI modes have eliminated the forced blanking period when the atrial escape interval completes if the atrial output had been inhibited. The blanking period now only occurs when an atrial stimulus is released.

In some pacemakers, either by design or manipulation of the programmer, hysteresis has been incorporated into the DDI mode. In this setting, the escape rate of the pacemaker following a sensed R wave will be significantly slower than the base rate of the system during stable pacing. The indication for this feature is the various neuroregulatory abnormalities that may require a relatively rapid AV sequential pacing rate when pacing is needed but the pacemaker is inhibited at times when it is not required. The one caution is that the AV interval not be too long, otherwise the conducted R wave will be sensed during the AV interval at the low rate and reset the hysteresis escape interval, locking the system into an inappropriately slow rate when pacing is required.

VDD Pacing

The first dual chamber pacing system ever developed was the VAT mode, which provided P wave synchronous ventricular pacing.[16,17] While there was atrial sensing, it could not sense in the ventricle, resulting in competition with ventricular ectopic beats as it triggered a ventricular output in response to either the sinus P wave, a retrograde P wave, or sensing of the far-field R wave. Improvements in technology resulted in sensing on both atrial and ventricular channels, and while there were a few dedicated VDD units introduced in the early 1980s, most of the present generation DDD devices can be programmed to the VDD mode.

At the base rate, the VDD mode provides effective single chamber ventricular pacing as it is not capable of atrial stimulation[18] (Fig. 9). In addition, there are two single-lead VDD systems that have been recently introduced, which are gaining popularity given that they only require implantation of a single, albeit unique, electrode. There are two slightly different timing designs with respect to lower rate limit behavior.

In the Pacesetter and older Cordis dual chamber pacemakers programmed to the VDD mode, a sensed R wave resets a ventricular escape

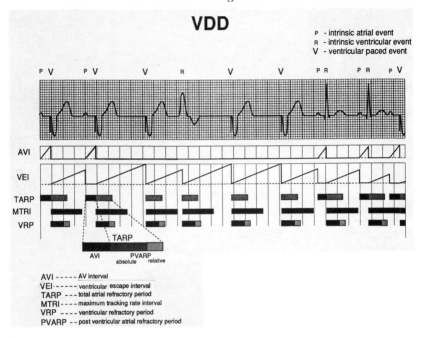

Figure 9. Detailed timing diagram of the VDD mode. An R wave that is sensed anywhere within the ventricular alert period will reset the ventricular escape interval. A P wave will terminate the ventricular escape interval and initiate an AV interval. As there is no atrial output, the VDD mode does not have a ventricular blanking period nor does it have safety pacing.

interval. If a P wave does not occur before the VEI completes, a ventricular output pulse will be released at the end of the VEI. A sensed atrial depolarization will terminate the VEI and initiate an AV interval, resulting in tracking of the intrinsic atrial signal. If an atrial event is sensed even one millisecond before completion of the VEI, this interval will be terminated and an AVI initiated (Fig. 10). Thus, the pacemaker can track atrial activity to rates that are lower than the programmed base rate. The degree to which this will occur will be dependent on the AV interval. If the base rate were 60 ppm (1000 ms ventricular escape interval) and the AVI were 200 ms, native atrial activity could be tracked down to a rate of 50 ppm (1200 ms). This is a form of hysteresis, and like hysteresis in a single chamber pacing system, it is designed to maintain AV syn-

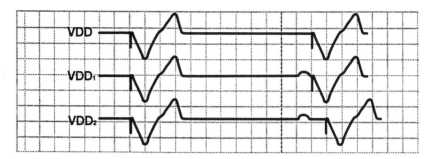

Figure 10. Schematic diagram of the VDD mode functioning at base rate when atrial activity is absent (top) or when native atrial activity occurs late, namely within the AV interval. The dashed vertical line identifies the end of the atrial escape interval. In one timing system (labeled VDD$_1$), the atrial channel refractory period begins with completion of the atrial escape interval. Thus, any P wave which occurs during the AV interval will be ignored and a ventricular output pulse will be released upon completion of the base rate timing interval in an effort to maintain the programmed base rate although sacrificing optimal AV synchrony. In the second timing design (labeled VDD), a P wave that is sensed just milliseconds before completion of the base rate pacing interval will inhibit the ventricular output, initiate an AV interval, and then release a ventricular output pulse upon completion of the AV interval which started with the sensed P wave. In this design, AV synchrony is maintained while the paced rate is allowed to fall below the programmed base rate.

chrony to lower rates than will occur during base rate pacing where AV synchrony is lost.

Other VDD systems do not have a ventricular escape interval as in the preceding discussion but utilize the design of ventricular-based lower rate limit DDD pacing. Following a ventricular event, an atrial escape interval is initiated. When the AEI completes, the AV interval timer is initiated as is an AVI atrial refractory period. Thus, during the AVI, the atrial sense amplifier is rendered refractory. A P wave that might otherwise be sensed during the AEI will not be sensed if it occurs during the AVI. This forces ventricular pacing at the programmed base rate while sacrificing AV synchrony.

Dual Chamber (DDD) Rate-Modulated Pacing

A sensor that is independent of intrinsic atrial activity might be looked upon as a mechanism to automatically adjust the lower rate limit of the pacing system on a temporary basis. Assuming that the sensor-input signal indicates that the base rate should be 90 ppm, in the absence of intrinsic atrial activity, there will be atrial or AV sequential pacing at the sensor-determined rate in the DDD mode. In a manner identical to that associated with DDD pacing, a sensed atrial event will terminate the sensor-defined atrial escape interval, initiate an AV interval, and assume control of the pacing system.[5,6]

In some systems, the maximum sensor rate and maximum tracking rate are independently programmable. For this purpose, the maximum tracking rate is the maximum paced ventricular rate that can occur in response to a sensed atrial event. The maximum sensor rate is the maximum paced ventricular rate that can occur in response to a sensor input signal. This can result in a number of unique rhythms that are all compatible with normal function of the pacing system. Assuming that the native atrial rate exceeds the programmed maximum tracking rate, the ventricular paced response will be limited to the maximum tracking rate. However, if there is concomitant sensor drive of sufficient strength and the maximum sensor rate is greater than the maximum tracking rate, the atrial output will be inhibited by the sensed P wave but a ventricular output will be controlled by the sensor-input signal, allowing for a paced ventricular stimulus occurring at a rate that exceeds the maximum tracking rate.[19,20] Thus, on the surface ECG, it will appear that the pacemaker is violating its maximum tracking rate limit, the paced ventricular pulse will appear to track the sensed P wave, but this is merely coincidence as the paced ventricular output will not actually be responding to the sensed atrial event. When the native atrial rate exceeds the maximum tracking rate but there is a sufficient sensor-input signal to drive the ventricular paced rate higher than the maximum tracking rate, the pacemaker will behave as if it were in the DDIR mode.

A second normal rhythm that might result will be functional DVI rate-modulated pacing with loss of atrial sensing at the higher rates resulting in atrial competition.[21] This may also result in potential functional noncapture if the atrial stimulus were released during the physioiogic refractory period of the atrium, a rhythm that has been termed AV desynchronization arrhythmia. The reason that this can be anticipated is that the refractory periods are often programmed for the base rate. The total atrial refractory period (TARP) is the sum of the AV interval and the postventricular atrial refractory period (PVARP). If a long TARP is programmed, this will limit the maximum atrial rate that can be sensed.

While this will impose an additional limitation on the maximum tracking rate of the pacemaker, it will not limit the sensor which might drive the pacemaker to even higher rates. At these higher rates, the atrial alert period will be either very short or nonexistent (functional DVI), allowing for atrial competition. Thus, one should program the AV delay and PVARP as short as possible in an attempt to maintain as long an atrial alert period as possible at the higher sensor rates. This is facilitated in those units that have rate-responsive AV delay and/or an adaptive PVARP allowing for longer intervals at the lower rates and shorter refractory periods at the higher rates. Similarly, the ventricular refractory period should be programmed as short as possible to minimize the chance of ventricular undersensing at the higher rate, whether under control of an atrial sensed event or the rate-modulated sensor.

Summary

The initial complexity of dual chamber timing has been increased by the introduction of two different timing systems: ventricular- and atrial-based timing. In a ventricular-based timing system, a sensed or paced ventricular event always resets the atrial escape interval, which then facilitates rhythm analysis. In an atrial-based timing system, a sensed R wave occurring during the usual atrial escape interval resets the base rate AA interval while a sensed R wave occurring during the AV interval is virtually ignored with respect to the timing circuits of the pacemaker. Rate-modulated pacing effectively repeatedly resets a temporary lower rate limit, but since this is based on an electrocardiographically invisible signal, analysis of the resultant rhythm may be confusing.

When considering lower rate limit function and specifically the atrial output pulse, one must be concerned with the various manifestations of crosstalk. There is crosstalk-mediated ventricular output inhibition which, in a ventricular-based timing system, can result in atrial paced rates that are either faster or slower than the programmed base rate. In both timing systems, safety pacing in the presence of crosstalk will result in AV pacing at an abbreviated AV interval.

To analyze a paced rhythm, it is essential to know the programmed parameters and timing system design of the pulse generator. Without these two basic building blocks, it would be very easy to misidentify a normal rhythm as reflecting an abnormality and an abnormal rhythm as normal.

References

1. Levine PA, Normal and abnormal rhythms associated with dual chamber pacemakers. Cardiol Clin 1985;3:595–616.
2. Barold SS, Falkoff MD, Ong LS, Heinle RA. Characteristics of pacemaker arrhythmias due to normally functioning atrioventricular demand (DVI) pulse generators. PACE 1980;3:712–723.
3. Furman S, Cooper JA. Atrial fibrillation during AV sequential pacing. PACE 1982;5:133–135.
4. Levine PA, Mace RC. Pacing Therapy: A Guide to Cardiac Pacing for Optimum Hemodynamic Benefit, Futura Publishing Co., Mt. Kisco, NY, 1983, pp 105–127.
5. Hayes DL, Levine PA. Pacemaker Timing Cycles. In: Ellenbogen KA (ed.), Cardiac Pacing, Blackwell Scientific Publishers, Cambridge, MA, 1991, pp 263–308.
6. Levine PA, Sholder JA. Interpretation of rate modulated dual chamber rhythms: The effect of ventricular-based and atrial-based timing systems on DDD and DDDR rhythms. Siemens-Pacesetter Inc, Sylmar, CA, March 1990.
7. Furman S, Reicher Reiss H, Escher DJW. Atrioventricular sequential pacing and pacemakers. Chest 1973;63:783–789.
8. Levine PA, Venditti FJ, Podrid PJ, Klein MD. Therapeutic and diagnostic benefit of intentional crosstalk mediated ventricular output inhibition. PACE 1988;11:1194–1201.
9. Levine PA, Mace RC. Pacing Therapy: A Guide to Cardiac Pacing for Optimum Hemodynamic Benefit, Futura Publishinc Co., Mt. Kisco, NY, 1983, pp 239–251.
10. Barold SS, Falkoff MD, Ong LS, Heinle RA. Interpretation of electrocardiograms produced by a new unipolar multiprogrammable "committed" AV sequential demand (DVI) pulse generator. PACE 1981;4:692–708.
11. Levine PA, Seltzer JP. Fusion, pseudofusion, pseudopseudofusion and confusion: Normal rhythms associated with atrioventricular sequential (DVI) pacing. Clin Prog Pacing Electrophysiol 1983;1:70–80.
12. Barold SS. The DDI mode of cardiac pacing. PACE 1987;10:480.
13. Floro J, Castellanet M, Fiorio J, Messenger J. DDI: A new mode for cardiac pacing. Clin Prog Pacing Electrophysiol 1984;2:255–260.
14. Erlbacher JA, Stelzer P. Inappropriate ventricular blanking in a DDI pacemaker. PACE 1986;9:519–521.
15. Bertusso J, Kapoor AS, Schafer J: A case of ventricular undersensing in the DDI mode: Cause and correction. PACE 1986;9:685–689.
16. Perhsson K, Lentell J, Levander-Lindgren M, et al. A new concept for atrial triggered pulse generators. PACE 1979;2:560–567.
17. Nathan DA, Center S, Wu CY, et al. An implantable synchronous pacemaker for long-term correction of complete AV block. Circulation 1963;22:682–686.

18. Levine PA, Seltzer JP, Pirzada FA. The "pacemaker syndrome" in a properly functioning physiologic pacing system. PACE 1983;6:279–282.
19. Hanich RF, Midei M, McElroy B, et al. Circumvention of maximum tracking limitations with a rate modulated dual chamber pacemaker. PACE 1989;12:392–397.
20. Levine PA, Hayes DL, Wilkoff BL, Ohman AE. Electrocardiography of Rate-Modulated Pacemaker Rhythms, Siemens-Pacesetter Inc, Sylmar, CA, 1990, pp 71–73.
21. Clinical Cases in Cardiac Pacing, Complex Dual Chamber Rhythms, Siemens-Pacesetter Inc, Sylmar, CA, 1991, 1, #3.

Chapter 9

DDDR Timing Cycles: Upper Rate Behavior

DAVID L. HAYES

Introduction

DDDR pacing is designed to restore rate responsiveness while maintaining atrioventricular (AV) synchrony. DDDR, by definition, indicates that there is pacing and sensing in both the atrial and the ventricular chambers, that the response to sensing includes both triggered pacing and inhibition by intrinsic activity in each chamber, and that the device has rate-adaptive capability. As with any DDD pacemaker, a DDDR pacemaker must have a programmed lower rate as well as an upper rate. All the basic rules that apply to DDD upper rate behavior must still be considered when the upper rate behavior of a DDDR pacemaker is interpreted[1-4] (Fig. 1). The major difference lies in understanding the interplay between P-tracking and sensor-driven pacing, either or both of which may determine upper rate behavior. Understanding this interplay allows optimal programming of rate-response parameters to achieve the upper rate response that is subjectively and objectively best for the patient. The type of lower rate timing system in a particular DDDR pacemaker, that is, atrial, ventricular, or a hybrid of both, may also have a direct effect on the upper rate behavior of the pacemaker. (For the purpose of this chapter, the term "upper rate limit" represents the maximum achievable paced ventricular rate regardless of whether it is accomplished by P-tracking or by sensor activation.)

At the upper rate limit, a DDDR device may display several be-

New Perspectives in Cardiac Pacing, Vol. 3, edited by S. Serge Barold and Jacques Mugica, Mount Kisco, NY, Futura Publishing Co., © 1993.

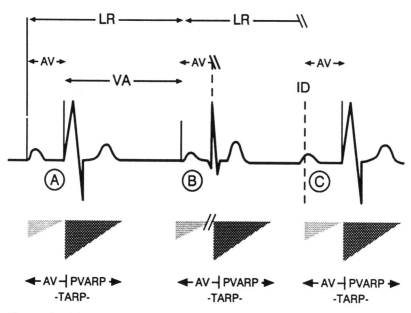

Figure 1. The DDD timing cycle consists of a lower rate (LR) interval, atrioventricular (AV) interval (AVI), ventricular refractory period (VRP), postventricular atrial refractory period (PVARP), and upper rate interval. The DDD timing cycle has three variations. If intrinsic atrial and ventricular activity occur before the LR limit times out, both channels are inhibited and no pacing occurs. If no atrial activity is sensed before the ventriculoatrial (VA) interval is completed, an atrial pacing artifact is delivered, which initiates the AVI. If no intrinsic ventricular activity occurs before the termination of the AVI, a ventricular pacing artifact is delivered, that is, AV sequential pacing (A). If intrinsic ventricular activity occurs before the termination of the AVI, ventricular output from the pacemaker is inhibited, that is, atrial pacing (B). If a P wave is sensed before the VA interval is completed (the LR interval minus the AVI), output from the atrial channel is inhibited. The AVI is initiated, and if no ventricular activity is sensed before the AVI terminates, a ventricular pacing artifact is delivered, that is, P-synchronous pacing (C). (From ref. 21, by permission of WB Saunders Company.)

haviors: pseudo-Wenckebach block, 2:1 AV block, AV sequential pacing, P-synchronous pacing, or a combination of these. In some DDDR devices, the maximum rate at which the sensor can drive the pacemaker is programmed independently from the maximum tracking rate, that is, the maximum rate at which there is 1:1 response between intrinsic atrial activity and paced ventricular activity. In other DDDR pacemakers, a single programmable value limits the upper rate regardless of whether it is reached by tracking of intrinsic atrial activity or by sensor-indicated activity. In addition, there are other upper rate behaviors unique to individual DDDR models.

Pseudo-Wenckebach Behavior

If the rate-response parameters of a DDDR pacemaker are programmed such that the sensor consistently indicates a slower rate than the intrinsic atrial rate, it is possible that sensor-driven pacing may never be seen, so that only DDD operation is seen. In DDD pacing, the upper rate limit is a function of the programmed AV interval (AVI) and the postventricular atrial refractory period (PVARP). A sensed or paced atrial event initiates an atrial refractory period (ARP) and also initiates the AVI (Fig. 1). During this portion of the timing cycle, the atrial channel is refractory to any sensed events and atrial pacing will not occur. A sensed or paced ventricular event also initiates a PVARP.[5,6] The PVARP prevents atrial sensing of a retrograde P wave that occurs within the PVARP and also prevents sensing of far-field ventricular events. The combination of the PVARP and the AVI forms the total atrial refractory period (TARP). The TARP, in turn, is the limiting factor for the maximum sensed atrial rate that the pacemaker can track on a 1:1 basis. For example, if the AVI is 150 ms and the PVARP is 250 ms, the TARP is 400 ms, which limits the maximum atrial tracking rate to 150 ppm. A paced ventricular event initiates the 250-ms PVARP, and only after this interval has been completed can an atrial event be sensed. If an atrial event is sensed immediately after the termination of the PVARP, the sensed atrial event initiates the AVI of 150 ms. On termination of the AVI, in the absence of an intrinsic R wave, a paced ventricular event occurs, resulting in a VV cycle length of 400 ms, or 150 ppm. Programming a long PVARP limits the upper ventricular pacing rate by limiting the maximum atrial rate that can be sensed.[5,6] (Fig. 2).

It is unlikely that P-synchronous pacing will be sustained at exactly the upper rate limit for prolonged periods. When the sinus rate exceeds the upper rate limit, pseudo-Wenckebach behavior is initiated. The appearance is that of group beating, progressive lengthening of the PV (intrinsic P wave followed by paced ventricular complex) interval, and

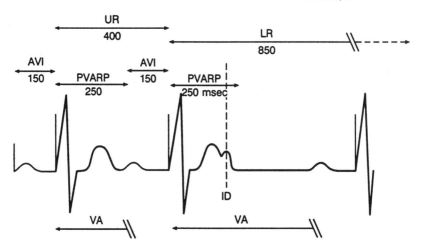

Figure 2. In the DDD pacing mode, the UR (upper rate) is limited by the atrioventricular interval (AVI) and the postventricular atrial refractory period (PVARP). In this example, the AVI is 150 ms and the PVARP is 250 ms, for a total atrial refractory period of 400 ms (corresponding to a rate of 150 ppm). As shown, after the first paced ventricular complex, a P wave occurs just after completion of the PVARP. This P wave is sensed, and after initiating the AVI, it is followed by another paced ventricular complex. The subsequent P wave occurs within the PVARP and is therefore not sensed. The DDD response is to wait for the next intrinsic P wave to occur, as in this example, or for the ventriculoatrial (VA) interval to be completed, whereupon atrioventricular sequential pacing occurs. ID = intrinsic deflection; LR = lower rate. (From ref. 22, by permission of the publisher.)

intermittent pauses on the ECG when the PP interval becomes shorter than the programmed upper rate interval (Fig. 3, upper panel). In DDD pacemakers, the AVI and the upper rate interval must be completed before a ventricular stimulus can be released. A sensed P wave initiates the AVI. On completion of the AVI, if the upper rate interval has been completed, or timed out, a pacemaker stimulus is released. If the upper rate interval has not yet been completed on completion of the AVI, the release of the ventricular output pulse is delayed until the upper rate interval has timed out. This delay has the functional effect of lengthening the PV interval. It also places the ensuing ventricular paced beat closer to the next P wave. The PVARP and the upper rate interval are each initiated by a paced or sensed ventricular event. During pseudo-Wenckebach upper rate behavior, a P wave eventually coincides with the

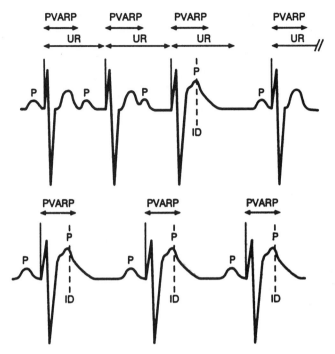

Figure 3. Upper panel: In the DDD pacing mode, the programmed upper rate (UR) interval cannot be violated regardless of the sinus rate. When a P wave is sensed after the postventricular atrial refractory period (PVARP), the atrioventricular interval (AVI) is initiated. If, however, at the termination of the AVI, delivering a ventricular pacing artifact would violate the UR interval, the ventricular pacing artifact cannot be delivered. The pacemaker waits until completion of the UR interval and then delivers the ventricular pacing artifact. This delay results in a prolonged AVI. Lower panel: If the sinus rate becomes so rapid that every other P wave occurs within the PVARP, effective 2:1 atrioventricular block occurs, that is, every other P wave is followed by a ventricular pacing artifact. ID = intrinsic deflection.

PVARP, is not sensed, and is therefore ignored by the pacemaker. A relative pause results. Depending on the atrial rate and programmed lower rate, one of two events occurs. Either the P wave that follows the unsensed P wave is tracked, restarting the cycle at the programmed AVI, or the pause is terminated by AV sequential pacing. If the native atrial rate is fast enough for every other P wave to occur in the PVARP, each

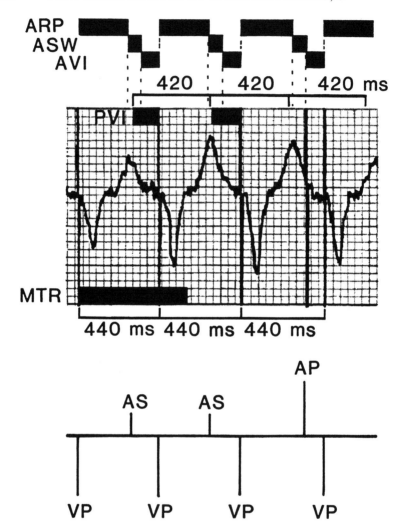

Figure 4.   Diagram showing how an appropriately timed P wave can inhibit the sensor-driven atrial pacing artifact and result in apparent P-wave tracking above the maximum tracking rate (MTR). In this example, the MTR is 100 ppm (upper rate interval = 600 ms) and the sensor rate is 136 ppm (sensor-driven interval = 440 ms). The intrinsic rate is 143 bpm (PP interval = 420 ms). The second and third complexes are preceded by an intrinsic P wave that occurred during the atrial sensing window (ASW). This resulted in inhibition of the atrial pacing artifact, or P-wave tracking above the MTR. The fourth complex was

P wave in the PVARP is not sensed and hence not tracked, and the result is a marked slowing of the paced rate[7] (Fig. 3, lower panel).

It should again be emphasized that pseudo-Wenckebach or 2:1 upper rate behavior (or both) is seen in a DDDR pacemaker only if the sensor-driven rate is slower than the patient's intrinsic atrial rate.

AV Sequential Pacing

Sensor-directed pacing predominates if the patient is chronotropically incompetent or if the sensor is programmed to indicate a faster rate than the intrinsic atrial rate. In a DDDR pacemaker, AV sequential pacing can be seen at any rate between the programmed lower and upper rate limits. If the pacemaker reaches the programmed upper rate limit via the sensor, AV sequential pacing continues at the upper rate limit even if the patient's exercise intensity increases.

In DDDR pacemakers that require independent programming of the maximum tracking and maximum sensor rates, it is possible to program these upper rates discrepantly. For example, the maximum tracking rate could be programmed to 100 ppm and the maximum sensor rate to 150 ppm, in which case P-wave tracking should not occur at sinus rates of greater than 100 bpm. It is possible, however, to see what appears to be P-wave tracking above the maximum tracking rate. The mechanism for this apparent P-wave tracking is inhibition of the atrial output because of precise timing of the intrinsic atrial beat. The atrial sensing window (ASW) is the period during which the atrial sensing channel is alert. The ASW can be defined as that portion of the pacing cycle other than the PVARP and AVI, because during both of these intervals there is no atrial sensing. If the PVARP or AVI (or both) is extended, there may effectively be no ASW. For example, at a programmed upper rate limit of 150 ppm,

---

initiated by atrial pacing, because the preceding native P wave occurred outside the ASW in the atrial refractory period (ARP, 275 ms). Note the short P stimulus interval produced by the subsequent atrial pacing artifact. Also shown are the ASW, 65 ms, atrioventricular interval (AVI, 100 ms), and variable PV (intrinsic P wave followed by paced ventricular complex) interval (PVI). A diagram in Marker Channel™ (Medtronic, Inc., Minneapolis, MN) fashion demonstrates the electrocardiographic findings. AP = atrial paced event; AS = atrial sensed event; VP = ventricular paced event. (From Hayes and Higano.[20] By permission of Futura Publishing Company, Inc.)

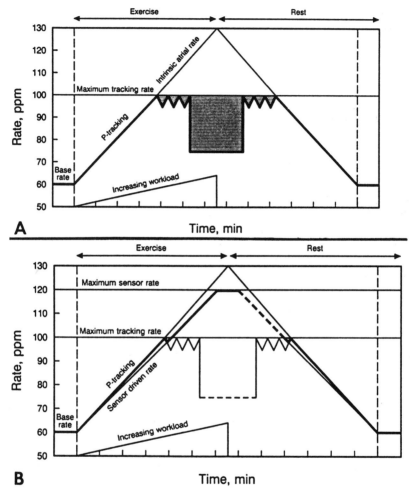

Figure 5. (A) Diagram illustrating the rate response of a DDD pacemaker with Wenckebach-type block at the upper rate limit (100 ppm). The heavy black line represents the ventricular paced rate, assuming complete heart block. Note the varying RR intervals during Wenckebach-type block as the atrial rate exceeds the maximum tracking rate. (The shaded area is meant to represent potential paced ventricular rates that may occur during DDD upper rate behavior.) After termination of exercise, if the patient's atrial rate had increased to the point that the pacemaker was responding to every other P wave, that is, 2:1 block, the paced ventricular rate will actually increase to the maximum tracking rate as the

the minimum VV cycle length is 400 ms. If the PVARP is 250 ms and the AVI is 150 ms, there is no ASW; that is, 250 + 150 = 400 ms, which is the same as the upper rate limit. However, if a DDDR pacemaker has exceeded the programmed maximum tracking rate and is pacing at faster rates on the basis of sensor activation, an appropriately timed intrinsic P wave can still inhibit sensor-driven atrial pacing artifacts and give the appearance of P-wave tracking at rates greater than the maximum tracking rate[8] (Fig. 4). The maximum tracking rate appears to be variable and equal to the sensor-driven rate when the sensor-driven rate exceeds the programmed maximum tracking rate if a P wave occurs during the ASW to inhibit output of an atrial pacing artifact. Although this behavior has the appearance of variable maximum tracking, the same behavior could theoretically be seen with DDIR pacing. In the DDIR mode, sensed atrial activity can only inhibit atrial pacing and not trigger ventricular pacing. Appropriately timed P waves could occur within the ASW and inhibit the subsequent A spike. Again, although this pacing mode is incapable of atrial tracking, this event would make it appear that the P wave were tracked at a rate equal to the current sensor rate.

Sensor-Driven Rate Smoothing

For an understanding of the combination of upper rate behaviors that can be observed with DDDR pacing, the fundamental difference between DDD and DDDR pacing must be emphasized (Fig. 5). In DDD pacing, two potential mechanisms achieve ventricular pacing. The first is the lower rate interval; for example, if the lower rate of the DDD pacemaker is programmed to 70 ppm (857 ms) and the AVI is 150 ms, the atrial pacing stimulus occurs at 707 ms after the previous ventricular

---

atrial rate slows and fewer P waves fall within the PVARP. (B) Diagram illustrating the rate response of the DDDR pacemaker and its behavior at both the maximum tracking and the maximum sensor rates. The heavy black line shows the ventricular paced rate, assuming complete heart block, as it progresses from the P-tracking mode to atrioventricular sequential pacing through a period of Wenckebach-type block. The rate may increase to the programmed maximum sensor rate. At termination of exercise, the ventricular paced rate gradually decreases to the base rate or lower rate limit unless activity resumes. Pseudo-Wenckebach activity can be minimized by optimal programming of the sensor rate response parameters.

event (857–150 ms) and the paced ventricular event occurs after the programmed AVI of 150 ms to maintain a lower rate limit of 70 ppm. The second mechanism of driving the ventricle is in 1:1 synchronization with the sinus rate; that is, if the sinus rate is greater than the programmed lower rate limit, 1:1 P-synchronous pacing occurs until the upper rate limit is reached and DDD upper rate behavior is imposed. However, a third mechanism is possible with DDDR pacing[9] (Fig. 6). The ventricle can be paced in an AV sequential fashion in response to sensor input. For example, if the sensor input at a given point of exercise corresponds to an appropriate heart rate of 100 bpm, the DDDR pacemaker paces AV sequentially at 100 ppm. The only exception is that if the sinus rate at that time is greater than 100 bpm, the sinus rate predominates and P-synchronous pacing occurs. If the sinus rate is less than 100 bpm, the sensor predominates. Either the sinus or the sensor may be wholly predominant at any point in time. It is possible, however, for control to be mixed: sensor-driven AV sequential pacing is seen for a few cycles and is followed by emergence of the sinus rate with P-synchronous pacing.[10] This interplay between sinus and sensor must be appreciated to understand DDDR behavior.[7]

Establishing an optimal interplay between sinus and sensor should be the goal of programming in an effort to maximize hemodynamic benefits of DDDR pacing. This is accomplished by achieving a smooth transition between sinus- and sensor-driven pacing. The transition has been designated "sensor-driven rate smoothing." "Rate smoothing" was introduced as an option in a dual chamber pacemaker manufactured by Cardiac Pacemakers, Inc. (St. Paul, MN) (see below). It is intended to eliminate large cycle-to-cycle variations in rate by preventing the paced rate from changing more than a certain percentage from one paced VV interval to the next. This option would eliminate large fluctuations in rate during fixed-ratio or pseudo-Wenckebach block that may occur at the upper rate limit. With DDDR pacemakers, fluctuations in cycle length can be prevented or significantly minimized by optimal programming of the pacemaker, resulting in sensor-mediated rate smoothing. If the rate-responsive circuitry is programmed to mimic the native atrial rate, the paced ventricular rate should not demonstrate 2:1 behavior and would demonstrate pseudo-Wenckebach behavior for only short periods or not at all. Conversely, if the rate-responsive circuitry is programmed to very low levels of sensor-driven pacing, little or no rate-smoothing takes place. This rate response is illustrated diagrammatically in Figure

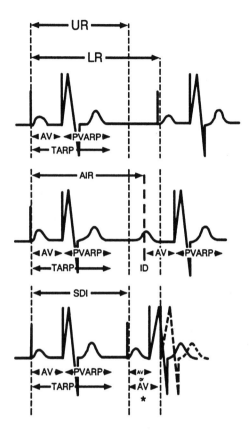

Figure 6. DDDR pacemakers are capable of all pacing variations previously described for DDD pacemakers (Fig. 1). When a DDDR pacemaker is functioning above the programmed lower rate (LR) limit, it may increase the heart rate on the basis of the atrial-indicated rate (AIR), middle panel, or the sensor-driven interval (SDI), bottom panel. In most currently available DDDR pacemakers, the postventricular atrial refractory period (PVARP) remains fixed regardless of cycle length. With a rate-responsive atrioventricular (AV) interval (AVI), the length of the AVI varies (asterisk) with the SDI; that is, as the SDI increases, the AVI shortens. Because a rate-responsive AV delay is incorporated, the total atrial refractory period (TARP) may shorten by virtue of the changing AVI. ID = intrinsic deflection; UR = upper rate.

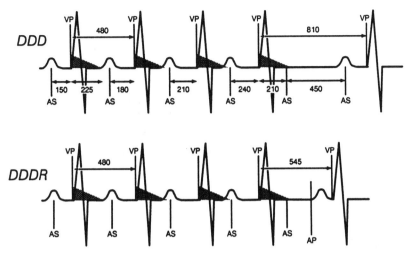

Figure 7.   This diagram illustrates the difference in DDD and DDDR behavior when the intrinsic atrial rate increases. In the upper panel, DDD pacing is shown. The sensed atrial events (AS) occur increasingly closer to the postventricular atrial refractory period (PVARP), which is programmed to 225 ms (shown by the triangles) until the fifth AS event occurs at 210 ms after the preceding paced ventricular beat (VP), or within the PVARP, and is not sensed. This event is followed by another AS and VP after the programmed atrioventricular interval (AVI) of 150 ms. The resultant cycle length is 810 ms, significantly longer than the preceding cycles of 480 ms. In the lower panel, DDDR pacing is illustrated. The intervals are programmed to the same values as those in the upper panel. When the fifth AS event occurs within the PVARP, it is, by definition, not sensed. However, the escape event is a sensor-driven atrial pacing artifact (AP) followed by a VP after the AVI. The sensor-indicated cycle length is 545 ms. Therefore, only a 65-ms difference exists between the programmed upper rate limit and the sensor-indicated rate, a minor difference in cycle lengths. (Modified from Markowitz.[9])

7. The upper panel in Figure 7 shows the DDD response, that is, sensor "off," or "passive," to exercise-induced increases in atrial rate, assuming complete heart block, a maximum tracking rate of 100 ppm, and pseudo-Wenckebach response at the maximum tracking rate. The ventricular and atrial rate responses to exercise are shown. As the maximum tracking rate is exceeded, there is a transition from 1:1 P-synchronous function to pseudo-Wenckebach upper rate behavior. The lower panel in Figure 7 shows the response that would occur with the sensor "on" (DDDR)

and a maximum sensor rate of 120 ppm. The ventricular rate response to exercise, along with the atrial and sensor rates, is shown. Below the maximum P-wave tracking rate, the ventricle is paced in a P-synchronous fashion, similar to DDD function. However, with the sensor "on" (DDDR), there is a transition from P-synchronous to AV sequential pacing through a period of pseudo-Wenckebach block as the atrial rate exceeds the maximum tracking rate. The cycle containing the unsensed P wave at the end of a Wenckebach sequence is shortened by sensor-driven pacing. Sensor-driven rate smoothing requires optimal programming of rate-response parameters. (When true "rate smoothing" is an option in DDDR pacing, other manifestations are possible; see below.) An example of sensor-driven rate smoothing is demonstrated in Figure 8.[11]

If the sensor-indicated rate and the intrinsic rates are not well matched, there will be greater cycle-to-cycle variation, which may result in suboptimal hemodynamics. Figure 9 demonstrates the electrocardiographic manifestations of programming that result in a slight difference

RR = 461 ms

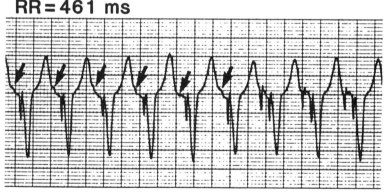

Maximum tracking rate = 130 ppm
Maximum sensor rate = 130 ppm

Figure 8. Electrocardiographic tracing from a patient with a DDDR pacemaker programmed to a maximum tracking rate of 130 ppm and maximum sensor rate of 130 ppm. There is essentially no difference in VV cycle length between P-synchronous pacing (arrows) and sensor-driven atrioventricular sequential pacing (the last three complexes).

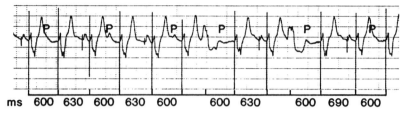

ms 600 630 600 630 600   600 630   600 690 600

Figure 9. Electrocardiographic tracing from a patient with a DDDR pacemaker programmed to a maximum tracking rate (MTR) of 100 ppm and maximum sensor rate of 150 ppm. Two VV cycle lengths are seen, 600 ms and 630 ms. The 600-ms cycle length corresponds to the MTR of 100 ppm. However, when the P wave occurs within the postventricular atrial refractory period, the pacemaker escapes by the sensor-driven rate, a sensed P wave, or the lower rate limit. In this example, the escape after the 600-ms cycle length is sensor-driven. The sensor indicates that the appropriate rate is 95 ppm (630 ms) at a time when the corresponding sinus rate is approximately 115 bpm.

between sensor-indicated and intrinsic rates. In this example, the pacemaker is in the DDDR mode with a lower rate of 60 ppm, maximum tracking rate of 100 ppm, maximum sensor rate of 150 ppm, AV interval of 175 ms, and PVARP of 250 ms. When the intervals are carefully measured, it is apparent that all but one of the VV cycles are either 600 ms or 630 ms. Each of the VV cycles that is P-synchronous, that is, without a sensor-driven atrial pacing artifact, is 600 ms, which is equivalent to a paced rate of 100 ppm. As noted before, the maximum tracking rate was programmed to 100 ppm, so that these cycles demonstrate normal behavior. The other predominant cycle length of 630 ms occurs when the intrinsic P wave occurs within the PVARP. The P wave, therefore, is not sensed, and before another intrinsic P wave occurs, the sensor-indicated interval of 630 ms, or a rate of 95 ppm, occurs. This is normal function in a DDDR pacemaker when the atrial rate exceeds the maximum tracking rate and there is concomitant sensor-driven pacing. Slowing of the rate from 100 to 95 ppm is a function of sensor programming. This minimal difference, 5 ppm, between atrial rate and sensor-indicated rate would not be clinically significant. The actual sensor input signal to the pacemaker cannot be ascertained from the electrocardiogram. Although the pacemaker is capable of a maximum sensor rate, 150 ppm, its actual sensor-controlled rate is based on the actual input signal. (Programming in this manner, a maximum tracking rate significantly lower than the maximum sensor rate, is somewhat unusual in a patient capable of achieving faster sinus rates. It may occasionally be useful in patients with paroxysmal supraventricular rhythm disturbances;[12] see below.)

Variations of DDDR Upper Rate Behavior

DDDR upper rate behavior may differ among devices from different manufacturers because of the lower rate timing system used, that is, ventricular-based or a combination of ventricular- and atrial-based timing behaviors as well as other design-specific characteristics.[13,14] Because upper rate behavior may be device-specific, it is necessary to refer to the specific pacemaker.

In a ventricular-based timing system, the VA interval, or atrial escape interval (AEI), which is the interval from a ventricular sensed or paced event to an atrial paced event, is fixed (Fig. 10, upper panel). A ventricular sensed event occurring during the AEI would reset this timer, causing it to start all over again. A ventricular sensed event occurring during the AVI would both terminate the AVI and initiate an AEI. If AV conduction is intact and the time from atrial pacing to intrinsic QRS (AR interval) is shorter than the programmed AVI, the AEI would be reset by the intrinsic ventricular event. The atrial cycle length, therefore, is slightly shorter than if the programmed AVI had been completed, resulting in a slight acceleration of the atrial pacing rate. By contrast, if a DDDR pacemaker operated on an atrial-based timing system, the AA interval would be fixed (Fig. 10, lower panel).

Although acceleration of ventricular rate in ventricular-based timing systems is minimal at the lower rate limit, it may become more significant as sensor-driven rates increase. In a ventricular-based timing system, the effective atrial paced rate could theoretically be significantly higher than the programmed upper rate limit if AR conduction were present[14,15] (Fig. 11, top panel). If it is assumed that the maximum sensor-controlled rate is 150 ppm (a cycle length of 400 ms), with a programmed AVI of 200 ms, the AEI is also 200 ms. If there is intact AV conduction such that the AR interval is 150 ms, the actual pacing interval is the AR interval + AEI, or 150 ms + 200 ms, or 350 ms. A cycle length of 350 ms is equal to 171 ppm, which is significantly higher than the programmed upper rate limit of 150 ppm.

If a DDDR pacemaker had a true atrial-based timing system, sensor-

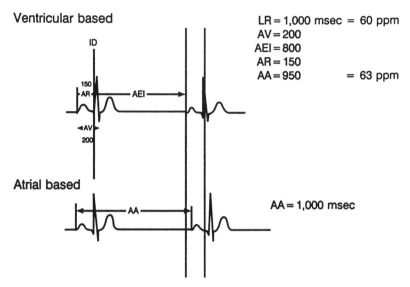

Figure 10.   Upper panel: With ventricular-based timing in patients with intact atrioventricular (AV) nodal conduction after atrial pacing (AR pacing), the sensed R wave resets the atrial escape interval (AEI). Because the base pacing interval is the sum of the AR and AEI, it is shorter than the programmed minimum rate interval. Lower panel: With true atrial-based timing in patients with intact AV nodal conduction after AR pacing, the sensed R wave would inhibit the ventricular output but would not reset the basic timing of the pacemaker. There would be AR pacing at the programmed base rate. ID = intrinsic deflection; LR = lower rate. (Modified from Levine et al.[11])

driven pacing could not exceed the programmed maximum pacing rate because the AA interval would be maintained (Fig. 11, middle panel). Therefore, intact AR conduction would not alter the basic timing. At present, there are no pure atrial-based DDDR pacemakers.

Rate acceleration can be minimized in a ventricular-based timing system with a rate-responsive AV delay (RRAVD).[14] As the sinus- or sensor-driven rate progressively increases, RRAVD causes the PV and AV intervals to progressively shorten (Fig. 11, bottom panel). Shortening the AVI with RRAVD results in a shorter TARP (shorter AVI + PVARP). This increases the intrinsic atrial rate that can be sensed, reducing the likelihood of both a fixed block upper rate response and functional atrial undersensing; that is, fewer P waves occur in the PVARP.

Ventricular-based timing--fixed AV delay

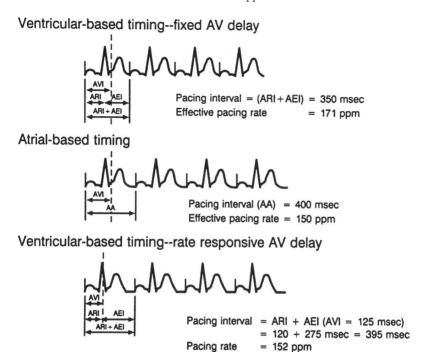

Pacing interval = (ARI + AEI) = 350 msec
Effective pacing rate = 171 ppm

Atrial-based timing

Pacing interval (AA) = 400 msec
Effective pacing rate = 150 ppm

Ventricular-based timing--rate responsive AV delay

Pacing interval = ARI + AEI (AVI = 125 msec)
= 120 + 275 msec = 395 msec
Pacing rate = 152 ppm

Figure 11. Effect of different timing systems on maximum sensor rate with intact, stable atrioventricular (AV) nodal conduction (AR [atrial paced event followed by intrinsic R wave] pacing). Top panel: In a ventricular-based timing system, in which the programmed AV interval remains constant at all rates, a significant increase in the paced atrial rate could exceed the programmed upper rate limit. In the example shown, even though the maximum sensor rate programmed is 150 ppm (upper rate interval of 400 ms, which is equal to the AV interval at 200 ms and the atrial escape interval of 200 ms), the effective pacing rate achieved is 171 ppm, because the effective pacing rate is a function of the AR interval (ARI) and the atrial escape interval (AEI), which remains constant in a ventricular-based timing system; that is, 150 + 200 = 350 ms (171 ppm). Middle panel: In a true atrial-based system, the R wave sensed during the AV interval (AVI) would not alter the basic timing during stable AR pacing. This would result in atrial pacing at the sensor-indicated rate. Bottom panel: The addition of rate-responsive AV delay to a ventricular-based timing system compensates for the difference between the AVI and the ARI and minimizes the increase in the paced atrial rate above the programmed sensor-indicated rate. In this example, the pacemaker is operating at the maximum sensor rate, and the rate-responsive AV delay shortens the AVI by 75 ms (AVI of 200 ms at lower rate interval − 75 ms = AVI of 125 ms). With an AR interval of 120 ms, there is now only a minimal difference between the AVI and the ARI. The 75 ms subtracted from the AVI is effectively added to the AEI (200 ms + 75 ms = 275 ms). (From ref. 21, by permission of WB Saunders Company.)

It also minimizes the chance of an inappropriately long PV interval at higher rates that may occur with a fixed AVI when the fixed AVI is programmed appropriately for lower rate behavior. When the Synchrony II DDDR pacemaker by Pacesetter Systems, Inc., is operating under sensor control with RRAVD programmed "on," as the AVI shortens, the ventricular rate is held to that governed by the sensor. The time subtracted from the AVI due to RRAVD is added to the AEI. Thus, if the programmed upper rate is 150 ppm, the pacing interval is 400 ms, and the RRAVD results in shortening of the AVI by 75 ms from an initially programmed AVI of 200 ms, the AVI shortens to 125 ms. Since the overall ventricular timing is held constant, the 75 ms subtracted from the AVI is added to the AEI, increasing it to 275 ms. In this example, the upper rate interval is 275 ms (AEI) + 125 ms (AVI), or 400 ms, corresponding to an upper rate limit of 150 ppm.

The RRAVD provides a more physiologic AVI at the faster rate, and if there is intact AR conduction, it minimizes the degree of rate increase over the programmed maximum sensor rate. Assuming that the upper rate limit is 150 ppm and the initial AVI is 200 ms, the RRAVD results in an AVI of 125 ms at the upper rate limit. If intact AR conduction is present at 120 ms, the overall shortening of the pacing interval is only 5 ms above that seen at 150 ppm, a rate of 152 ppm (Fig. 11, bottom panel).

The META (Telectronics, Inc., Englewood, CO) DDDR pacemaker uses a conventional ventricular-based timing cycle and determines the sensor-driven rate and metabolic-indicated rate (MIR) by minute ventilation. The META DDDR allows the programming of a baseline PVARP, which is the PVARP that exists when the MIR is indicating a resting or minimum rate. As the MIR increases because of an increase in workload or emotional stress, the pacemaker has the capability of not only an RRAVD but also a rate-adaptive PVARP. The PVARP shortens in a linear fashion, so that at maximum rate, the AVI plus the PVARP is equal to the maximum interval.[16,17] The shortening of the AVI and the PVARP prevents the upper rate limit from being restricted by fixed values of the AVI and PVARP. The pacemaker monitors the atrial rate or, more specifically, the PP interval. When the PP interval is less than the operational TARP, the atrial rate is considered to be a nonphysiologic atrial tachyarrhythmia, for example, atrial fibrillation, atrial flutter, or paroxysmal atrial tachycardia. If what the pacemaker has determined to be a nonphysiologic atrial rhythm is present, the pacing mode auto-

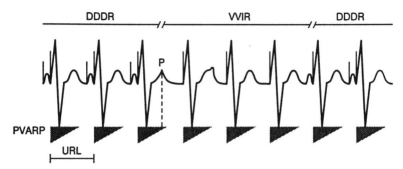

Figure 12. Electrocardiographic appearance of Automatic Mode Switching (AMS) when the pacemaker is programmed to an upper rate limit (URL) of 150 ppm. The first three cardiac cycles are due to sensor-driven atrioventricular (AV) sequential pacing, that is, DDDR pacing. After the third paced ventricular complex, a P wave occurs during the postventricular atrial refractory period (PVARP) (triangles) and initiates AMS to the VVIR mode because the atrial rate has exceeded the URL. The pacing mode reverts to DDDR when the atrial rate falls below the programmed URL; that is, P waves fall outside the PVARP. (From ref. 21, by permission of WB Saunders Company.)

matically changes to VVIR until the criteria for nonphysiologic atrial rhythm are no longer met, at which time DDDR pacing resumes (Fig. 12).[12] This feature can obviously affect the upper rate limit behavior. The upper rate response during a physiologic atrial rate increase is based on the Automatic Mode Switching mechanism described. During a physiologic increase in the atrial rate, that is, increased sinus rates based on increasing workload or stress, the TARP shortens as the MIR increases to the programmed upper rate limit, at which TARP equals the maximum rate interval. When the atrial rate exceeds the programmed maximum rate, the PP interval is less than the TARP and the device reverts to VVIR pacing.

To overcome the potential rate variability of ventricular-based DDDR devices already described, modified AA timing regimens have been developed for several DDDR pacemakers. The Relay (Intermedics, Inc., Angleton, TX) DDDR pacemaker is considered atrial-based, but it incorporates some features of ventricular-based timing. Whenever the time from the atrial event, whether sensed or paced, to the ventricular event, whether sensed or paced, is less than the programmed AVI, AA timing exists. Whenever the time from an atrial sensed event to the ventricular event, be it sensed or paced, is greater than the programmed

AVI, ventriculoatrial timing (ventricular-based) occurs. (This would also include a ventricular sensed event not preceded by an atrial event, for example, premature ventricular contractions.)

The Relay pacemaker also incorporates a modified tracking limit scheme to prevent inappropriate upper rate ventricular pacing in response to atrial tachyarrhythmias[18] (Fig. 13).[13] In this device, a programmable option exists with which the sensor output is cross-checked against the sensed atrial rate. A "conditional tracking limit" set to 35 ppm above the lower pacing rate is in effect if the sensor output indicates that the patient is at rest. This limits the ventricular pacing rate if any atrial sensed events occur faster than 35 ppm above the lower pacing rate. This "con-

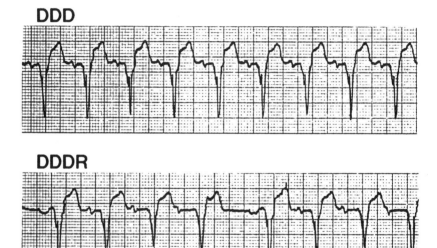

Figure 13. Electrocardiographic tracings from a patient with a DDDR pacemaker with "conditional tracking limit." In both tracings, the patient is at rest despite the rapid sinus rate. In the upper panel, P-wave tracking occurs with a sinus rate of 100. In the lower panel, the pacemaker is programmed DDDR, lower rate 70 ppm. Because the patient is resting, the sensor indicates that a slower ventricular rate is appropriate. Because the atrial sensed events are more than 35 bpm faster than the lower rate limit, the pacemaker operates in pseudo-Wenckebach behavior. (An artifact is present during the fifth T wave.)

ditional tracking limit" is deactivated when the sensor detects a period of exercise, or it can be programmed off.

In the PRECEPT DR and VIGOR DR (Cardiac Pacemakers, Inc., St. Paul, MN), the upper rate behavior may be altered by rate smoothing.[19] "Rate smoothing" is the term used to describe a feature capable of differentiating between abrupt changes in sensed atrial or ventricular events. Rate smoothing is designed to minimize cycle-to-cycle rate variations and is programmable to a fixed percentage value of the cycle-to-cycle pacing interval. This value defines for the pulse generator

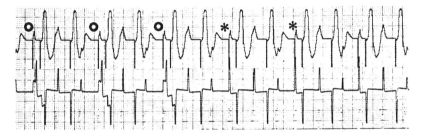

Figure 14. Electrocardiographic tracing from a DDDR pacemaker (VIGOR DR, Cardiac Pacemakers, Inc., St. Paul, MN) with rate smoothing as a programmable option. In this example, the pacemaker is programmed to 60 ppm, upper rate limit of 100 ppm, and maximum sensor rate of 150 ppm with rate smoothing "on" at 21%. The electrocardiogram (ECG) is shown in the upper portion of the tracing, and the event markers immediately below the ECG identify the various electrocardiographic events. (On the event marker recording, atrial events are noted by upward deflections and ventricular events by downward deflections.) For the atrial events noted, there are three different sizes of upward deflections. The largest deflection, approximately 15 mV, represents a paced atrial event, the 10-mV deflection represents a sensed atrial event, and the 5-mV deflection represents an atrial event that has occurred in the postventricular atrial refractory period. If the deflection representing a paced atrial event has a step-shaped deformity, the paced atrial event occurred because of rate smoothing, denoted by the circles above the ECG. If there is no indicator of rate smoothing, denoted by the asterisks, the paced atrial event was sensor-driven. Without the event marker recording, it may be very difficult to determine which paced atrial events are sensor-driven and which are the result of rate smoothing. Had rate smoothing not been programmed "on" in this example, there would have been greater variation in paced ventricular cycle length because the pacemaker would have responded with pseudo-Wenckebach behavior until the time that enough activity was present to activate the sensor.

what is a physiologic rather than a pathologic change for the patient; rate changes less than the programmed percentage are considered physiologic and changes greater than the percentage are considered pathologic. When a sensed event exceeds this percentage of the previous cycle's interval, either faster or slower, the AEI is allowed to increase or decrease up to the programmed percentage for each cycle. As always, if a P wave is not sensed by the end of the rate-smoothing-calculated AEI, atrial pacing occurs. This prevents sudden changes in cycle length while maintaining AV synchronous operation.

In a DDDR pacemaker with rate smoothing programmed "on," even if rate-response parameters are suboptimally programmed, that is, "sensor-driven rate smoothing" is suboptimal or minimal, there should not be any sudden alterations in cycle length, because they are prevented by rate smoothing (Fig. 14).[14] Rate smoothing will continue to prevent RR or VV cycle interval alterations until a steady state is reached with the sinus rate or until the workload has increased to the point at which sensor-driven pacing predominates.

DDDR Upper Rate Behavior With Paroxysmal Supraventricular Tachyarrhythmia

As with DDD pacing, if a paroxysmal supraventricular tachyarrhythmia (PSVT) occurs in a patient with a DDDR pacemaker, the pacemaker may track the supraventricular rhythm.[4,12] Tracking may be irregular and may result in paced ventricular rates that remain at the upper rate limit or vary between the lower and upper rate limits. The sensor will most likely not come into play, because the PSVT controls the rate and inhibits sensor activity. In a discussion of DDDR upper rate behavior, this subject warrants inclusion because tracking of PSVT while maintaining the capability of rate responsiveness is possible in a DDDR pacemaker. Several DDDR pacemakers currently available can be programmed to the DDIR mode. In this mode, "tracking" of the atrial rate is not possible. Therefore, whether the patient has normal sinus rhythm or PSVT, atrial activity is not tracked. However, in the DDIR mode, rate responsiveness can still be achieved by the sensor. If the DDIR pacing mode is not available, there are alternatives. If the maximum tracking rate and maximum sensor rate are independently programmable, the maximum tracking rate can be programmed to a lower rate, for

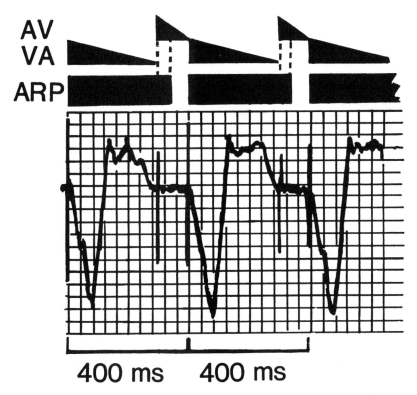

Figure 15. In this electrocardiographic example from a DDDR pacemaker, the maximum sensor rate is 150 ppm (400 ms), the atrial refractory period (ARP) is 350 ms, and the atrioventricular (AV) interval (AVI) is 100 ms. As illustrated in the block diagrams above the electrocardiogram, the two sensor-driven atrial pacing artifacts both occur during the terminal portion of the postventricular atrial refractory period (PVARP). Even though no atrial sensing can occur during the PVARP (as can be seen in this example by the intrinsic P wave that occurs immediately after the first paced ventricular depolarization), a sensor-driven atrial pacing artifact is not prevented by the PVARP. Whether a sensor-driven atrial pacing artifact is delivered depends on the sensor-indicated rate at that time and not the PVARP. VA = ventriculoatrial. (From Hayes and Higano.[20] By permission of Futura Publishing Company, Inc.)

example, 100 ppm, and the maximum sensor rate can be programmed to a higher rate, such as 150 ppm. If PSVT occurs, tracking is limited to a rate of 100 ppm. During exertion, rates to 150 ppm can be achieved through the sensor. If the upper rate limit is a single programmable value, the maximum rate desired through the sensor can be programmed as the upper rate limit. Tracking can in turn be limited by programming of the TARP (AVI + PVARP). If the AVI is 150 ms and the PVARP is 350 ms, the TARP is 500 ms and tracking is limited to 120 ppm. This outcome is possible because even though the PVARP prevents sensing of atrial activity, it does not prevent pacing the atrium on the basis of sensor activation[20] (Fig. 15).

Summary

DDDR upper rate behavior is more complex than upper rate behavior with any other pacing mode. The additional complexity is justified by the potential clinical advantages of DDDR pacing, the greatest of which is the avoidance of large cycle-to-cycle variations at the upper rate limit. Design-specific differences that exist among DDDR pacemakers from various manufacturers make it necessary to know the capabilities of the specific DDDR pacemaker to understand its upper rate behavior.

References

1. Barold SS, Falkoff MD, Ong LS, et al. Upper rate response of DDD pacemakers. In: Barold SS, Mugica J (eds.). New Perspectives in Cardiac Pacing, Futura Publishing Company, Mount Kisco, NY, 1988, pp 121–172.
2. Furman S. Dual chamber pacemakers: upper rate behavior. PACE 1985;8: 197–214.
3. Barold SS, Falkoff MD, Ong LS, et al. Timing cycles of DDD pacemakers. In: Barold SS, Mugica J (eds). New Perspectives in Cardiac Pacing, Futura Publishing Company, Mount Kisco, NY, 1988, pp 69–119.
4. Levine PA. Normal and abnormal rhythms associated with dual-chamber pacemakers. Cardiol Clin 1985 Nov;3:595–616.
5. Barold SS. Management of patients with dual chamber pulse generators: central role of the pacemaker atrial refractory period. Learning Center Highlights 1990 Summer;5:8–16.
6. Levine PA. Postventricular atrial refractory periods and pacemaker mediated tachycardias. Clin Prog Pacing Electrophysiol 1983;1:394–401.

7. Higano ST, Hayes DL, Eisinger G. Sensor-driven rate smoothing in a DDDR pacemaker. PACE 1989;12:922–929.
8. Higano ST, Hayes DL. P wave tracking above the maximum tracking rate in a DDDR pacemaker. PACE 1989;12:1044–1048.
9. Markowitz HT. Dual chamber rate responsive pacing (DDDR) provides physiologic upper rate behavior. PhysioPace 1990;4:1–4.
10. Hayes DL, Higano ST, Eisinger G. Electrocardiographic manifestations of a dual-chamber, rate-modulated (DDDR) pacemaker. PACE 1989;12:555–562.
11. Levine PA, Hayes DL, Wilkoff BL, Ohman AE. Electrocardiography of Rate-Modulated Pacemaker Rhythms. Siemens-Pacesetter, Inc., Sylmar, CA, 1990, pp 12–31.
12. Higano ST, Hayes DL, Eisinger G. Advantage of discrepant upper rate limits in a DDDR pacemaker. Mayo Clin Proc 1989;64:932–939.
13. Barold SS, Falkoff MD, Ong LS, et al. A-A and V-V lower rate timing of DDD and DDDR pulse generators. In: New Perspectives in Cardiac Pacing. 2. Barold SS, Mugica J (eds.). Futura Publishing Company, Mount Kisco, NY, 1991, pp 203–247.
14. Levine PA, Sholder JA. Interpretation of rate-modulated, dual-chamber rhythms: the effect of ventricular based and atrial based timing systems on DDD and DDDR rhythms. Pacesetter Systems, Inc., A Siemens Company, March, 1990.
15. Hanich RF, Midei MG, McElroy BP, et al. Circumvention of maximum tracking limitations with a rate modulated dual chamber pacemaker. PACE 1989;12:392–397.
16. Vanerio G, Patel S, Ching E, et al. Early clinical experience with a minute ventilation sensor DDDR pacemaker. PACE 1991;14:1815–1820.
17. Lau C-P, Tai Y-T, Fong P-C, et al. Clinical experience with a minute ventilation sensing DDDR pacemaker: upper rate behavior and the adaptation of the PVARP (abstr). 1990; PACE13:1201.
18. Lee MT, Adkins A, Woodson D, et al. A new feature for control of inappropriate high rate tracking in DDDR pacemakers. PACE 1990;13:1852–1855.
19. van Mechelen R, Ruiter J, De Boer H, et al. Pacemaker electrocardiography of rate smoothing during DDD pacing. PACE 1985;8:684–690.
20. Hayes DL, Higano ST. DDDR pacing: follow-up and complications. In: Barold SS, Mugica J (eds.). New Perspectives in Cardiac Pacing. 2. Mount Kisco, NY, Futura Publishing Company, 1991, pp 473–491.
21. Hayes DL. Timing cycles of permanent pacemakers. Cardiol Clin, in press.
22. Hayes DL, Levine PA. Pacemaker timing cycles. In: Ellenbogen KA (ed). Cardiac Pacing. Blackwell Scientific Publications, Cambridge, MA, 1992, pp 263–308.

Chapter 10

AV Delay Optimization in DDD and DDDR Pacing

CLAUDE DAUBERT, PHILIPPE RITTER,

PHILIPPE MABO, CORINNE VARIN,

CHRISTOPHE LECLERCQ

Introduction

A few manufacturers and many physicians still ignore the need for individual and permanent optimization of AV delay in DDD and DDDR pacing. Experience has demonstrated, however, the importance of the opinion expressed by Wish[1] in 1987: "The benefit of dual chamber pacing has been generally underestimated by lack of an appropriately programmed AV delay."

There are two main objectives for individual optimization: first, optimizing cardiac performance cycle by cycle while guaranteeing the maximal contribution of the atrial systole, and second, maintaining 1:1 AV synchrony during all the patient's daily activities, that is, even up to the highest heart rates acceptable for the patient's physiologic and/or pathologic situation.

Cycle to Cycle Optimization of the Left Atrial Contribution

Physiological Basis

An optimal AV delay means that in every cardiac cycle, the AV interval produces exactly the delay required for the left atrial systole to

New Perspectives in Cardiac Pacing, Vol. 3, edited by S. Serge Barold and Jacques Mugica, Mount Kisco, NY, Futura Publishing Co., © 1993.

make its maximum contribution to stroke volume, either at rest or during exercise.

Optimal AV Delay at Rest

The optimal electrical AV interval is the one that gives the best timing of left atrial systole. Unfortunately, there is no correlation between this electrical interval, applied at the pacing sites usually in the right heart, and the optimal mechanical delay that concerns the left heart. This lack of correlation results from important interindividual differences in electrical and electromechanical intervals both in atria (electromechanical delay within the right atrium (RA), interatrial conduction time, electromechanical delay within the left atrium (LA), and in ventricles (especially the interventricular conduction time).[2] An important consequence is the definite, but quite variable, extension of the mechanical delay when a DDD pacemaker switches from a sensed atrial cycle to a paced atrial cycle. Many factors affect this extension. They include not only the electromechanical delay within the right atrium (which depends on the position of the lead in the atrium, the atrial size, and the functional quality of the myocardium), but also the delay of interatrial conduction. The electromechanical delay in the right atrium is easily measured as the interval between the atrial spike, or the beginning of the spontaneous sinus P wave, to the beginning of the A wave on the right atrial pressure curve or on the transtricuspid echo Doppler flow. In an earlier study,[2] we found this interval to lie between 40 and 90 ms in sensed cycles (VDD mode) and between 70 and 140 ms in paced cycles (DDD mode) in patients who were going to be permanently paced in the DDD mode. There was an average difference of 43 ± 11 ms between atrial sensed and atrial paced cycles. The interatrial conduction time must then be added to this interval in order to obtain the real electromechanical delay separating the electrical event initiating in the right atrium and the effective mechanical action of the left atrium. In patients selected for their lack of atrial conduction disorder on the surface ECG,[2] there is little interindividual variation in interatrial conduction time; pacing mode has little effect (57 ± 23 ms in VDD mode and 74 ± 18 in DDD mode, an extension of 17 ms) and the rate of permanent atrial pacing has no effect. However, about 25% of the patients considered for permanent DDD pacing have high degree intra- and interatrial conduction disorders.[3]

When Wish et al.[4] included such patients in their series, they found an average value of 144 ± 82 ms at spontaneous rate, with extreme values of 70 and 380 ms. In addition, during paced cycles in patients with advanced interatrial blocks, there appeared to be a significant extension of the interatrial delay over that observed in healthy hearts.

The wide variability of the electrical and electromechanical delays explains the important interindividual differences observed for the "extension of the AV delay."

Optimal AV Delay During Exercise

In DDD pacing, the dynamic nature of the optimal AV delay should come as close as possible to the physiologic adaptation of the PR interval to heart rate (HR) in the normal individual. It is well known that the PR interval shortens progressively as the HR increases.[5,6] Despite this fact, precise measurements of this physiologic behavior using endocardial ECG recordings are rare. Atterhog[7] studied 27 normal subjects, most of them young (average age 26), during maximum exercise tests either in the supine or in a sitting position (n = 12). In some patients, the test was run again after IV injection of atropine or propranolol in order to study the effect of the autonomic nervous system on PR interval behavior.[8] In a more recent study,[8] we investigated the behavior of the PR interval in a setting corresponding to permanent DDD pacing in 10 healthy volunteers (aged 17–65 yrs). Recordings were made from two temporary bipolar electrode leads: one positioned in the right atrium (J-shaped atrial lead) and the other at the apex of the right ventricle. The two leads were connected to a computer that automatically calculated, cycle by cycle, the AA, AV, and VA intervals with a precision of ±1 ms. Continuous measurements were made for 10 minutes at rest then during a cycloergometer exercise test in supine position starting at 20 watts with increments of 10 watts every minute to exhaustion, and finally for the first 5 minutes of the recovery period. During the exercise test, HR increased from an average of 81 ± 23 bpm to 167 ± 21 bpm (133–194) at peak exercise, or 97.5% (91–109) of the maximal predicted heart rate. As had already been noted by Atterhog,[7] the PR interval shortened during exercise in all the patients, moving from an average of 169 ± 21 ms (134–191) at rest to 141 ± 20 ms (100–160) at peak exercise, an average decrease of 28 ± 11 ms (11–43) or 16 ± 7%.

These results are similar to those found by other authors. In Atterhog's study[7] of exercise in supine position, the PR interval shortened from an average of 174 ms at rest to 136 ms at a rate of 140 bpm. He did not find any further significant shortening above this limit. Luceri[9] studied 437 subjects, mean age 43 years, taking no cardiodepressor drugs, with surface ECG recordings, and found an average shortening of 31 ms in the PR interval between rest (168 ms) and peak exercise (137 ms).

Whatever the actual values, in all cases, the percentage of shortening was significantly smaller for the PR interval than for the RR interval. This gives a constant and progressive increase in the PR/RR ratio during exercise. In our study,[8] this value increased from an average of 25 ± 4% at rest to 38 ± 7% at peak exercise. This suggests that there is a particular physiologic regulation of the ideal atrial depolarization time in the cardiac cycle, controlling the chronologic relationship between atrial systole and ventricular contraction and consequently the effectiveness of atrial function. It is remarkable that in both Atterhog's and our study,[7,8] the AV interval never fell below a minimal threshold of 100 ms, even for the younger patients and for the highest heart rates.

Our methodology[8] produced a mathematical formula linking the PR and RR intervals during exercise. In nine of the ten patients (Fig. 1), there was obviously an almost perfect linear relationship ($y = ax + b$), the r coefficient comprised between 0.94 and 0.99. We found an exponential curve in only one patient.

These findings correlate with those of Atterhog,[7] who found a linear relationship only between the resting heart rate and a "high" rate of 130–140 bpm. Above this level, shortening of the PR interval was minimal and not statistically significant. However, Atterhog did find considerable differences depending on the technical methodology used for the exercise test. Performed in a sitting position, the variation was, on the contrary, least significant at low rates; then the shortening became linear up to the highest rates when the slope paradoxically accelerated. In a preliminary study analyzing the surface ECG recordings of 20 normal subjects during exercise, Barbieri et al.[10] described a five-phase model with an initial phase (zone 0), corresponding to low rates where the PR interval remained constant. Zone 1 is for rates up to 90 bpm where the PR shortened very slowly, zone 2 between 90 and 120 bpm with a rapid and linear shortening of PR, and finally, zones 3 and 4 corresponding to higher rates (120–150 bpm, then >150 bpm) where the PR interval behaved in the same way it did in zones 1 and 0.

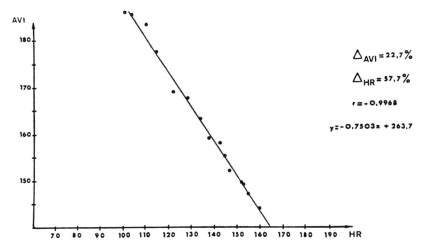

Figure 1. Physiological relationship between AV interval (AVI) and heart rate (HR) during exercise. In this healthy subject aged 21 years, there is an almost perfect (R = 0.98) linear relationship between the AV interval (endocardial recordings) and HR during a maximum exercise test.

Thus, apparently at least for physiologic ranges of HR, the PR-RR relationship is usually linear, but the slope normally remains small since the average shortening of PR was 4 ± 2 ms for an acceleration of 10 bpm in our study and 4.7 ms in Atterhog's series.[7] Nevertheless, there were large interindividual differences in both studies and we do not know much about their causes. Several questions remain unanswered: what is the effect of age, of the baseline PR value, of an eventual organic heart disease, its nature and severity, of cardiodepressor drugs? The results of our study[8] tend to give some insight but without any statistical significance due to the small number of subjects in the series. It would appear that the shortening of the PR interval during exercise could be of greater importance in middle-aged persons and in elderly subjects than in young individuals. The most significant shortening was observed during exercise in the patients with the longest PR intervals at rest.

The effects of cardiodepressor drugs has been studied by several authors. Atterhog[7] found no significant modification of the PR interval adaptation to exercise after IV propranolol. Luceri[9] also found adaptation to be nearly normal in patients treated with β-blockers or class I antiarrhythmic drugs, but only for submaximal exercise levels. This contrasts with an adaptation much less sensitive than in normal subjects at higher levels of exercise. Luceri also found the same results in patients with congestive heart failure.

Algorithms for Automatic Optimization and Rate Modulation of the AV Delay in DDD and DDR Pacing

The algorithms available in modern pacemakers naturally result from the physiologic data mentioned above. There are essentially two types of algorithms.

AV Delay Hysteresis

Most of the DDD pacemakers presently implanted have an AV delay hysteresis that automatically reduces the basic programmed AV interval by a fixed or programmable value when the unit switches from a paced atrial cycle (AV sequential mode) to a sensed atrial cycle (VDD mode). The switch occurs automatically whenever the sinus rate exceeds the programmed lower rate. A wide range of programmable values is required for this algorithm because of the wide interindividual variability in the optimal value of the AV delay hysteresis. Most of the devices (Biotronik Diplos, Intermedics Cosmos II, Medtronic Elite) have two different AV intervals: a "sensed AV interval" and a "paced AV interval," which can be programmed independently within large ranges from 15 to 30 ms to 300 ms, by 10–20 ms increments (Fig. 2). In the ELA Chorus, the basic AV delay is a sensed AV delay with an algorithm of automatic AV delay extension programmable within a range from 0 to 90 ms, by increments of 15–16 ms.

Automatic Rate-Adaptative AV Delay

The complexity and thus the level of performance of this algorithm vary greatly from one device to another.

Some models can only shorten the AV interval by an automatic fixed value when the spontaneous atrial rate exceeds a "threshold" value. In the Medtronic Elite model (Fig. 2), when this feature is programmed

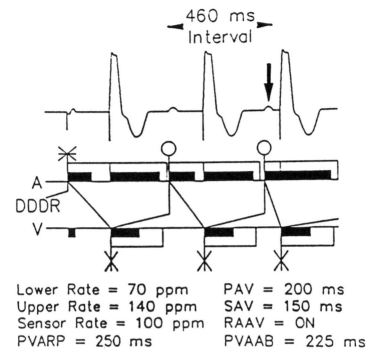

Lower Rate = 70 ppm   PAV = 200 ms
Upper Rate = 140 ppm   SAV = 150 ms
Sensor Rate = 100 ppm   RAAV = ON
PVARP = 250 ms   PVAAB = 225 ms

Figure 2. AV delay hysteresis (AVDH) and rate-adaptative AV delay (RAAVD) in the Medtronic Elite DDD/DDDR pacemaker (with permission of Medtronic Inc., USA). AVDH results from programming two different values of AVD: an AVD on paced atrial cycles (PAV) and an AVD on sensed atrial cycles (SAV). AVDH automatically shortens AVD by the difference between PAV and SAV when the unit switches form a paced cycle to a sensed cycle. RAAVD corresponds to an automatic and abrupt shortening at a fixed value of 65 ms when the AA interval (intrisic atrial rate) decreases below 500 ms.

"ON," any AA interval ≤500 ms (HR = 120 bpm) initiates a sensed AV delay of 65 ms after the atrial event. This rudimentary algorithm has the disadvantage of maintaining a fixed and sometimes long AV interval up to relatively high HR. It also induces wide variability in the length of the delay from one cycle to the next.

Most of the modern DDD pacemakers automatically adapt the AV delay step by step each time the HR rises by a certain increment. This usually produces a more or less linear adaptation, in an approximation of physiologic behavior. In the Siemens-Pacesetter models, when the spontaneous atrial rate accelerates, the PV interval (or sensed AV delay) is shortened by 25-ms steps within the limit of 75 ms less than the programmed value of the basic (or paced) AV delay. As a result, the PV interval can be 25, 50, or 75 ms less than the programmed AV delay. If these devices are programmed in a rate-responsive dual chamber (DDDR) pacing mode, the AV delay will shorten as the pacing rate increases in response to patient activity detected by the sensor. For pacing rates above the programmed basic rate and <90 bpm, no shortening of the AV interval will occur. The AV delay will shorten successively by 25-ms steps at pacing rates above 90, 110, and 130 bpm.

In the Biotronik system (Fig. 3), the sensed AV delay may be programmed at five different values within a specified range of intrinsic rates: <70, 70–90, 90–110, 110–130, and >130 bpm.

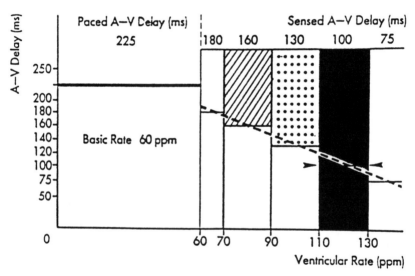

Figure 3. "Dynamic AV delay" (AVD) in the Biotronik Diplos 06 DDD pacemaker; an example of nearly linear adaptation. AVD can be programmed at six different values: a maximum value (basic AV delay) after a paced atrial event (solid line), and five different programmable values after a sensed atrial event occurring within specific ranges of intrisic rates beyond the programmed basic pacing rate: 60–70, 70–90, 90–110, 110–130, and >130 bpm. This produces a more or less linear adaptation of the AV delay to HR (broken line). (With permission of Biotronik Gmb H, Germany.)

In the Intermedics Cosmos II, when the "rate-adaptative AV delay" is programmed "ON", the pacemaker adapts the AV delay after a sensed event to changes in the preceding AA interval, in a 1:8 ratio (minimum change = 2.56 ms). Thus, for every 20.48 ms change in the AA interval, the subsequent AV delay after a sensed event will change by 2.56 ms. The minimum value, below which the AV delay will not be shortened, is calculated on the basis of the programmed pacing rate and the ventricular tracking limit and is displayed by the programmer; in no case can it be less than 75 ms.

The Vitatron algorithm (Fig. 4) has a distinguishing feature producing an exponential adaptation curve. It automatically decreases the sensed AV delay as the atrial rate increases according to the algorithm:

$$AVD_x = \left(AVD_p - 38.4 - \frac{VLRL \text{ ms}}{8}\right) + \frac{X \text{ ms}}{8}$$

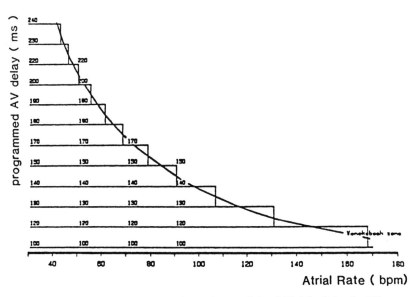

Figure 4. Algorithm for "rate dependence of the AV delay" in the Vitatron Quintech DDD pacemaker (with permission of Vitatron Medical, the Netherlands). This algorithm produces a nonlinear shortening in AVD. The exponential relationship between AVD and atrial rate results in a rapid shortening at lower HR but in a minor shortening at medium and higher HR.

where AVD_x corresponds to the real AV interval obtained from the instantaneous atrial rate, AVD_p is the programmed basic AV delay, VLRL ms is the pacing interval at the lower rate limit, and X ms the pacing interval for the HR being considered. As previously shown (Fig. 4), this algorithm decreases the AV delay exponentially with a variable curve depending on the programmed values of VLRL, VURL (pacing interval at the upper rate limit), and AVD, which causes rapid shortening in the AV interval at low and medium HR but a slow decrease at higher HR.

The ELA Chorus algorithm (Fig. 5) mimics physiology perfectly by adapting   the sensed AV delay to HR, cycle by cycle, from a lower limit of 78 bpm to an upper limit of 142 bpm, with a true linear shortening between a maximum and a minimal programmable value (Fig. 5).

Another way to mimic physiologic behavior is to vary the AV delay as a function of exercise level instead of the instantaneous HR. This can only be achieved by DDDR pacemakers. The Telectronics Meta DDDR unit, responsive to minute ventilation, uses the metabolic indicated rate (MIR) to automatically set the AV delay. The AV interval equals $\frac{1}{16}$th

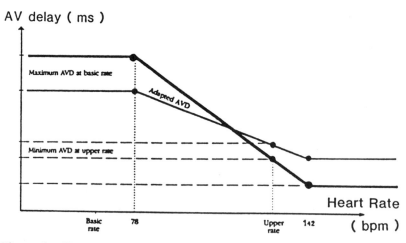

Figure 5. "Rate responsive AV delay" algorithm in the ELA Chorus DDD pacemaker (with permission of ELA Médical, France). This algorithm gives a linear beat-by-beat interpolation of the AV delay between two programmable values: a minimum value for HR $\leq$78 bpm and a maximum value for HR $\geq$142 bpm.

of the MIR interval (ms) plus a constant C, which can be programmed at a "normal" value of 80 ms or a "long" value of 100 ms. Unfortunately, this algorithm gives only very small variations in the AV delay.

Methodology: How to Measure the Optimal AV Delay in the Individual Patient

Many investigational methods have been used to determine the optimal AV delay at rest and during exercise. The invasive methods are still the gold standard because they alone can give a direct measurement of cardiac output, right heart pressures, and arterial pressure.[11,12] Noninvasive methods have different objectives. Some are used to study heart function (LV diameters and volumes, LV global and regional ejection fractions (EF), LV filling) while giving an indirect measurement of cardiac output. These methods include radionuclide angiography[13,14] and Doppler echocardiography.[2,4,15,17,18] Other methods give data on the quality of cardiorespiratory adaptation to exercise and allow measurements of VO_2max and the anaerobic threshold. Such methods include cardiopulmonary exercise testing.[19-21] Other methods included plethysmography impedance[29] and plasma c-AMP and atrial natriuretic peptide assays.[23]

In everyday clinical practice, one must rely on a single, simple, noninvasive method that is reproducible, inexpensive, widely available, and applicable to rest and exercise. When rigorously performed and interpreted, Doppler echocardiography best meets these requirements. To measure the optimal AV delay on a sensed atrial cycle at rest, the basic pacing rate first has to be programmed below the spontaneous atrial rate. Then the required sensed AV delay can be identified by determining the delay that gives the best synchronization of the A wave on the transmitral flow and the best ejection indices (Vmax; time velocity integral and calculated cardiac output) for LV ejection flow. To measure the optimal AV delay for a paced cycle, and at the same time the optimal AV delay hysteresis, the basic pacing rate is simply programmed slightly faster than the spontaneous atrial rate in order to obtain consistent atrial capture. The operator then searches for the programmed AV delay that yields the same interval between the peaks of E and A waves on the transmitral flow as the optimal interval previously measured on a sensed cycle. Finally, the development of exercise Doppler echocardiography should make it possible to determine the optimal slope of adaptation for the AV delay to HR.

Normal Range of "Optimal AV Delays"

The Basic AV Delay

Many studies have shown that in healthy individuals, the optimal AV delay in AV sequential pacing lies between 150 and 200 ms.[24] Nevertheless, under identical conditions, its value may vary greatly from one patient to another as a function of several physiologic and pathologic factors, including age (the optimal AV delay is shorter in young people) and the status of LV function. In cases of LV dysfunction, a long AV delay, 200–250 ms, is often more effective. Recent studies[25] have shown, however, a paradoxical benefit from programming very short AV delays (100 ms) in patients with drug-resistant congestive heart failure due to idiopathic dilated cardiomyopathy.

AV Delay Hysteresis (Fig. 6)

Several authors have used Doppler echocardiography to measure the individual values of AV delay extension when switching from a sensed atrial cycle to a paced atrial cycle. Wish et al.[4] found extensive interindividual variation, from 35 to 260 ms with an average of 90 ms, but his study included some patients with major intra- or interatrial conduction defects. The results of two other series[2,18] are more in agreement with mean values of 70 ± 12 and 70 ± 26 ms, respectively, and extremes of 42–83 and 16–94 ms, respectively. These findings strongly suggest the need to evaluate each individual patient's own AV delay extension. This can easily be done with noninvasive techniques. In general, however, an estimated value of about 70 ms would appear to be reasonable.

Rate-Adaptative AV Delay

Carleton[26] was the first to establish in man the presence of a beat-by-beat linear correlation between the optimal value of the PR interval, that giving the maximal atrial contribution to stroke volume, and heart

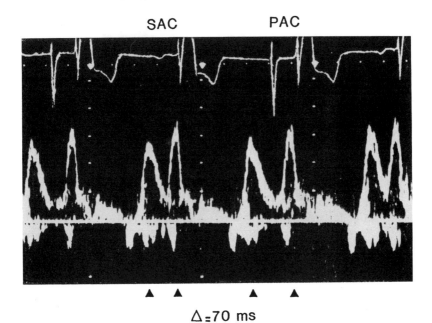

Figure 6.   The mechanical importance of AV delay hysteresis. A study of the transmitral flow by Doppler echocardiography in a patient implanted with a DDD pacemaker programmed at a fixed AVD of 156 ms. 1:1 alternance of paced atrial cycle (PAC) and sensed atrial cycle (SAC) clearly shows a constant delay of 70 ms in the peak of the A wave between SAC and PAC.

rate. By cycle-to-cycle analysis of recordings in patients with complete AV block, he demonstrated that in a given individual, there is a specific value of AV delay that is appropriate for each level of heart rate. This evidence is an additional argument in favor of AV delay rate modulation in DDD pacing aimed at optimizing the mechanical delay between atrial systole and ventricular contraction at each cycle, thus offering the patient the most efficient hemodynamic performance.

In the 1980s, several studies were performed to demonstrate the potential benefit of rate adaptation of the AV delay in patients implanted with DDD pacemakers. Due to the lack of automatic algorithms, these studies were based on comparisons of different programmed values of the AV delay that remained constant all along the protocol in the same patient.[19,20] Except for the study of Mehta et al.,[17] the results were disappointing and led to negative conclusions as to the interest of such adaptation.

In 1989 we published[11] the results of a hemodynamic study in 10 patients with complete AV block who were temporarily paced in DOO mode at rates progressively increasing, by 10 bpm per minute steps, from 90 to 150 bpm. This study was designed to come as close as possible to the situation of spontaneous rate adaptation during an exercise test. Three different modes were tested in random order: fixed AV delay of 200 ms, fixed AV delay of 150 ms, and AV delay adapted to HR by reducing by 20 ms every 10 bpm acceleration between a maximum value of 220 ms at 90 bpm and a minimum value of 100 ms at 150 bpm. Thus, the procedure gave a variation in AV delay four to five times greater than the physiologic variation in PR.[8] Significant differences were observed in favor of rate-adapted AV delay (RAAVD) for the two principal hemodynamic parameters studied, i.e., cardiac index (Fig. 7) and pulmo-

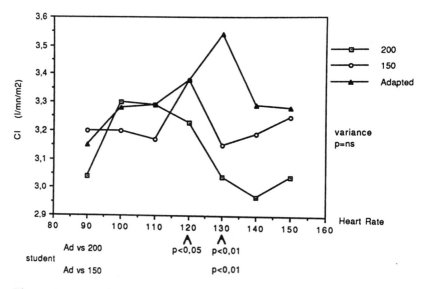

Figure 7. Hemodynamic benefit of a rate-adapted AV delay in DOO Pacing at increasing rates: behavior of cardiac index (CI). Rate-adapted AV delay (Ad) significantly improves the cardiac performance in comparison with a 200 ms fixed AVD at 120 bpm, and with 200 and 150 ms fixed AVD at 130 bpm.

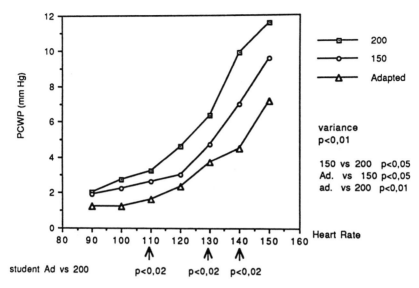

Figure 8. Hemodynamic benefit of a rate-adapted AV delay in DOO pacing at increasing rates: behavior of pulmonary capillary wedge pressure (PCWP). Rate-adapted AV delay (Ad) significantly reduces LV filling pressure in comparison with 200 and 150 ms fixed AV delay at pacing rates ranging from 110 to 140 bpm.

nary capillary wedge pressure (Fig. 8). For cardiac index, the best curve was observed with RAAVD, but, as is logical, the level of performance was identical to that obtained with the 200 ms fixed AVD at the lowest rate of 90 bpm, and to that obtained with the 150 ms fixed AVD at the medium rate of 120 bpm. On the contrary, at 130 bpm and beyond, the performance was significantly better with RAAVD. This study can, however, still be criticized because it was conducted at rest and did not take into account the hemodynamic and metabolic modifications of exercise.

The advent of implantable DDD pacemakers with automatic RAAVD mimicking physiology has allowed such studies in exercising patients. Two studies[12,21] were designed with similar experimental protocols aimed at comparing a fixed AV delay (156 ms) with an RAAVD based on a linear reduction between a maximal value of 156 ms at a low rate of 78 bpm and a minimal value of 63 ms at a high rate of 142 bpm during standard exercise tests. The patients received an ELA Chorus DDD pacemaker for high degree AV block. In the first study,[12] hemodynamic performance was studied and the upper rate limit (URL) was programmed at 120 bpm in all patients. At peak exercise, the ventricular rate (p = 0.008) and the rate × pressure product (p = 0.005) were significantly higher with RAAVD, while the pulmonary capillary wedge pressure (p = 0.03; Fig. 9) and the cycle-to-cycle arterial pressure variability (0.001 < p < 0.02) were lower. There was a tendency towards increased cardiac output (Fig. 10) and decreased atrial rate. This study demonstrates a slight but unquestionable hemodynamic benefit with RAAVD compared with the fixed AVD.

The second study[21] evaluated cardiopulmonary performance without limitation of URL. Exercise duration was significantly longer with RAAVD (224 ± 111 vs. 187 ± 97 sec; p < 0.01). At anaerobic threshold, VO_2 (757 ± 263 vs. 664 ± 290 mL/min, p < 0.02) and VCO_2 (634 ± 236 vs. 549 ± 249 mL/min, p < 0.002) were significantly higher, and the differences remained significant at peak exercise in favor of RAAVD. These results suggest that cardiopulmonary performance during exercise is significantly improved by RAAVD.

The problem of optimizing this algorithm for each individual re-

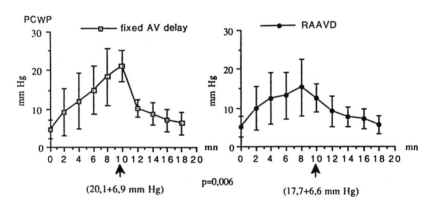

Figure 9. Comparison of an automatic rate-responsive AV delay (RAAVD) and of a fixed AVD (156 ms) during exercise in patients chronically implanted for complete AV block (n = 11). At peak exercise (arrows) (cycloergometer sitting), the average pulmonary capillary wedge pressure (PCWP) was significantly decreased with RAAVD, compared with the fixed value.

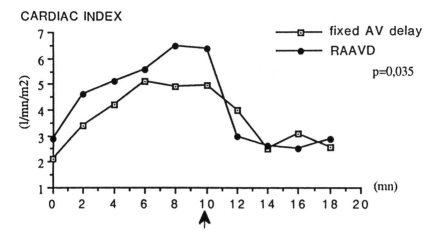

Figure 10. Comparison of an automatic rate-responsive AV delay (RAAVD) and a fixed but individually optimized (Doppler echocardiography) AVD in a patient chronically implanted for complete AV block. At each exercise level, and especially at peak exercise (arrow), RAAVD produced significantly higher cardiac index (CI) compared with the fixed value.

mains to be solved. It is very likely that there is an optimal adaptation slope for each individual patient as well as a critical minimal value for the AV delay below which it would be best not to shorten. Further work, in particular with Doppler echocardiography is needed to find the answer to these questions. Until such results are available, it appears advisable to program near the "physiologic" slope of a mean variation of 4 ms per a 10 bpm acceleration in HR.[8]

Nonphysiologic Situations

The most characteristic example is high degree interatrial blocks. Although this situation is rare in the general population,[27] the prevalence of interatrial blocks is relatively high in pacemaker patients and has been estimated (personal data) at 12% of patients with high degree AV block and 35% of patients with atrial disease. Even in the latter, high degree interatrial block is often associated with AV conduction disorders requiring the DDD mode for permanent pacing. If a "classic" 150–200 ms

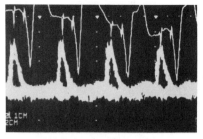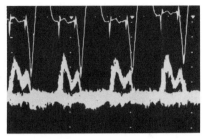

AV Delay = 150 msec   AV Delay = 250 msec

Figure 11.   Doppler echocardiographic demonstration of the deleterious consequences of advanced interatrial block in patients paced in the DDD mode. No A wave can be seen on the transmitral flow when the AV delay is programmed at a "usual" value of 150 ms. It is necessary to prolong AVD at 250 ms for recovering a correctly synchronized A wave.

AV delay is programmed in these patients, the greatly extended interatrial conduction time (mean $= 145 \pm 32$ ms in our series) results in a very delayed left atrial systole. The atrial kick then occurs during ventricular contraction when the mitral valve is closed, thereby losing the hemodynamic efficacy of atrial systole (Fig. 11). Restoration of effective atrial systole requires programming a very long AV delay of 250–300 ms. But this has two major disadvantages. First, the interatrial asynchrony remains untouched, with the resultant risk of arrhythmia (atypical atrial flutter).[27] Second, the pacemaker must have a very long total atrial refractory period (TARP) that substantially lowers its upper rate limit (URL) and reduces the capacity for exercise adaptation. In order to solve this twofold problem, we have proposed resynchronizing the electrical and mechanical activity of the two atria by pacing them simultaneously.[3] The system uses two atrial leads: one placed in the usual position in the right atrium and the other in the coronary sinus to pace and sense the left atrium at its inferior wall. A "triple chamber pacemaker" paces the two atria simultaneously, in synchrony with the ventricular stimulus. The effectiveness of this system in preventing atrial arrhythmias[28] and optimizing cardiac performance[3] has been demonstrated with traditional programmed values for AV delay and a significantly shorter TARP. The hemodynamic benefit is illustrated in Figure 12 and in Table 1. For a mean optimal AV delay of 175 ms, dual atrial pacing increases cardiac

TABLE *1*

Hemodynamic Benefits of Permanent Atrial Resynchronization in Patients with Advanced Interatrial Blocks Paced in the DDD Mode

Patient No.	Cardiac Output (L/mm)			Optional AV Delay (ms)		
	Uni	Dual	Δ	Dual	Uni	Δ
1	5.7	6.5	+14%	150	250	100
2	4.6	5.9	+28%	200	?	?
3	5.1	6.8	+33%	150	200	50
4	4.9	6	+23%	150	250	100
5	4.3	5	+16%	250	?	?
6	6.6	8.1	+23%	150	250	100
m ± SD	5.2 ± 0.8	6.4 ± 1	23 ± 6%	175 ± 30		

Patient No.	Pulmonary Capillary Wedge Pressure			Optional AV Delay (ms)		
	Uni	Dual	Δ	Dual	Uni	Δ
1	14	12	−14%	200	?	?
2	22.5	15	−33%	200	?	?
3	15	7.5	−50%	125	250	125
4	12	8.5	−30%	100	200	100
5	20	18	−10%	250	?	?
6	12	9	−25%	150	250	100
m ± SD	16 ± 3	12 ± 3	27 ± 13%	171 ± 45		

Comparison of a single right atrium pacing mode (Uni) and a simultaneous dual atrium pacing mode (Dual) at identical pacing rates in six patients. Δ = difference (%) between Dual and Uni; ? = nondeterminable.

output by 23 ± 10% and decreases pulmonary capillary wedge pressure by 27 ± 13% in comparison with single right atrial DDD pacing. Indeed, to reach a similar degree of performance with the DDD mode, the AV delay has to be lengthened by 100 ms (mean) as compared to the dual atrial mode.

This new concept of permanent atrial resynchronization illustrates the importance in these particular situations of preserving fully effective atrial function without altering pacemaker behavior at high atrial rates.

TRANSMITRAL FLOW   LV EJECTION FLOW

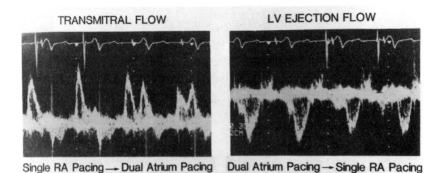

Single RA Pacing → Dual Atrium Pacing   Dual Atrium Pacing → Single RA Pacing

Figure 12.   Mechanical benefit of permanent atrial resynchronization in patients with advanced interatrial block paced in DDD mode. Doppler echo study of the transmitral flow and of the LV ejection flow. Though AVD remains constant at 150 ms, switching from a single right atrium pacing mode to a simultaneous dual atrium pacing mode produces the recovery of a well-synchronized A wave and increases significantly Vmax and the time velocity integral of the ejection flow.

The Relative Importance of AV Synchrony and the Ventricular Activation Sequence

The hemodynamic benefit of permanent cardiac pacing, independent of the basic heart function (nature and stage of any underlying cardiopathy) depends on two main parameters: first, effective atrial function through optimal AV synchrony, and second, the ventricular activation sequence.

Three recent studies underline the importance of the ventricular activation sequence. The results of these three studies are in perfect agreement, though each used a different method: radionuclide angiography at rest, and Doppler echocardiography at rest and during exercise,[14] cardiopulmonary exercise testing,[29] and hemodynamics and radionuclide angiography in our own work.[30] In patients implanted with a DDD or DDDR pacemaker for isolated sinus node dysfunction (intact AV conduction and narrow QRS), three different pacing modes were evaluated at rest and during exercise: AAI mode maintaining AV synchrony and a normal ventricular activation sequence, DDD mode with complete ventricular capture but preserving AV synchrony, and VVI mode lacking both. In the three studies, the AAI mode produced a significant benefit over DDD pacing, both at rest and during exercise. This benefit was observed for all the parameters measured: cardiac output and pulmonary pressures[30] (Figs. 13 and 14), global and regional (septal) LV ejection fractions,[14,30] and VO_2 and O_2 pulse at peak exercise.[29] No significant difference was observed between the DDD mode and the VVI mode in Rosenqvist's series,[14] but in our personal study,[30] we found a significant benefit with the DDD mode, although the effect was observed only for hemodynamic parameters[30] (Figs. 13 and 14).

The deleterious effects of apical pacing in the right ventricle are similar to those encountered with left bundle branch block.[31] Inversion of the ventricular activation sequence creates major activation asynchrony between the two ventricles and within the left ventricle, disrupting septal motion.

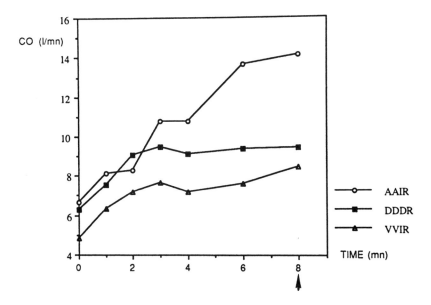

Figure 13.   Hemodynamic importance of preserving a normal sequence of ventricular activation. Comparison of three pacing modes (AAI, VVI, and DDD) at identical pacing rates during exercise in a patient chronically implanted for sinus node disease with intact AV conduction and narrow QRS. Cardiac output (CO) is significantly higher in the AAI mode than in the DDD and VVI modes at each exercise level and especially at peak exercise (arrow).

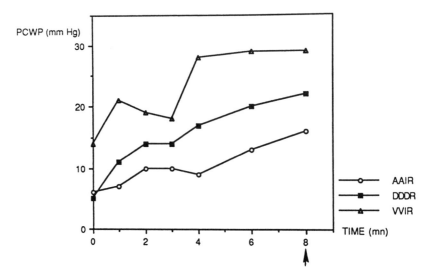

Figure 14. Hemodynamic importance of preserving a normal sequence of ventricular activation. Comparison of three pacing modes (AAI, VVI, and DDD) at identical pacing rates during exercise in a patient chronically implanted for sinus node disease with intact AV conduction and narrow QRS. Pulmonary capillary wedge pressure (PCWP) is significantly lower in the AAI mode than in the DDD and VVI modes at each exercise level, and especially at peak exercise (arrow).

These observations suggest that the normal ventricular activation sequence should be preserved and the ventricle should not be paced except for inadequate AV or intraventricular conduction. Ventricular pacing could thus be avoided in many cases of isolated sinus node dysfunction as well as in most cases of carotid sinus syndrome and vasovagal syndrome and in certain circumstances of paroxysmal AV block. This objective can be obtained with many available techniques: programming in the AAI mode, programming in the DDD or DDI mode with a basic AV delay longer than the spontaneous PR or the stimulus-R interval, and use of an automatic algorithm that maintains the AAI mode as long as AV conduction is normal and switches to the DDD mode when the PR interval increases beyond a critical value or when a nonconducted P wave occurs (ELA Medical Chorus II).

Thus it appears that in certain circumstances, the optimal AV delay is not actually the delay that would guarantee maximal left atrial contribution, but rather the delay that provides the best hemodynamic compromise between AV conduction time (which might be lengthened) and a normal ventricular activation sequence.

Conversely, abnormally long AV delays cannot be accepted simply to maintain the normal ventricular activation sequence. This point has been clearly demonstrated in a series of patients with a very long spontaneous PR interval in whom DDD pacing provides functional and he-

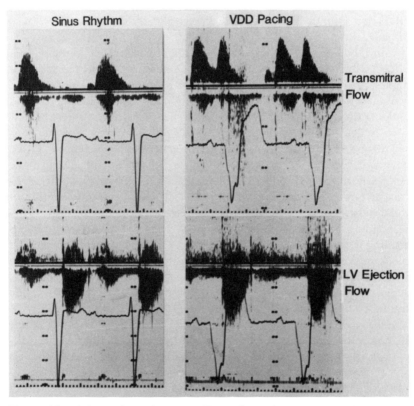

Figure 15. Adverse hemodynamic effects of very long PR intervals: Doppler echocardiographic demonstration. No A wave is seen on transmitral flow in sinus rhythm. Temporary DDD pacing with a 150 ms AVD produces recovering of a well-synchronized A wave and significantly increases Vmax and the time velocity integral of the LV ejection flow.

modynamic benefit by restoring an effective left atrial function despite obligatory ventricular pacing (Fig. 15).[32]

Optimization of AV Synchrony in Daily Life Activities

A complementary and major advantage of the AV delay rate-modulation algorithms (AV delay hysteresis and automatic rate-adaptive AV delay), but also of atrial resynchronization in the particular case of high degree interatrial blocks, is to optimize the upper rate response of DDD and DDDR pacemakers, and consequently the exercise tolerance of patients.

In DDD pacing, exercise tolerance depends above all on the highest HR at which 1:1 AV synchrony may be sustained. Theoretically, the highest possible upper rate limit should be programmed not only to guarantee normal AV synchrony up to high sinus rates, but also to avoid undesirable triggering of the algorithms for ventricular protection, especially 2:1 block and Wenckebach behavior. The hemodynamic consequences of such algorithms have not been investigated extensively. We have recently studied[33] eight patients chronically paced in the DDD mode (ELA Chorus pacemaker) for complete AV block. Atrial rate (AR), ventricular rate (VR), and arterial pressure (AP) were continuously monitored during four consecutive exercise tests at a constant workload corresponding to the maximum workload achieved during a previous training test. Each test lasted 2 minutes. 1:1 AV synchrony, Wenckebach block response (W), 2:1 AV synchrony, and fallback (F) were tested in random order. Results (Table 2) show that AR was the lowest with 1:1, suggesting a lower metabolic demand. A time of 1:1 AV reassociation during recovery was significantly (p = 0.001) shorter with W (35 ± 20 sec) than with F (97 ± 24 sec) and 2:1 (85 ± 35 sec). 1:1 provided the highest VR, diastolic AP, mean AP, and rate pressure product. In comparison, the worst mode was 2:1, and the less deleterious was W. This study clearly shows that algorithms for ventricular protection are hemodynamically deleterious and that a high URL has to be programmed as often as possible to avoid their triggering. However, the tracking rate must remain compatible with the physiologic and pathologic status of the individual patient, taking into account age, physical activity, the presence of ischemic heart disease or congestive heart failure, and especially the potential risk for atrial tachyarrhythmias.

TABLE *2*

Hemodynamic Consequences of Triggering Ventricular Protection Algorithms During Exercise in DDD Pacing (n = 9 pts.)

	1:1	*W*	*2:1*	*F*	*Variance (p)*
VR (bpm)	138 ± 12	95 ± 12	72 ± 6	86 ± 11	0.0001
AR (bpm)	138 ± 12	148 ± 13	146 ± 14	144 ± 21	0.0025
Syst. Art P (mm Hg)	226 ± 12	205 ± 29	206 ± 25	210 ± 34	ns
Diast. Art P (mm Hg)	92 ± 10	70 ± 17	63 ± 10	68 ± 10	0.0001
Mean Art P (mm Hg)	144 ± 14	121 ± 23	116 ± 16	121 ± 18	0.0001
Rate Pres. Product	3126 ± 371	2098 ± 445	1502 ± 217	1793 ± 246	0.0001
AV Reassociation (sec)		35 ± 20	85 ± 35	97 ± 24	0.001

1:1 = 1:1 AV conduction; W = Wenckebach association; 2:1 = 2:1 AV block; F = fallback; VR = ventricular rate; AR = atrial rate; Syst. Art P = systolic arterial pressure; Diast. Art P = diastolic arterial pressure; Mean Art P = mean arterial pressure; Rate Pres. Product = heart rate × SAP product; AV Reassociation = time delay to 1:1 AV reassociation during recovery.

In DDD pacing, URL cannot exceed the 2:1 point corresponding to the TARP, which is the sum of the AV delay and of the postventricular atrial refractory period (PVARP). Unfortunately, most of the presently available units have to be programmed with long or relatively long PVARP, such as 300 ms or more, because (except some models) they do not have reliable algorithms to prevent PMTs. Such programming decreases dramatically the 2:1 point, holding down URL and potentially the patient's exercise capacity. Looking at a practical example (Table 3) shows that programming a fixed AV delay of 200 ms and a PVARP of 300 ms would limit the tracking rate to 120 bpm. AV delay rate modulation algorithms make it possible to raise URL significantly by shortening TARP. This can be done either abruptly from one cycle to the next by the AV delay hysteresis, or progressively by tracking the spontaneously increasing atrial rate with an automatic RAAVD. These two algorithms can be combined in perfect synergy to achieve optimized adaptation. Thus, by programming an AVDH of 70 ms, the sensed AV delay can be reduced to 130 ms and URL can be raised by 20 bpm, giving 1:1 AV synchrony up to rates of 140 bpm. Now combining this 70 ms AVDH with an automatic rate-adaptive AV delay mimicking the physiologic adaptation of the PR interval gives a significant amplification of this benefit (URL = 154 bpm) while preserving an acceptable value for the minimal AV delay (90 ms).

TABLE *3*

Optimization of the Upper Rate in DDD Pacing by AV Delay Rate Modulation Algorithms

PVARP (ms)	Fixed AV Delay			AV Delay Hysteresis (70 ms)			AVDH + RAAV (70 ± 40 ms)		
	AVD	TARP	URL	AVD	TARP	URL	AVD	TARP	URL
250	150	400	150	150	330	182	150	290	207
	200	450	133	200	380	158	200	340	176
300	150	450	133	150	380	158	150	340	176
	200	500	120	200	430	140	200	390	154
350	150	500	120	150	430	140	150	390	154
	200	550	109	200	480	125	200	440	136

PVARP = postventricular atrial refractory period; AVD = AV delay; TARP = total atrial refractory period; URL = upper rate limit; AVDH = AV delay hysteresis; RAAV = rate-adaptive AV delay.

As previously seen, these theoretical considerations were confirmed by clinical studies demonstrating significant improvement in ergometric and respiratory performances with RAAVD.[21] Moreover, we can emphasize that these algorithms may optimize the upper rate response even when programming a low value of URL in order to protect against rapid atrial rates. In a study where URL was intentionally limited to 120 bpm,[12] we observed that despite a low level of exercise, RAAVD delayed the onset of Wenckebach block response or of 2:1 AV block during exercise by an average of 38 seconds and inversely shortened the time to 1:1 AV reassociation during recovery by an average of 17 seconds, compared with a fixed AV delay. Moreover, a 2:1 block occurred at peak exercise in only two patients in the rate-adaptative mode compared to 6/10 with the fixed AV delay. And finally, RAAVD significantly decreased the Wenckebach ratio and the subsequent escape interval for the Wenckebach cycle by increasing the difference between TARP and URL interval.

Conclusion

Individual tuning of the AV delay is fundamental to optimize both hemodynamic benefit offered by DDD and DDDR pacing and the behavior of these pacemakers at upper rates that is the principal factor limiting the physical capacity of the patient. This objective may be achieved by an optimal programming of the basic AV delay that can be individually determined by Doppler echocardiography and by the optimal use of AV delay rate modulation algorithms with, when possible, the wise combination of an AV delay hysteresis and of an automatic rate-adaptative AV delay, thus mimicking the physiologic linear relationship between the PR interval and heart rate during exercise.

References

1. Wish M, Fletcher RD, Cohn A. Hemodynamics of AV synchrony and rate. J Electrophysiol 1989;3:170–175.
2. Ritter P, Mabo P, Cereze P, et al. Interest and assessment of the atrioventricular hysteresis function in dual chamber pacing. Eur Heart J 1992 (in press).
3. Daubert C, Mabo Ph, Berder V, et al. Simultaneous dual atrium pacing in high degree interatrial blocks: Hemodynamic results (abstr). Circulation 1991;84:II-453.
4. Wish M, Fletcher RD, Gotdiener JS, et al. Importance of left atrial timing in the programming of dual chamber pacemaker. Am J Cardiol 1987;60: 566–571.
5. Lepeschkin E. Modern Electrocardiography. Williams & Wilkins Baltimore, 1951, p 151.
6. Bengtsson E. The exercise electrocardiograpm in healthy children and in comparison with adults. Acta Med Scand 1956;154:225.
7. Atterhog JH, Loogna E. PR interval in relation to heart rate during exercise and the influence of posture and autonomic tone. J Electrocardiology 1977; 10:331–336.
8. Daubert C, Ritter P, Mabo P, et al. Physiological relationship between AV interval and heart rate in healthy subjects: applications to dual chamber pacing. PACE 1986;9:1032–1039.
9. Luceri R, Brownstein SL, Vardeman L. PR interval behavior during exercise: implications for physiologic pacemaker. PACE 1990;13:1719–1723.
10. Barbieri D, Percoco GF, Toselli T, et al. AV delay and exercise stress tests: behavior in normal subjects. PACE 1990;13:1724–1727.
11. Ritter P, Daubert C, Mabo P, et al. Hemodynamic benefit of a rate adapted AV delay in dual chamber pacing. Eur Heart J 1989;10:637–646.
12. Mabo P, Ritter P, Varin C, et al. Intérêts d'un algorithme d'adaptation automatique du délai AV à la fréquence atriale instantanée en stimulation cardiaque DDD. Arch Mal Coeur 1992;85:1001–1009.
13. Videen JS, Huang SK, Bazgan ID, et al. Hemodynamic comparison of ventricular pacing, atrioventricular sequential pacing and atrial synchronous

ventricular pacing using radionuclide ventriculography. Am J Cardiol 1986; 57:1305–1308.

14. Rosenqvist M, Isaaz K, Botvinick EH, et al. Relative importance of activation sequence compared to atrioventricular synchrony in left ventricular function. Am J Cardiol 1991;67:148–156.

15. Iwase M, Sotobata I, Yokota M, et al. Evaluation by pulsed Doppler echocardiography of the atrial contribution to left ventricular filling in patients with DDD pacemakers. Am J Cardiol 1986;58:104–109.

16. Lascault G, Bigonzi F, Frank R, et al. Non-invasive study of dual chamber pacing by pulsed Doppler. Prediction of the hemodynamic response by echocardiographic measurements. Eur Heart J 1989;10:525–531.

17. Mehta D, Gilmour S, Ward DE, et al. Optimal atrioventricular delay at rest and during exercise in patients with dual chamber pacemakesr: a non-invasive assessment by continuous wave döppler. Br Heart J 1989;61:161–166.

18. Rey JL, Slama MA, Triboulloy C, et al. Etude par écho-dôppler des variations hémodynamiques entre modes double-stimulation et détectio de l'oreillette ches des patients porteurs d'un stimulateur double-chambre. Arch Mal Coeur 1990;83:961–966.

19. Ryden L, Kerlsson O, Kristensson BE. The importance of different atrioventricular intervals for exercise capacity. PACE 1988;11:1051–1062.

20. Haskell RJ, French WJ. Physiological importance of different atrioventricular intervals to improved exercise performance in patients with dual chamber pacemaker. Br Heart J 1989;61:46–51.

21. Ritter P, Vai F, Bonnet JL, et al. Rate adaptative atrioventricular delay improves cardiopulmonary performances in patients implanted with a dual chamber pacemaker for complete heart block. Eur J CPE 1991;1:31–38.

22. Eugene M, Lascault G, Frank R, et al. Assessment of the optimal atrioventricular delay in DDD paced patients by impedance plethysmography. Eur Heart J 1989;10:250–255.

23. Theodorakis G, Kremastinos D, Mardianos M, et al. C-AMP and ANP levels in VVI and DDD pacing with different AV delays during daily activity and exercise. PACE 1990;13:1773–1778.

24. Daubert C, Ritter P, Mabo P, et al. Hemodynamic response to cardiac pacing in DDD mode. In: Barold SS, Mugica J (eds.). New Perspectives in Cardiac Pacing 1, Futura Publishing Co, Mount Kisco, NY, 1988, pp 27–43.

25. Hochleitner M, Hörtnagl H, Choi-Keung Ng, et al. Usefulness of physiological dual chamber-pacing in drug-resistant idiopathic dilated cardiomyopathy. Am J Cardiol 1990;66:198–202.

26. Carleton RA, Passovoy M, Graettinger JS. The importance of the contribution and timing of left atrial systole. Clin Sci 1966;30:151–154.

27. Bayès de Luna A, Cladella M, Oter R, et al. Interatrial conduction block with retrograde activation of the left atrium and paroxysmal supraventricular tachyarrhythmia. Eur Heart J 1988;9:1112–1118.

28. Mabo P, Berder V, Ritter P, et al. Prevention of atrial tachyarrhythmias related to advanced interatrial block by permanent atrial resynchronization (abstr). PACE 1991;14:648.

29. Harper GR, Pina IL, Kutalek SP. Intrinsic conduction maximizes cardio-pulmonary performance in patients with dual chamber pacemakers. PACE 1991;14:1787–1791.
30. Leclercq C, Mabo P, Le Helloco A, et al. Hemodynamic interest of pre-serving a normal sequence of ventricular activation in permanent cardiac pacing (abstr). J Am Coll Cardiol 1992;19:66A.
31. Grines C, Bashore T, Boudoulas H, et al. Functional abnormalities in isolated left bundle branch block; the effect of interventricular asynchrony. Circu-lation 1989;79:845–853.
32. Mabo P, Cazeau S, Forrer A, et al. Isolated long PR interval as only indi-cation of permanent DDD pacing (abstr). J Am Coll Cardiol 1992;19:150A.
33. Ritter P, Mabo P, Varin C, et al. Effects of 1:1 Wenckebach, 2:1 AV as-sociations and fallback on arterial pressure and cycle to cycle arterial pressure variability during exercise in DDD pacing (abstr). PACE 1991;14:682.

Chapter 11

Advances in Sensor Technology for Activity Rate-Adaptive Pacemakers: Traditional Piezoelectric Crystal Versus Accelerometer

ECKHARD ALT

Introduction

While rate-adaptive pacing was considered a rather esoteric form of treatment in the early or even the late 1980s, it is now utilized routinely in clinical practice. The popularity of rate-adaptive devices stems from their relatively simple clinical applicability and follow-up, as well as the lack of additional risks associated with implantation. These basic requirements are best exemplified by activity-controlled rate-adaptive (i.e., dependent on body activity) pacemakers, now by far the most widely used rate-adaptive devices.

There are now two ways of using body activity for rate control of pacemakers. The traditional way involves the detection of vibrational forces and pressure on the pacemaker can according to the activity of the patient (Activitrax principle). The more recently developed approach utilizes acceleration forces detected by a small accelerometer integrated into the pacemaker's electronic circuitry. This chapter focuses on the technological advances and potential clinical benefits of new accelerometer-driven, rate-adaptive pacemakers.

New Perspectives in Cardiac Pacing, Vol. 3, edited by S. Serge Barold and Jacques Mugica, Mount Kisco, NY, Futura Publishing Co., © 1993.

Functional Characteristics of Vibration and Acceleration Sensors

The purpose of any activity or motion sensor is to convert mechanical forces detected within the patient's body into electrical signals. Therefore, all activity sensors can be described as mechanoelectrical converters. The sensors used in pacemakers for conversion of mechanical phenomena into electrical signals are based on piezo effects (i.e., piezoelectric crystals, piezoresistive structures, and piezocapacitive sensors). A typical piezoelectric sensor is a self-generating source and produces voltages in the range of 50 to 100 mV in response to mechanical forces and therefore consumes virtually no battery power.

Comparison of Sensors for Detection of Vibration and Acceleration

Mechanoelectrical sensors are currently used in two different ways for rate control in pacemakers. Traditionally they act as transducers of vibration, shock, and pressure applied to the pacemaker can. Thus, in pacemakers such as the Activitrax, Legend, Synergyst, Elite (Medtronic), Sensolog, Synchrony (Pacesetter-Siemens), or Ergos (Biotronik), the sensor is cemented or bonded to the inner side of the pacemaker (or housing) can (Fig. 1, top). The piezoelectric sensor must make a tight contact with the pacemaker housing to transduce the mechanical phenomena to the piezoelectric sensor. Accelerometers detect mechanical phenomena in a somewhat different way and therefore do not need tight contact with the pacemaker housing. The acceleration forces are transmitted by a small seismic mass attached to the piezo structure. With body movement in an anterior-posterior direction, the small mass is accelerated and decelerated and exhibits a mechanical force that produces a voltage output at the piezoelectric sensor. These sensors are very small and the one used in the Intermedics accelerometer-controlled pacemakers (Relay and Dash) is 4.6 × 3.8 × 1.5 mm in size while the one used in CPI's accelerometer-controlled devices (Excel and Vigor) is 6 × 2 × 1.5 mm (Fig. 1, bottom). Since an accelerometer responds to body movements, but is not dependent on local pressure and force against the pacemaker can, it can detect walking activities with a good (linear) correlation with true energy expenditure (Fig. 2). Figure 2 shows the acceleration forces

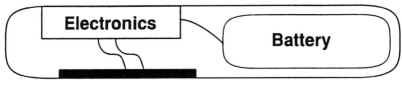

Piezoelectric Device

ACCELEROMETER TECHNOLOGY

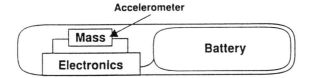

The accelerometer is mounted on the hybrid circuit and monitors body motion rather than vibration

Figure 1. Vibration accelerometer sensors. Top: Piezoelectric sensor glued to the inner case of a pacemaker. Bottom: The size and weight of accelerometers are small, allowing easy incorporation into the electronic hybrid circuitry without the need of pacemaker housing contact.

in g-values detected from a volunteer in the three axes: vertical, lateral, and horizontal. With walking, continual low frequency acceleration and deceleration signals can be recorded in all three axes. During treadmill exercise, signal amplitude increases with increasing speed and also increases considerably with an increase in the slope of the treadmill because walking uphill produces more vigorous movement of the upper body compared to level walking. This response represents an advantage over conventional vibration piezoelectric-driven devices in which the signal detected by the sensor depends mostly on how hard the foot hits the ground. Conventional vibration-controlled activity pacemakers typically

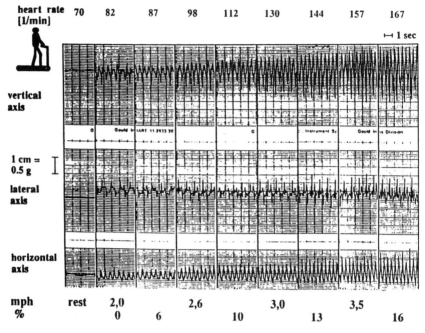

Figure 2. Acceleration signals in the vertical, lateral, and horizontal (anterior-posterior) direction recorded from a healthy volunteer undergoing treadmill exercise. The protocol[23] starts with 3.2 km (2 miles) per hour, 0% incline, and then calls for increases in speed and then slope (alternately) up to a maximum speed of 3.5 mph and a 16% incline. The heart rate increased from 70 bpm to 167 bpm in a linear fashion. Note that frequency and amplitude of the acceleration signals also increase linearly with greater speed and also with greater incline.

tend to increase the pacing rate less with walking uphill compared to level walking.

The typical frequency spectrum of acceleration forces for walking and for everyday exercise falls in the low frequency range between 1 and 4 Hz.[1-6] in contrast to forces centering around 10 Hz generally detected by vibration-sensitive rate-adaptive devices.[7,8] With the new type of accelerometer-based devices, a 4-Hz low pass filter is required to enhance the differentiation of noise signals from true exercise signals.[1,5] Better signal discrimination based on selective frequency sensing of acceleration signals appears to be an important advantage of acceleration-controlled devices.

Clinical Experience with Vibration Controlled Pacemakers

Several studies investigating the behavior of rate-adaptive pacemakers controlled by piezoelectric sensors during a variety of physical activities[8–14] have demonstrated that the speed of reaction of these systems corresponds closely to that of the normal sinus node. In this regard, no important difference was found between Medtronic or Pacesetter-Siemens vibration-controlled activity pacemakers. Several studies evaluating the capability of various activity-controlled devices to discriminate different levels of workload[8–10,15–17] found that an increase in walking speed results in a correct increase of the pacing rate with all vibration-sensitive devices manufactured by Medtronic or Pacesetter-Siemens. A better response to graded treadmill activities has been reported with the Pacemaker-Siemens Sensolog pacemaker,[8,10] while the Medtronic activity-controlled devices have generally demonstrated a weaker discrimination of varying workloads related to different slopes on the treadmill.[8,13] Each time the foot hits the ground, a mechanical (vibration) wave travels through the body. Vibration-controlled devices, therefore, sense the forces emanating mainly from impact of the feet on the ground. With walking uphill or on a treadmill with an incline, the foot is set to the ground from a lower altitude and a somewhat smoother movement results. Therefore, when walking uphill or going up stairs, the mechanical forces detected by vibration-sensitive sensors seem to be weaker compared to the shock and mechanical waves that travel through the body during level walking or when going downhill or down stairs. Several studies have confirmed this assumption by comparing the pacemaker response when going up stairs and down stairs. Walking down stairs generally resulted in a 10–15 beat higher pacing rate than walking up stairs,[12,17] reflecting the importance of the power used in hitting the ground.[13,17] In this respect, the new acceleration-controlled devices generally provide a more satisfactory response to various activities (Fig. 3). Accelerometer-based devices generate a better response walking up stairs (103 bpm) vs. walking down stairs (98 bpm) compared to the weaker response of vibration-sensitive devices when walking up stairs (83 bpm) vs. walking down stairs (89 bpm) at 80 steps per minute (Fig. 3).[15,16]

Several studies have addressed the susceptibility of activity-controlled pacemakers to environmental noise. With regard to vibration-controlled devices, riding in a car or other everyday activities have shown

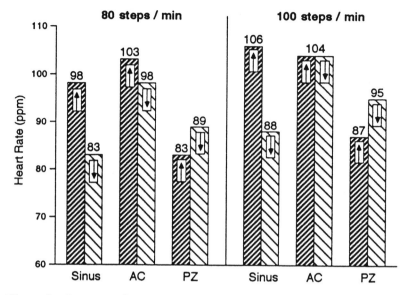

Figure 3. Response of 10 asymptomatic, healthy subjects walking up stairs and down stairs at two different speeds. A vibration-sensitive piezoelectric device and an accelerometer-controlled device were both strapped to the subjects in the midpectoral area. Both pacemakers were programmed to nominal settings as stated by the manufacturers. A metronome was employed to help the subjects keep a steady rate. The accelerometer-controlled devices more closely mimic the intrinsic rate response. The vibration-sensitive piezoelectric devices exhibited a less satisfactory overall response and produced a paradoxical increase in the rate when walking down stairs. (Sinus = sinus rate of the healthy volunteers; AC = accelerometer-controlled devices; PZ = vibration piezoelectric-controlled devices. (Reproduced with permission.[25])

no major effect on the pacing rate, but dental drilling can drive a vibration-controlled device to the upper rate,[18]

Clinical Experience with Accelerometer Controlled Pacemakers

In accelerometer-controlled devices, pedal impact has much less influence on pacing rate compared to piezoelectric vibration-sensitive devices. Since the accelerometer is oriented in an anterior-posterior direction (horizontal), motion of the upper body in an anterior–posterior direction produces the main activity signal for accelerometer function. When walking uphill, the upper body moves in a more anterior–posterior direction to accomplish a higher workload. There are only a few reports on the performance of accelerator-based, rate-adaptive systems because they were only recently introduced. Lau et al. reported the first results of the Intermedics devices Dash (VVIR) and Relay (DDDR) pacemakers.[19,20] Lau et al. compared the behavior of accelerator-driven with conventional piezoelectric-controlled activity devices and found that accelerometer-controlled devices showed a better response to walking, jogging, and standing. Lau et al. also indicated that the type of footwear worn produced virtually no effect on the response of accelerometer-driven devices in contrast to traditional piezoelectric-driven devices that are influenced by the type of shoe worn by the patient.[19] As might be assumed already from looking at Figure 2 (showing a linear increase in acceleration signals with linearly increasing workload), increasing the incline on the treadmill during exercise produced a significant increase also in pacing rate with accelerometer devices while there was little or no change in the pacing rate with traditional piezoelectric-driven pacemakers. Lau et al. concluded that compared with the piezoelectric-driven pacemakers, accelerometer-driven pacemakers exhibit a more appropriate rate response with effort and are less susceptible to direct pressure or tapping on the device. Lau et al. also emphasized that the use of the triphasic rate-responsive curves generated by the Intermedics Relay and Dash pacemakers (and accompanying programmers) have a stabilizing effect during ordinary exercise.[19]

We recently conducted a study at our institute[21,22] comparing the response of accelerometer-controlled to vibration-sensitive devices during treadmill exercise with increasing and decreasing speed and slope (Fig. 4). To avoid bias by different initial settings of the various devices, the external pacemakers strapped on the chest were calibrated in 10 patients and in 10 volunteers to the same basic conditions. The baseline pacing rate was set in each volunteer and in each patient to 70 bpm. The individual systems were tailored to yield a response of 95 bpm when the subjects were walking on a treadmill with a speed of 3.2 km (2 miles per hour) and 0% grade. The sinus rate of the volunteers was recorded and compared to the pacemaker-generated rate. Our previously described protocol guarantees a smooth and linear increase and decrease in workload.[23] The correlation of natural sinus rate with increasing and decreas-

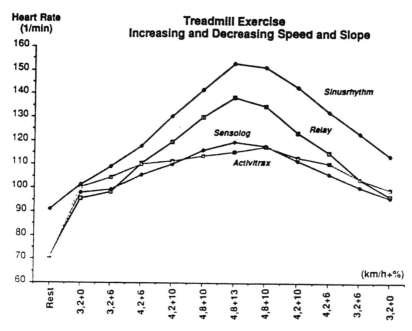

Figure 4. Comparison of rate response on exercise with vibration-controlled devices (Sensolog and Activitrax) with that of an accelerometer-driven device (Relay) in 10 healthy subjects and 10 pacemaker patients with implanted vibration-sensitive piezoelectric pacemakers. All three devices (Activitrax, Sensolog, and Relay) were taped to the midpectoral region of the patients and volunteers. There was no difference in the rate response between the implanted and external devices at the same settings. In each subject, all three external devices were individually calibrated to the same basic parameters. The pacing rate at rest was set at 70 beats per minute and the rate response was individually adjusted to generate a pacing rate of 95 per minute with an initial speed on the treadmill of 3.2 km per hour and 0% grade. With increasing and decreasing workload, the rate response of the accelerometer-driven pacemaker remains far more parallel to the natural sinus rate than other devices. The intrinsic sinus rate at the beginning of exercise was already 20 bpm higher than the lower pacing rate of the activity-controlled devices, and the difference persisted throughout the study.

ing treadmill grades was also very high (r = 0.97), reflecting the linear changing workload of the exercise protocol. The accelerometer-controlled Relay pacemaker exhibited a similar rate increase and decrease with increasing and decreasing workloads as shown in Figure 4. The resting rate was 70 bpm from the pacemakers and 90 bpm in the volunteers, a difference of about 20 bpm that persisted at rest and on effort throughout the entire trial. Thus, if the accelerometer-driven devices had started at a higher rate, the rate response of the pacemakers would have been very close to that of normal sinus rhythm. Correlation of the accelerometer pacemaker rate generated with exercise versus sinus response was also good (r = 0.90). Also, the slope of the increase of the atrial sinus rate (x = 8.96) was similar to that of the accelerometer (accelerometer x = 7.22) compared to the more flat increase in pacing rate of the Activitrax (x = 3.92) and Sensolog devices (x = 5.51). (The x factor indicates by how many beats per minute the heart or pacing rate changes when the workload is increased according to the protocol used. When x = 1, it indicates no change in the pacing rate.)

Other studies comparing accelerometer-controlled devices with conventional piezoelectric vibration-controlled devices have also shown a more straight and linear correlation with the performed workload (Fig. 5).[15,16] The correlation coefficient of the pacing and intrinsic rates in the accelerometer-controlled devices (Excel VR from CPI) was found to be 0.8. The average rate variation determined by the root mean square (rms) was 11 bpm. In the same study, the performance of the piezoelectric vibration-driven devices during treadmill exercise showed a more variable response with a considerably smaller correlation coefficient (r = 0.27), while the average rate variation determined by the root mean square was measured at 26 bpm. (Root mean square, rms, is a measurement to determine the variation of the individual data points from the mean value. The smaller the rms, the closer the individual data points are centered around the mean.)

New Features of Acceleration-Controlled Devices

An interesting feature for the control of nonphysiologic (i.e., unrelated to physical exercise) rapid ventricular paced rates secondary to atrial tachyarrhythmias was incorporated by Intermedics in their Relay and Stride accelerometer-controlled DDDR devices.[20,24,25] I believe that

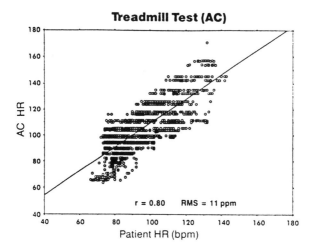

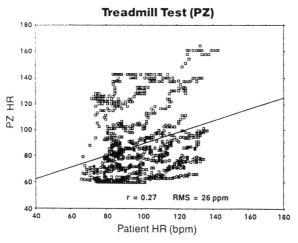

Figure 5.   Clinical results obtained with the CPI accelerator-based rate-adaptive system (Excel). Same database and methodology as in Figure 3. The heart rate of individuals with normal chronotropic function was compared to the calculated pacing rate obtained from an external device taped on the chest. The correlation was found to be r=0.80, and the average rate variation noted by the root mean square (rms) was 11 ppm (top). The performance of the vibration-sensitive devices during treadmill testing showed a more variable response (bottom). This variation depended on the individual subject and the correlation coefficient for the rate of traditional piezoelectric-controlled devices compared to the intrinsic heart rate was 0.27, and the average rate variation noted by the root mean square was 26 bpm. (Reproduced with permission.[25])

the use of different upper rate limits (one limit for atrial-triggered upper rate ventricular rate and another for sensor-controlled upper ventricular rate) does not provide a satisfactory way of dealing with inappropriate atrial tachyarrhythmias. Furthermore, programming two disparate rates carries the theoretical risk of precipitating atrial arrhythmias. In the Intermedics devices, there is a common upper rate for sensor-controlled and atrial-triggered ventricular pacing. Aside from controlling the pacing rate according to patient activity, the accelerometer sensor in Intermedics devices forms part of a mechanism that prevents tracking of fast atrial rates secondary to atrial tachyarrhythmias when physical exercise is absent. In order to control the maximum ventricular pacing rate triggered by sensed atrial events, a conditional ventricular tracking limit (CVTL) is established when the sensor-indicated rate is not sufficiently high to confirm the presence of physical exercise. In such a case, the maximum achievable ventricular pacing rate is limited to the CVTL 35 bpm above the baseline lower rate, i.e., a Wenckebach upper rate response occurs at the CVTL. In practical terms, with a lower rate limit of 60 bpm and excessively high atrial rate, the maximum ventricular pacing rate would be limited to only 95 bpm if there is no confirmation of physical exercise by the sensor. This response is important in patients with paroxysmal atrial flutter/fibrillation, not an uncommon current indication for dual chamber pacing. Another feature of clinical importance in the Intermedics DDDR pulse generators is the so-called redraw function of the rate-responsive setting. A built-in rate profile memory records either the sensor-calculated rate or the patient's actual rate over selectable periods of time from as short as 15 minutes up to 24 hours. This feature offered by the Intermedics accelerometer-controlled devices allows the operator to redraw the rate response under different settings on the programmer screen. After reading the memory, the display on the programmer (Fig. 6) enables the physician to adjust the rate response according to patient need. If, for example, a target rate of 120 bpm is believed to be appropriate with the type of exercise performed, the exercise rate response can be simulated by means of new and different settings of the rate-response slope until the desired target rate is achieved. This feature minimizes the time required to optimize the rate-responsive settings in the individual patient as only one exercise trial is required.

Conclusion

Activity-controlled pacing is currently the most widely used form of rate adaptation for implanted pacemakers. The easy clinical applica-

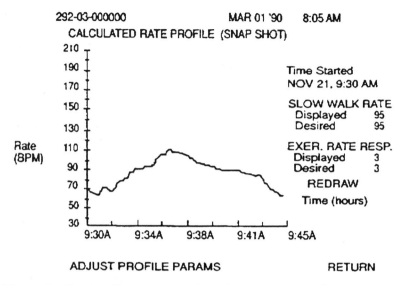

Figure 6. Rate profile demonstrated on the programmer of accelerometer-based pacemakers from Intermedics. The rate profile provides the record of either the sensor-calculated rate or the actual patient's heart rate for selectable durations of 15 minutes to 24 hours. The curve can be redrawn with different settings to evaluate the exercise response, thereby providing an important tool for the selection of the appropriate rate-adaptive settings for the need of individual patients. This process allows rapid optimization of pacemaker settings and takes only a few minutes.

bility of activity-controlled pacemakers and their high sensitivity to the onset and termination of exercise have made these pacemakers very popular with now more than 300,000 implants worldwide. Activity-controlled pacemakers based on acceleration forces introduced clinically within the last year (CPI: Excel VR, Vigor DR; Intermedics: Relay, Dash, Stride, Dart) have thus far shown promising results. Accelerometer-controlled devices have certain advantages over conventional vibration-sensitive systems in terms of a higher sensitivity to varying workloads, higher specificity to the type of exercise performed, and less susceptibility to environmental noise. Some accelerometer-controlled devices offer attractive new features such as the conditional ventricular tracking limit (that minimizes nonphysiologic ventricular pacing rates during paroxysmal supraventricular tachycardia) and redraw functions that facilitate follow-up. Because both activity sensors—vibration and acceleration—work on the same principle, they have similar limitations in that they are nonmetabolic sensors. Nevertheless, their easy clinical applicability and reliability represent distinct advantages over nonactivity sensors used in other rate-adaptive pacemakers.

The clinical applicability of activity-controlled devices will undoubtedly become even more appealing by designing more automatic functions such as (1) automatic slope selection of the activity sensor, (2) automatic capture verification (with resultant enhanced battery life), (3) automatic AV adaptation, and (4) automatic refractory period adaptation, and also by refining the role of sensor input in automatically limiting the ventricular pacing rate in response to inappropriate paroxysmal supraventricular tachyarrhythmias.

References

1. Alt E, Heinz M, Theres H, Matula M, Blöjmer H. A new body motion activity based rate responsive pacing system: PACE 1987;10:422.
2. Matula M, Alt E, Theres H, Heinz M, Völker R. Rate responsive pacing based on a new activity sensing principle. PACE 1987;10:1220.
3. Lau CP, Stott RR, Toff WD, Zetlein M, Ward DE, Camm J. Vibration sensing: new design of activity sensing rate responsive pacemaker. PACE 1987;10:1217.
4. Alt E, Matula M, Theres H, Heinz M. Grundlage aktivitätsgesteuerter frequenzvariabler Herzschrithnacher: Analyse von belastungs und umweltbedingten mechanischen Eintliissen am menschlichen Körper. Z Kardiol 1989;78:587–597.
5. Alt E, Matula M, Theres H, Heinz M, Baker R. The basis for activity controlled rate variable cardiac pacemakers: an analysis of mechanical forces on the human body induced by exercise and environment. PACE 1989;12:1667–1680.
6. Lau CP, Stott JR, Toff WD, Zetlein MB, Ward DE, Camm AJ. Selective vibration sensing: a new concept for activity-sensing rate-responsive pacing. PACE 1989;11:1299–1309.
7. Bunge T, Thompson D. Sensing internal and external body activities. In: Perez-Gomez F (ed.). Cardiac Pacing, Editorial Gronz, Madrid 1985, p 786–791.
8. Stangl K, Wirtzfeld A, Lochschmidt O, Heinze R, Blömer H. Möglichkeiten und Grenzen eines "aktivitätsgesteuerten" Schrittmachersystems. Herz/Kreisl 1987;19:351–357.
9. Mond H, Line P, Hunt D. A third generation activity pacemaker: is the rate response algorithm superior? PACE 1990;13:1204.

10. Lau CP, Tse WS, Camm J. Clinical experience with Sensolog 703: a new activity sensing rate responsive pacemaker. PACE 1988;11:1444.
11. Schuchert A, Kuck KH, Bleifeld W. Einfluss der Schrittfrequenz und Muskelcraft auf die Stimulationsfrequenz aktivitätsgesteuerter Herzschrittmacher. Z Kardiol 1991;82:463–467.
12. Candinas RA, Gloor HO, Amann FW, Schoenbeck M, Turina M. Activity-sensing rate responseive versus conventional fixed-rate pacing: a comparison of rate behaviour and patient well-being during routine daily exercise. PACE 1991;14:204–213.
13. Lemke B, van Dryander St, Lawo T, Barmeyer J. Is there an adequate rate response during marching with an activity sensing pacemaker? PACE 1987;10:1218.
14. Stangl K, Wirtzfeld A, Lochschmidt O, Basler B, Mittnacht A. Physical movement sensitive pacing: comparison of two "activity"-triggered pacing systems. PACE 1989;12:102–110.
15. Bacharach DW, Hilden RS, Millerhagen JO, Westrum BL, Kelly JM. Activity-based pacing: comparison of a device using an accelerometer versus a piezoelectric crystal. PACE 1992;15:188–196.
16. Millerhagen J, Bacharach D, Street G, Westrum B. A comparison study of two activity pacemakers: an accelerometer versus piezoelectric crystal device. PACE 1991;14:665, A191.
17. Lau CP, Wong CK, Leung WH, Cheng CH, Lo CW. A comparative evaluation of a minute ventilation sensing and activity sensing adaptive-rate pacemakers during daily activities. PACE 1989;12:1514–1521.
18. Rahn R, Zegelman M, Brief I, Kreuzer J, Frenkel C. Störanfälligkeit frequenzadaptiver Herzschrittmacher bei zahnärztlichen Behandlungsmassnahmen. Dtsch Zahnärztl Z 1989;44:244–247.
19. Lau CP, Tai YT, Fong PC, Li JPS, Leung SK, Chung FLW, Song S. Clinical experience with an activity sensing DDDR pacemaker using an accelerometer sensor. PACE 1992;15:334–343.
20. Lau CP, Tai YT, Fong PC, Li JPS, Chung FLW, Song S. The use of implantable sensors for the control of pacemaker mediated tachycardias: a comparative evaluation between minute ventilation sensing and acceleration sensing dual chamber rate adaptive pacemakers. PACE 1992;15:34–44.
21. Matula M, Alt E, Schrepf R, Hölzer K, Blömer H. Response of activity pacemakers controlled by different motion sensors to treadmill testing with varied slopes. PACE 1992;15:523, A75.
22. Matula M, Alt E, Fotuhi P, Hölzer K, Blömer H. Influence of varied types of exercise to the rate adaption of activity pacemakers. PACE 1992;15:578, A280.
23. Alt E. A protocol for treadmill and bicycle stress testing designed for pacemaker patients. Stimucoeur 1978;15:33–35.
24. Goy J, Vogt P, Kappenberger L. Activity sensing for prevention of macemaker mediated tachycardia in DDD pacing. PACE 1988;11:531,A194.
25. Lau CP. Sensors and pacemaker mediated tachycardias. PACE 1991;14:495–498.

26. Alt E. Theres H, Heinz M, Matula M, Thilo R, Blömer H. A new rate-modulated pacemaker system optimized by combination of two sensors. PACE 1988;11:1119–1129.
27. Alt E, Heinz M, Theres H, Matula M. Function and selection of sensors for optimum rate-modulated pacing. In: New Perspectives in Cardiac Pacing, Barold S, Mugica J (eds.). Futura Publishing Co, Mt. Kisco, NY, p 163, 1991.
28. Schroeppel EA. Current trends in cardiac pacing technology. I. Bradycardia pacing. Biomed Sci Tech, in press.
29. Mugica J, Barold S, Ripart A. The smart pacemaker. In: New Perspectives in Cardiac Pacing, Barold S, Mugica J (eds.). Futura Publishing Co, Mt. Kisco, NY, p 545, 1991.

Chapter 12

Do We Really Need Multiple Sensors for Optimal Rate-Adaptive Pacing?

Harry G. Mond

Introduction

Rate-adaptive pacing has become firmly established as the preferable pacing option in appropriate patients with chronotrophic incompetence.[1-5] Although many sensors have been employed, only a small number have achieved success in the clinical arena.[6] Much has been learned during the last few years about these sensors and the manufacturers have attempted to improve pacing algorithms to overcome some of the deficiencies of earlier models. Despite these improvements, most pacemaker manufacturers have now initiated work on sensor combinations in an attempt to create the optimal sensor-based pacing system.

The question being posed is whether such combinations are really necessary. Can any one sensor stand alone and be incorporated into a single sensor-based pacing system appropriate for the vast majority of patients requiring single or dual chamber pacemakers? In order to answer these questions, this chapter will investigate the advantages and deficiencies of current single sensor-based pacemakers with particular emphasis on the recent algorithm changes in established systems.

The Search for the Optimal Sensor

The early and rapid success of the piezoelectric crystal as an activity sensor demonstrated the clinical value of incorporating sensors other than

New Perspectives in Cardiac Pacing, Vol. 3, edited by S. Serge Barold and Jacques Mugica, Mount Kisco, NY, Futura Publishing Co., © 1993.

the atrial electrogram into a pacing system in order to increase the pacing rate of patients with chronotropic incompetence. These sensor-based pacing systems are particularly valuable in patients with an abnormal sinus mechanism where reestablishment of atrioventricular synchrony alone is inadequate. Despite early enthusiasm with activity sensors, a number of limitations and deficiencies with this sensor became apparent. In particular, the programmed upper rate is rarely achieved and the sensor is sensitive to external vibrational forces.[7] Because of this, other more physiologic sensors have been investigated and developed into rate-adaptive cardiac pacing systems.

As seen in Table 1, at least 10 different sensors have undergone clinical evaluation. For practical reasons, these can be divided into two groups: those requiring a standard pacing lead and those systems where a special sensor is incorporated into the pacing lead. In general, the special lead systems are physiologic and thus theoretically highly desirable. Despite this, none of these sensors have become established in rate-adaptive cardiac pacing. Although most pacemaker implanters would prefer not to use a sensor-dedicated pacing lead, there are other more important reasons why such systems have not been widely accepted. Despite relatively large financial and research commitments, pacemaker manufacturers found that the pacing systems are complicated and poorly understood by physicians. In patients with normal cardiac function, the systems work admirably. However, the role of physiology in the presence of cardiac and other system pathologies becomes cloudy and obscure. In particular, pacemaker patients with congestive cardiac failure have abnormal right heart pressures, volumes, and flow patterns. This results in abnormal and occasionally inappropriate pacing responses to changes in sensor input.

TABLE 1
Sensors for Rate-Adaptive Pacing

Standard Pacing Lead	Special Pacing Lead
Activity	Central venous temperature
QT interval	Right ventricular dP/dt
Respiratory rate	Central venous O_2 saturation
Minute ventilation	Right ventricular stoke volume/pre-ejection period
Paced depolarization integral	Central venous pH

The sensor-based systems utilizing standard pacing leads are a heterogenous group. Physiologic sensors dependent on autonomic stimulation include the QT interval and paced depolarization integral. The former, which depends on the shortening of the paced QT interval with autonomic stimulation, has been widely studied, modified, and improved but still has a low response time limiting its widespread use.[8,9] The paced depolarization integral is a new sensor-based system that has not been widely investigated.[10] The sensor analyses the integral of the paced QRS complex, which alters with autonomic stimulation. The response time, ability to achieve the programmed upper rate, the sensitivity to emotional stimuli and interference with drugs, electrolyte imbalance, and myocardial ischemia all need to be investigated further.[10-12]

The two remaining sensors, although different, depend on movement: activity with the piezoelectric crystal, and respiration measured by changes in transthoracic impedance with chest wall movement. Respiratory rate alone is physiologically suspect and requires a special auxillary sensor implanted in the anterior chest wall[13] or, more recently, as a special lead.[14] Minute ventilation, however, is more physiologic and requires only a standard bipolar lead.[15,16] The activity and minute ventilation sensors have both withstood the test of time. They require a standard pacemaker implantation, are simple to program, and can be used with single and dual chamber pacing.

The question remains whether either or both of these sensors can stand alone or whether they must be combined with other sensors or each other to create the ideal sensor-based pacing system.

Activity Sensor

Activity sensor-based rate-adaptive pacing systems are clearly the most popular pacemakers sold today. Any unipolar or bipolar lead can be utilized, and successful pacing can be achieved in both the atrium and the ventricle.

Despite a rapid response time, the activity sensor is limited in its ability to achieve the programmed upper rate with exertion. The original activity algorithm used in both single chamber (Medtronic Activitrax® [Medtronic, Inc., Minneapolis, MN]) and dual chamber (Medtronic Synergyst,®) rate-adaptive pacing systems had three activity threshold levels and a family of 10 rate-response curves. Vibratory signals obtained from the sensor were required to exceed the programmed activity thresh-old level set at low (L or sensitive), medium (M), or high (H or insen-sitive). The rate-response curves can be likened to a preselected gain on electronic equipment. The curves determine the acceleration and pacing level achieved in response to incoming activity counts. The higher the value of the response curve, the more dramatic the rise in pacing rate (Fig. 1). In clinical practice, the most frequently used programmable settings have been a medium activity threshold and a rate response be-tween 5 and 8. Within these limits, a satisfactory pacing rate response occurs for the majority of pacemaker-dependent patients who require a

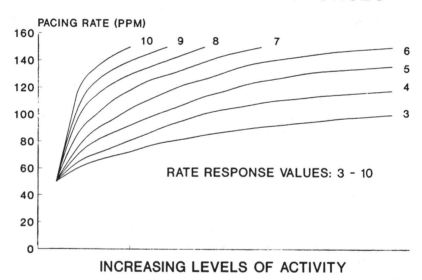

ACTIVITRAX
NON LINEAR RATE RESPONSES

Figure 1.   Graph to demonstrate the theoretical rate-response curves and upper rate limit of the first-generation activity rate-adaptive pacemaker (Activitrax). With increasing activity, the pacing rate increases toward the upper rate limit. With the rate response at low values (1–6), the upper rate is not achieved. With the high values (7–10) the response is rapid, reaching the upper rate limit soon after activity commences. In practice, however, these upper rates are rarely if ever achieved.

rapid response to modest exercise with a maximum pacing rate of about 110 pulses per minute. The ability to reach the programmed upper pacing rate of either 120 or 150 pulses per minute was rarely achieved with normal activities such as walking, jogging, or running (Fig. 2). This deficiency in the algorithm has been found to be clinically important in the young and active person, where with continuing exercise a high maximum pacing rate is desirable. This cannot be achieved unless inappropriately sensitive programs are used, which result in distressing palpitations with minor activities and are highly sensitive to extracorporeal vibratory forces.

In an attempt to overcome this deficiency, a second-generation ac-

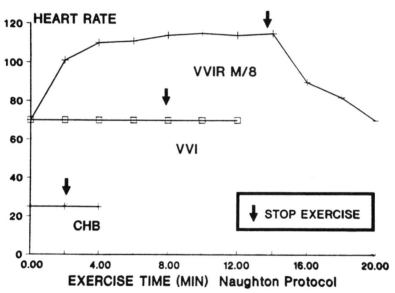

AB MALE/74

Figure 2. Three treadmill exercise stress tests in the same patient before and after the implantation of an single chamber ventricular Activitrax rate-adaptive pacing system. Prior to implantation (CHB = complete heart block), the exercise time was only 2 minutes. In the nonrate-adaptive mode (VVI), after 3 months, the exercise time was 8 minutes. After 3 months in the rate-adaptive mode (VVIR), medium activity threshold, rate response 8, the exercise time increased to 14 minutes. Note that with exercise, the heart rate rises rapidly to about 110 bpm, and despite ongoing activity, does not rise any further.

tivity pacing system has been developed that has a programmble acceleration and a larger range of activity threshold levels, and the rate-response curves have been replaced with a linear response (Fig. 3). Single chamber (Medtronic Legend®) and dual chamber (Medtronic Elite®) models are available. Provided vibratory forces increase, the pacing rate rises to the programmed upper limit. This can be demonstrated in Figure 4, where unlike the Activitrax, it is possible with the Legend to achieve the programmed upper rate with high workloads. This study was performed in the same control subject during the same exercise using external activity pulse generators securely strapped to the chest wall. Prior to performing the study, the most appropriate settings of the externally attached activity pulse generator were determined by comparing the rate

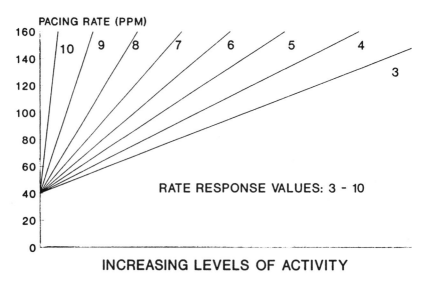

Figure 3.   Graph to demonstrate the theoretical linear rate response of the second-generation activity rate-adaptive pacemaker (Legend). Regardless of the rate-response value, the upper rate can be achieved provided the level of activity or vibrational forces continue to increase.

ACTIVITRAX/LEGEND
RATE RESPONSE 9

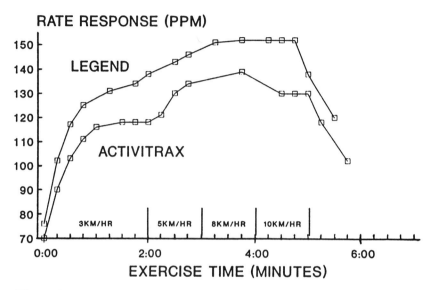

Figure 4. Exercise testing using external Activitrax and Legend pulse generators firmly attached to the anterior chest wall of a normal volunteer. Both pulse generators were programmed to the low activity threshold level and a rate response of 9. The workload was increased until the upper rate limit of 150 ppm was achieved with the Legend, whereas the rate of the Activitrax remains well below this level. This confirms that the linear response of the Legend will allow the upper rate to be achieved provided the workload is sufficient.

response with implanted activity pulse generators. For an implanted pulse generator set at M 7, a virtually identical rate response could be obtained with the external pulse generator set at L 7.[17] Consequently, the L 7 programmed setting was used in all external activity pulse generator studies.

The further addition of a programmable acceleration function (Fig. 5) and a wider range of activity threshold levels, but within the original range of the Activitrax, can be used to fine tune the patient's rate response to exertion.

In a more practical sense, studies were designed to prove whether

RATE ACCELERATION
LEGEND

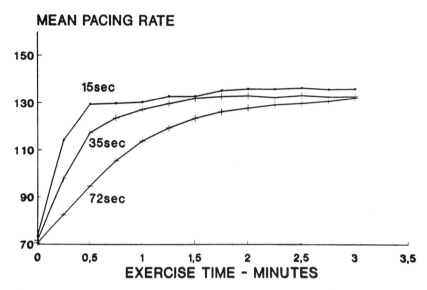

Figure 5.   Programmable rate acceleration of the Legend rate-adaptive pacing system. The treadmill exercise data were obtained using external Legend pulse generators securely strapped to the anterior chest wall of 10 normal volunteers. Three separate exercise tests (modified Bruce protocol, no incline) were performed on each subject using the three programmable acceleration times: 15, 35, and 72 sec. This is the time required to reach 90% of the difference between the start of sensor-driven pacing and the upper rate. The time required to reach the upper pacing rate was dependent on the acceleration time, and in each case virtually identical upper rates were achieved.

at normal patient exercise workloads, the linear rate response was superior to the original nonlinear slope. With the external pulse generators programmed to upper rates of 150 ppm, no difference in the achieved high rate was noted between the first- and second-generation activity pulse generators using a conservative treadmill exercise program both with[17] and without an incline (Fig. 6). This is not surprising as the vibratory forces in these studies were low and differences in the pacing rates cannot be expected. This, however, would be the anticipated work-

ACTIVITRAX/LEGEND 150

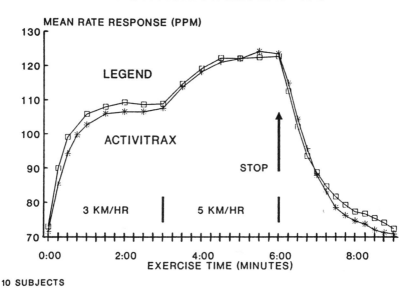

10 SUBJECTS

Figure 6. Exercise testing (modified Bruce protocol, no incline) using external Activitrax and Legend pulse generators firmly attached to the anterior chest wall of 10 normal volunteers. The pulse generators were programmed to the low activity threshold level, with a rate response of 7 and an upper rate of 150 ppm. Provided the exercise activity is low and the acceleration times identical, Activitrax and Legend pulse generators will respond in a similar manner and achieve identical upper rates.

load for the vast majority of activity rate-adaptive pacing system recipients.

Can, then, the exercise-achieved pacing rate be improved in patients undergoing these low level exercise protocols without resorting to inappropriate programming? On reviewing the linear rate-response graphs, the slope of a given value is dependent on the differential between the programmed upper and lower rates (Fig. 7). The slope, therefore, becomes more acute as the upper rate is increased in the presence of a fixed low rate. This hypothesis can be tested clinically using treadmill exercise and increasing the programmed upper rate. Using the external pulse generator technique in control subjects as already described, both

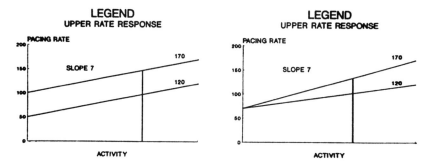

Figure 7. The programmed slope of a Legend pulse generator is also dependent on the programmed upper and lower rates. Left: Two identical slopes with a value of 7 are demonstrated. Although the upper and lower rates are different, there is a 50 ppm difference between each of these limits. Right: The low rates are identical, but there is a difference of 50 ppm at the upper rate. Thus, although both slopes are 7, the actual slopes are quite different.

the first- and second-generation activity pulse generators were studied. There was, as expected, no difference in the achieved high rate response with the Activitrax, which had a maximum programmable upper rate of 150 ppm (Fig. 8). The Legend, however, showed a consistent increase in the high rate achieved with exercise, despite the same settings for the activity threshold, rate response, and acceleration (Fig. 9).

Thus, in the second-generation activity rate-adaptive pacing system, it is possible with appropriate programming to achieve acceptable pacing rates with both conservative and demanding workloads. There is, however, still some concern that if too high an upper rate is selected, then occasionally inappropriate pacing rates and hence palpitations may occur.

Despite this, across a large spectrum of pacemaker recipients, activity appears acceptable as a single sensor rate-adaptive system obviating the necessity to link it with other sensors to improve the rate response to exercise. This fact is substantiated by the enthusiasm other pacemaker companies have had in adopting activity as a sensor for rate-adaptive pacing systems.

Minute Ventilation

Minute ventilation, the product of respiratory rate and tidal volume, is a highly physiologic variable that closely reflects the metabolic de-

ACTIVITRAX: 120, 150

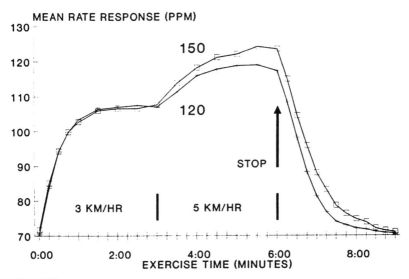

Figure 8. Exercise testing (modified Bruce protocol, no incline) using an external Activitrax pulse generator firmly attached to the anterior chest wall of 10 normal volunteers. The pulse generator was programmed to the low activity threshold level and a rate response of 7. Exercise tests were performed on two occasions with the upper rate set at 120 and 150 ppm. There was no difference between the pacing rates achieved in the two exercise studies.

mands of exercise.[18] The increase in minute ventilation with exercise closely parallels changes in oxygen uptake, cardiac output, and heart rate. In contrast to several other sensors, minute ventilation also varies in response to stress and pyrexia. It was not surprising, therefore, that minute ventilation was investigated and developed as a physiologic sensor for rate-adaptive pacing.

The single chamber minute ventilation rate-adaptive pacing system (Telectronics META® MV [Telectronics Pacing Systems, Denver, CO]), utilizes changes in measured transthoracic impedance as the sensed variable for adjusting pacing rate. In turn, changes in transthoracic impedance have been shown to strongly correlate with changes in minute ventila-

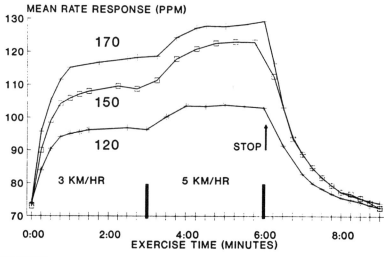

LEGEND: 120, 150 AND 170

Figure 9. Exercise testing (modified Bruce protocol, no incline) using an external Legend pulse generators firmly attached to the anterior chest wall of 10 normal volunteers. The pulse generators were programmed to the low activity threshold level and a rate response of 7. Exercise tests were performed on three occasions with the programmed upper rate set at 120, 150, and 170 ppm. Because of the variations in the rate response slope due to the differing programmed upper rates, there is a marked difference in the pacing rates achieved in the three exercise studies, with the programmed upper rate of 170 ppm achieving the highest pacing rate.

tion. The first generation minute ventilation rate-adaptive pacing system is suitable for both atrial and ventricular use. In addition to the SSI and SSIR pacing modes, an "adaptive SSI" mode is used to determine the most desirable programmable rate-adaptive parameters by providing an analysis of changes in minute ventilation without rate-adaptive pacing.

The system used a tripolar system; a standard bipolar lead and the pulse generator casing. Low energy pulses (1 mA for 15 μs at 20 Hz) are used for measurement of transthoracic impedance and are generated between the ring electrode of the lead and the pulse generator casing. Impedance measurements are performed each 50 ms between the tip electrode of the lead and the pulse generator casing. Transthoracic impedance increases with inspiration and decreases with expiration, with the amplitude representing tidal volume and the cyclical pattern, respiratory rate. The pulse generator circuitry identifies the two signals and processes them to yield minute ventilation. Two signal-averaging processes operate within the pulse generator; one with a short time constant of 36 seconds, which allows for smooth rate changes, and the other with a long time constant of approximately 1 to 2 hours. The difference between these two signal averages is then used to monitor the changes in minute ventilation, which is continually updated.

Programming the minute ventilation rate-adaptive system includes the upper and lower pacing rates, as well as the rate-response factor or slope, which determines the change in pacing rate in response to changes in minute ventilation. Fifty-nine slope values are available from 2 to 60, with the higher slope values producing marked changes in pacing rate for only small changes in minute ventilation (Fig. 10). The optimal slope value can be determined for each patient using a simple exercise test and the "peak exercise function." The implanted pulse generator is programmed to the adaptive mode and the patient is asked to rest for at least 1 hour prior to exercise testing. In this mode, the rate-adaptive sensing circuit adapts to the patient's individual respiratory impedance characteristics. With the pulse generator still in the adaptive mode, a near-maximal exercise test is performed. Using the peak exercise function, the suggested optimal slope value based on the patient's respiration characteristics during exercise is calculated by the implanted pulse generator and programmer and is displayed by the programmer.

Unlike the activity sensor, appropriate changes in minute ventilation will always allow the pacing rate to reach the programmed upper rate limit. However, the commencement in rate response and subsequent acceleration are slower than the activity sensor, which has an almost immediate response to vibration (Fig. 11). Although the delayed rate response and acceleration of the minute ventilation pacing system appear physiologic, in practice, however, most pacemaker recipients, being elderly, perform short exercise times and thus require a rapid rate response. How, then, can the minute ventilation rate-adaptive pacing system overcome this apparent deficiency in some patients?

As in the algorithm change with the activity rate-response curves to a linear response, a similar change was incorporated into the second-generation minute ventilation rate-adaptive single chamber (Telectronics

META   MV

COMPARISON OF RATE RESPONSE FACTORS

MIN.RATE 70.   MAX. RATE 100.

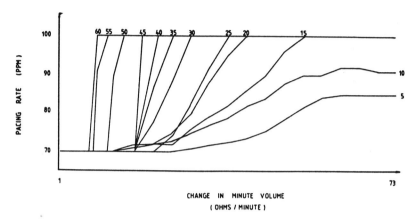

Figure 10.   Minute ventilation sensor. Examples of slope values comparing the pacing rate response to changes in minute ventilation (volume). At a programmed slope, there is a specific change in pacing rate for a given change in minute ventilation as determined by changes in transthoracic impedance.

META II®) and dual chamber (Telectronics META® DDDR) models (Fig. 12). The rationale for this, however, was different for the two sensors. With activity, the primary objective was to reach the programmed upper rate with exertion. With minute ventilation, the purpose was to create a more rapid acceleration in rate response. Such a change in the slope pattern, however, does not alter the initiation of the pacing rate change with alteration of minute ventilation at the commencement of (Fig. 12).

The solution to this lay in the data aquisition circuit which transfers the transthoracic impedance measurements to a microcontroller, which then calculates minute ventilation. As stated, the short–term data aquisition circuit has a constant of 36 seconds. This is the time required to reach 50% of the metabolically indicated rate in response to an instantaneous change in the measured minute ventilation. Revising this constant would therefore alter the rate response or the time of onset of pacing

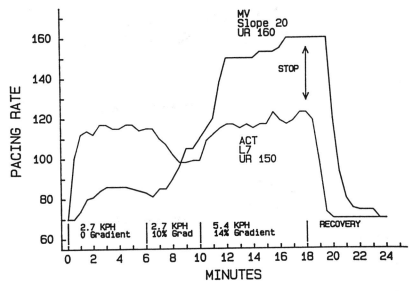

Figure 11. Graphs comparing the pacing rate responses to exercise of the external Activitrax (ACT) with an implanted META MV (MV) in the same patient at the same time using a modified Bruce protocol. The Activitrax responds very rapidly to exercise, reaching a maximum rate of about 115 ppm. During the second stage of exercise, a gradient is introduced resulting in a transient fall in pacing rate due to the slower more deliberate walking up the incline. The rise in pacing rate of the META MV with exercise is much slower, and at peak exercise, the programmed upper rate is achieved.

rate changes. The META II has two programmable response times: 36 seconds (medium) and 18 seconds (fast). As documented in Figure 13, a rapid response time program has an earlier onset and faster pacing rate acceleration with exercise, equivalent to the activity sensor.

Both the second-generation single and dual chamber minute ventilation rate-adaptive models are highly sophisticated programmable systems. The dual chamber model allows high upper rates to be achieved by automatically shortening the atrioventricular delay and postventricular atrial refractory period with increasing atrial rates. The pacing system will also sense the atrial electrogram in the postventicular atrial refractory period and revert to VVIR pacing. This will allow DDDR pacing to be used in patients with intermittent atrial tachyarrhythmias.

MINUTE VENTILATION SENSOR
RATE RESPONSE FACTORS

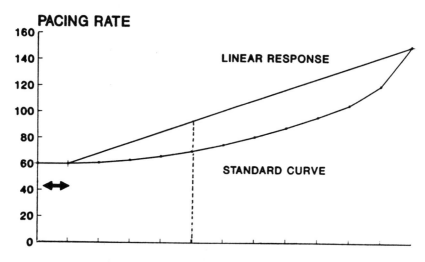

CHANGE IN MINUTE VENTILATION (IMPEDANCE)

Figure 12. By altering the standard rate-response curve of the META MV to a linear response, there is a more marked rate response to a fixed change in transthoracic impedance or minute ventilation (broken line). The initiation of the pacing rate change with changes in minute ventilation, however, does not alter (double arrow).

A number of limitations of the original VVIR model have been corrected in the second-generation single chamber minute ventilation rate-adaptive system. Prior to programming the rate-adaptive mode, a 3-minute rest period rather than an hour is now all that is required. To obviate the necessity for exercise testing to choose the most appropriate rate-response factor, an built-in automatic rate histogram will rapidly determine if the chosen slope is appropriate with normal exercise. Such histograms, with varying levels of complexity and sophistication, are also available with the activity-based sensor systems.

There are very few negative features with the minute ventilation rate-adaptive pacing systems. For the rate-adaptive system, a bipolar lead

META II VS META MV

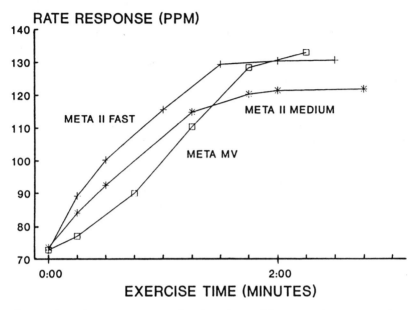

Figure 13. The pacing rate acceleration phase of three exercise tests: one in a patient with an implanted META MV and two in a patient with an implanted META II to demonstrate the improved pacing rate of the linear rate-response factor and the earlier response time when programmed to fast (see text for details).

is mandatory, but because of polarity programming, either unipolar or bipolar pacing and sensing can be used. For rate-adaptive pacing, the pulse generator must be implanted in the anterior chest wall. The system is highly physiologic, and with appropriate programming, can be used in patients with airways disease and within limitations in the pediatric age group. Despite being physiologic, significant pacing rate changes may occur with rapid shoulder movements. This is not necessarily a negative feature, as in some cases the movements enhance the pacing rate response with exercises such as walking and swimming. However, if the patient experiences palpitations with certain shoulder movements, the problem can be easily overcome with reprogramming of the rate-response factor and/or the upper rate.

The single and dual chamber minute ventilation rate-adaptive pacing systems can be used across the entire spectrum of pacemaker recipients. Like activity, the value of incorporating this sensor with others in a dual or multisensor system is questionable. Despite this, dual sensor systems will be or have already been developed. In most cases, it is to overcome the well-recognized deficiencies of some sensors such as activity, central venous temperature, QT interval (ventricular endocardial paced evoked response) or central oxygen saturation.[19-21] In other cases, companies with more than one sensor have combined these into a single product, hoping to rationalize their product range. Such are the examples of activity/minute ventilation (Medtronic), activity/QT interval (Vitatron [Vitatron, The Netherlands]),[22] and minute ventilation/paced depolarization integral (Telectronics). The sensors may be separated within the same product or have combined complex algorithms. Their value has yet to be proven. With the correct programming of current sensor-based systems, and in particular activity and minute ventilation, dual sensor systems may not be necessary.

References

1. Lau CP, Camm AJ. Role of left ventricular function and Doppler-derived variables in predicting haemodynamic benefits of rate-responsive pacing. Am J Cardiol 1988;62:906–911.
2. Buckingham TA, Woodruff RC, Pennington DG, et al. Effect of ventricular function on the exercise hemodynamics of variable rate pacing. JACC 1988;11:1269–1277.
3. Tyers GFO. Current status of sensor-modulated rate-adaptive cardiac pacing. J Am Coll Cardiol 1990;15:412–418.
4. Otto MA, Muderrisoglu H, Ozin MB, et al. Quality of life in patients with rate-responsive pacemakers: a randomized cross-over study. PACE 1991;14: 800–806.
5. Griffin JC. The optimal pacing mode for the individual patient: the role of DDDR. In: Barold SS, Mugica J (eds.). New Perspectives in Cardiac Pacing. 2. Futura Publishing Co, Inc, Mount Kisco, NY, 1991, pp 325–338.
6. Mond HG. Rate responsive cardiac pacing: a perspective. PACE 1989;12: 1309–1311.
7. Mond HG, Kertes PJ. Rate responsive cardiac pacing. Telectronics Pacing Systems, Sydney, 1987, pp 13–28.
8. Boute W, Gebhardt U, Begemann MJS. Introduction of a new generation of QT driven rate responsive pacemakers. PACE 1987;10:1208.
9. den Heijer P, VanWoersem RJ, Nagelkerke D, et al. Improved algorithm in TX pacemakers. Preliminary clinical experience. PACE 1987;10:1210.

10. Singer I, Olash J, Brennan AF et al. Initial clinical experience with a rate responsive pacemaker. PACE 1989;12:1458–1464.
11. Lasarides K, Paul VE, Katritsis D, et al. Influence of propranolol on the ventricular depolarization gradient. PACE 1991;14:787–792.
12. Singer I, Brennan AF, Steinhaus B, et al. Effects of stress and beta blockade on the ventricular depolarization gradient of the rate modulating pacemaker. PACE 1991;14:460–469.
13. Rossi P, Plicchi G, Canducci G et al. Respiratory rate as a determinant of optimal pacing rate. PACE 1983;6:502–507.
14. Rossi P. The birth of the respiratory pacemaker. PACE 1990;13:812–815.
15. Mond H, Strathmore N, Kertes P, et al. Rate responsive pacing using a minute ventilation sensor. PACE 1988;11:1866–1874.
16. Vanerio G, Patel S, Ching E, et al. Early clinical experience with a minute ventilation sensor DDDR pacemaker. PACE 1991;14:1815–1820.
17. Strathmore N, Mond H, Cheong S, Hunt D. Rate responsive pacing: comparison of a minute ventilation pacemaker with an external activity-sensing pacemaker. Aust NZ J Med 1989;19:576(Suppl).
18. Alt E, Volker R, Wirtzfeld A. Directly and indirectly measured respiratory parameters compared with oxygen uptake and heart rate. PACE 1985;8:A-21.
19. Stangl K, Wirtzfeld A, Heinze R, et al. A new multisensor pacing system using stroke volume, respiratory rate, mixed venous oxygen saturation, and temperature, right atrial pressure, right ventricular pressure, and dP/dt. PACE 1988;11:712–724.
20. Sugiura T, Kimura M, Mizushina S, et al. Cardiac pacemaker regulated by respiratory rate and blood temperature. PACE 1988;11:1077–1084.
21. Alt E, Theres H, Heinz M, et al. A new rate-modulated pacemaker system optimized by combination of two sensors. PACE 1988;11:1119–1129.
22. Landman MAJ, Senden PJ, van Rooijen H, et al. Initial clinical experience with rate adaptive cardiac pacing using two sensors simultaneously. PACE 1990;13:1615–1622.

Chapter 13

Sensor Combinations: Which, How and Why?

DEREK T. CONNELLY,

ANTHONY F. RICKARDS

Introduction

The quest for a single sensor that provides the ideal rate characteristics under all circumstances continues to be the unattainable "Holy
Grail" of rate-adaptive pacing. Such an "ideal" sensor[1] would have to
respond not only to exercise (including those forms of exercise that do
not involve much movement of the upper body) but emotional and psychologic stresses of various types, and have a rate response that was
appropriately rapid in onset and resulted in a pacing rate proportional to
the metabolic demand. Furthermore, the technical aspects of implantation
and follow-up of such a pacemaker should not be significantly more
complex than those for more straightforward devices, and the sensor
should have a stable response and should function reliably throughout
the lifetime of the unit (Table 1).

Why Combine Sensors?

The limitations of currently available sensors mean that none of them
is suitable for every patient under all circumstances[1,2] and any choice of
a single sensor rate-responsive pacemaker of necessity makes several
compromises. Activity-sensing pacemakers provide an appropriately

New Perspectives in Cardiac Pacing, Vol. 3, edited by S. Serge Barold and Jacques Mugica,
Mount Kisco, NY, Futura Publishing Co., © 1993.

TABLE *1*
Characteristics of Ideal Sensor*

Sensitive to exercise of all types and to other physiological and psychological stresses
Specific response; no inappropriate responses
Accurate rate response; proportional to metabolic demand
Speed of rate response should be appropriate
Technically reliable and stable over time, with simple implantation and programming

* Adapted from Lau and Camm[1]

rapid increase in pacing rate at the onset of exercise, but the pacing rate is not proportional to physiologic demand.[3-6] They respond to external sources of vibration (such as traveling in a car) and they do not respond well to isometric exercise or mental stress. Furthermore, certain types of activity, such as ascending and descending stairs or hills, can lead to pacing rate changes of inappropriate magnitude. For example, since most people walk downstairs faster than they walk upstairs, activity-based sensors tend to produce a faster pacing rate on walking downstairs,[3,4] although walking upstairs requires more effort. The inadequate rate response on ascending often leads to tiredness and a slowing of the rate of ascent, resulting in a nonphysiologic *decrease* in pacing rate.[7] In contrast, "physiologic" sensors, such as the QT interval, respiratory activity, temperature, oxygen saturation or pH, and right ventricular pressure or volume changes, may vary their pacing rate in accordance with physiologic demand, but their rate of increase in pacing rate at the onset of exercise is often poor in comparison to that produced by activity-sensing devices.[3,4,6]

Some individual sensors may have inappropriate responses to certain stimuli. The paced depolarization integral (or "ventricular depolarization gradient") responds well to most changes in physiologic demand[8-11] and has been incorporated in a "closed loop" pacing system. However, unlike most physiologic sensors, it does not respond appropriately to postural changes, producing an inappropriate rise in pacing rate when the patient assumes a horizontal position.[11] It also responds inappropriately to beta blockade, increasing the pacing rate in response to esmolol[12] or propranolol[13] infusion. The pacing system that senses respiratory minute ventilation by changes in thoracic impedance is designed to filter out impedance changes at a frequency of 1 Hz or faster, in order to ignore the effects of cardiac ejection on thoracic impedance. This makes it unsuitable for children, who often have rapid respiratory rates during activity or stress. In addition, the respiratory changes during speech may be inadvertently disregarded by this pacemaker, so that patients with this pacemaker may experience an inappropriate fall in pacing rate if they talk while exercising.[14]

Given these limitations of each individual sensor, the physician faced with the decision to implant a rate-responsive pacemaker must assess the patient's pattern of daily activities. Some physicians prefer to implant an activity-sensing device in the elderly and in relatively inactive patients who usually only exercise for brief periods, but they choose a more physiologic sensor for patients who are more likely to undertake more prolonged activities.[1] The actual choice of pacemaker may depend on local expertise and familiarity with certain pacing systems.[1]

Which Sensors?

Some currently available rate-adaptive pacemakers have "dual sensor" function by accident rather than by design. Two types of respiratory-sensing pacemakers (Biorate and Meta) have been shown to produce an increase in pacing rate with movement of the arm ipsilateral to the generator site,[15-17] even when the respiratory rate and minute volume remain constant. This fortuitous lack of specificity of the respiratory sensor may help to account for the fact that the response of respiratory-dependent pacemakers at the onset of exercise tends to be more rapid than that of most other "physiologic" sensors.

Dual chamber rate-responsive (DDDR) pacemakers effectively make use of two sensors in order to determine the ventricular pacing rate: the sensed atrial rate, and an additional sensor such as motion (vibration or acceleration) or minute ventilation. The earliest DDDR pacemakers were appropriate for patients with atrioventricular block and chronotropic incompetence: the resulting paced rate was simply whichever rate was higher—the sensed atrial rate or that indicated by the rate response sensor. Newer units incorporate a more refined pacing algorithm, so that the ventricular pacing rate will not necessarily be increased

TABLE *2*

Factors Influencing Choice of Sensor Combinations

1. Combining appropriate features of two sensors, e.g., activity sensor for rapid response at onset of exercise and physiologic sensor to regulate rate during exercise.
2. Offsetting an "inappropriate" response of one sensor by combination with another sensor.
3. Use of two sensors that have their maximum sensitivities at different levels of exercise.
4. Hardware requirements, e.g., additional sensing leads.
5. Expertise of individual manufacturers.

inappropriately in cases of atrial tachyarrhythmias if the rate response sensor does not indicate a need for an increase in ventricular rate. Similar "cross-checking" functions may also prove useful in the prevention and/or termination of pacemaker-mediated tachycardia in patients with DDDR pacemakers.

The factors that are likely to influence the choices of sensor combinations are listed in Table 2. Ideally, a dual sensor pacemaker would combine the best features of two or more sensors in an appropriate fashion, for example, by using an activity sensor to effect a rapid increase in pacing rate at the onset of activity, and a physiologic sensor to regulate the pacing rate during different levels of activity in accordance with metabolic demand. Such a system could also employ a "cross-checking" algorithm in order to limit any changes in pacing rate that might be produced by an inappropriate response of one of the sensors. For example, the inappropriate rate increase signaled by the paced depolarization integral (PDI) sensor when a patient lies down could be offset by coupling it with a physiologic sensor such as respiratory minute volume. On the other hand, coupling the PDI with an activity sensor may be inappropriate, since activity sensors may also respond inappropriately to postural changes in some patients.

Another potential application for sensor combinations is the use of two or more sensors that have their maximum sensitivities at different levels of exercise. For example, measurement of mixed venous oxygen saturation may be useful for rate response during low-level exercise or for exercise of recent onset, whereas mixed venous temperature measurements may help to ensure a sustained increate in rate with increasing levels of activity.

Since several rate response parameters require additional sensing hardware (e.g., specially constructed leads or additional leads for sensing pressure, temperature, etc.), it is obviously important that any combination of sensors be technically compatible. Ideally, the sensors should be compatible with a standard unipolar or bipolar pacing lead, and the dual sensor system should be implantable with ease at the time of a generator change; in practice, not more than one of the sensors should require a special lead or an additional lead. Finally, the expertise of individual pacing companies in the development and implementation of particular sensor systems may provide the incentive for the development of combinations of those sensors.

How Do They Work?

There have been several small-scale studies in which the effects of combinations of two or more sensors on pacing rate during exercise have been studied. Most of these have involved patients with an implanted VVI or single sensor VVIR pacemaker reprogrammed on a beat-to-beat basis in accordance with information from another sensor. Heuer et al.[18] studied 20 patients with an implanted ventricular pacemaker, an activity sensing pacemaker strapped to the chest wall, and a temperature sensing electrode inserted into the right atrium. The implanted pacemaker was programmed to the VVT mode. Signals from the activity and temperature sensors were processed by computer and the implanted pacemaker triggered by chest wall stimulation at a rate determined by the combination of the two sensors. They showed that the activity sensor responded well at the onset of exercise, and after the first 2 minutes of exercise, the change in mixed venous temperature was the dominant factor in inducing further changes in pacing rate. Subsequent studies in eight patients with an implanted QT-sensing pacemaker and an external activity-sensing pacemaker were largely unsuccessful because of difficulties in programming.

Stangl et al.[19] described a multisensor pacing system using stroke volume, respiratory rate, mixed venous oxygen saturation, temperature, right atrial pressure, right ventricular pressure, and right ventricular dP/dt. Using a multisensor catheter in 12 healthy volunteers, they studied the characteristics of each sensor during exercise testing on a bicycle ergometer. Of these parameters, they showed that oxygen saturation was the fastest to respond and was sensitive to workload during low-level exercise. Temperature responded slowly, but had the highest sensitivity at workloads above 75 watts. Respiratosy rate was slow to respond, but accurate at higher exercise levels. Stroke volume changes were rapid but poorly correlated with workload. They concluded that oxygen saturation and temperature might be a suitable combination of sensors, especially since both can be measured using the same semiconductor sensor.

Sugiura et al.[20] studied the effect of a combination of respiratory rate and blood temperature in an anesthetized dog with complete atrioventricular block. They demonstrated an increase in pacing rate and cardiac output in response to a pyrogenic drug which increased both respiratory rate and temperature. More recently,[21] they have used a "fuzzy logic" approach in order to combine data from these two sensors in canine studies.

Alt et al.[22] used a combination of activity and central venous temperature in five healthy volunteers in order to develop an external rate-responsive pacing system. Using a temporary pacing lead with integral thermistor and an externally attached activity-sensing device, they measured the outputs of both these sensors, individually and in combination during graded treadmill exercise tests, and developed a pacing algorithm that combined data from the two sensors. Onset of exercise was sensed by the motion sensor, resulting in an appropriate rapid increase in pacing rate. Unless exercise was confirmed by an increase in central venous blood temperature within 2 to 3 minutes, the pacing rate would return to baseline. If exercise continued, the pacing rate would be regulated according to the rise in temperature.

Res and Boute[23] studied 14 patients with implanted QT sensing pacemakers in order to determine whether useful additional information could be obtained from measurement of the endocardial T-wave amplitude. They studied the effects on evoked T-wave amplitude (measured with the pacemaker programmer) of various pacing rates (50 to 120 beats per minute) at rest and of exercise at a fixed pacing rate. They showed that increasing the pacing rate did not affect T-wave amplitude, but graded exercise at a fixed pacing rate resulted in a linear increase in T-wave amplitude, beginning within 30 seconds of onset of exercise. Whether these data can be incorporated into a rate-modulation algorithm remains to be determined.

The combination of evoked QT interval and activity has been shown to be beneficial as a sensor combination for rate-modulated pacing, Landman et al.[24] studied nine patients with implanted QT-sensing pacemakers and externally attached activity-sensing devices, and developed an algorithm to combine data from the two sensors. They performed three treadmill exercise tests on each patient, the internal pacemaker being programmed on a beat-to-beat basis according to signals from the QT interval, the activity sensor, or the combination. They demonstrated that the sensor combination provided a rate response more similar to the atrial rate than each individual sensor, with an appropriately rapid increase in rate (triggered by the activity sensor) at the onset of exercise, and a continuing rise in pacing rate (triggered by the QT interval) as workload increased.

An implantable pacemaker that incorporates QT and activity sensing (Topaz, Vitatron BV, Velp, Netherlands) has been developed and is now commercially available in Europe. As well as incorporating the functions

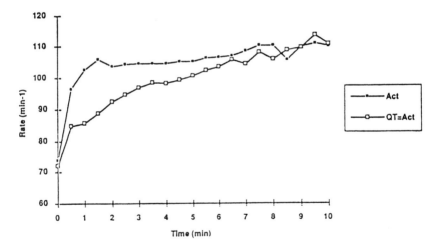

Figure 1. Average rate response during treadmill exercise testing in 15 patients with an implanted Topaz dual sensor pacemaker. With the rate response programmed to respond to activity alone, there is a rapid rise in pacing rate at the onset of exercise, but little further change in pacing rate as the workload increases. When the rate response is programmed to a combination of QT and activity, there is an appropriate increase in pacing rate within the first 30 seconds (triggered by activity) and a more gradual rate increase with increasing metabolic demand.

of the algorithm developed by Landman et al.[24] (Fig. 1), it includes a Sensor Blending™ (Vitatron BV, Velp, The Netherlands) function, whereby the relative contributions of activity and QT interval to the overall pacing rate are programmable for each patient. Furthermore, Sensor Cross-Checking helps to ensure that inappropriate responses of one sensor (such as tapping or vibration over the pacemaker generator) do not lead to an inappropriately high pacing rate for a prolonged period (Fig. 2). The evoked T wave is sensed from a standard unipolar lead, and activity sensing is achieved via a piezoelectric crystal in the generator.

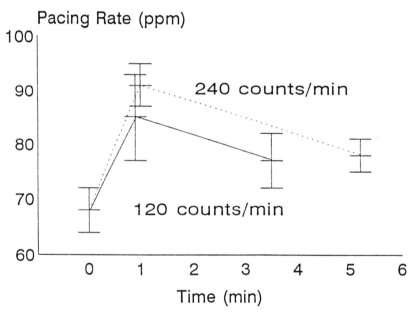

Figure 2.   Sensor cross-checking in a dual sensor VVIR pacemaker. Effect of false-positive activity sensing on the rate response of the Topaz dual sensor pacemaker. Continuous light tapping over the pacemaker generator at a rate of 120 per minute (solid line, n = 10) resulted in an increase in the pacing rate to 85 ± 8 pulses per minute (triggered by activity sensing). More vigorous tapping produced a doubling of the activity counts (dotted line, n = 3) and a maximum pacing rate of 91 ± 4 pulses per minute. As the QT interval signal did not confirm the requirement for a high pacing rate, the pacing rate gradually declined towards the baseline over the next few minutes despite the persistence of the high activity signal.

The pacemaker, therefore, does not require any additional hardware, and can be attached to a chronically implanted lead at the time of a generator change. Initial experience with the first 90 implants of this device[25] suggests that it functions well, is relatively easy to program, and that the algorithm for combining data from two sensors functions satisfactorily.

Conclusions

Several companies are now actively developing devices that utilize a combination of two or more rate-response sensors. It remains to be seen which of these new combinations will function appropriately in the long term. In particular, the benefits of sensor combinations need to be assessed not only on treadmill or bicycle ergometers, but during everyday activities and on a long-term basis in a wide range of patients. Future studies must determine whether a more "physiologic" profile of heart rate changes during activity equates with an improvement in symptoms or exercise tolerance, and if so, whether or not these advantages are gained at the expense of increased complexity in implantation, programming, and follow-up. Such complexities need not necessarily be the case; currently, optimal pacing with a single sensor device requires appropriate sensor and individualized programming of the rate-response parameters. If the "default" settings of a universally applicable dual sensor system perform as well as the highly individualized optimal settings of a carefully chosen single sensor device, dual sensor technology may actually simplify both the choice of rate-responsive pacemaker and the programming. Physicians and manufacturers should set their sights on the conquest of these challenges in the new era of dual sensor rate-responsive pacing.

References

1. Lau C-P, Camm AJ. Rate responsive pacing. In: El-Sherif N, Samet P (eds.). Cardiac Pacing and Electrophysiology, 3rd ed. 1991, pp 524–544.
2. Furman S. Rate-modulated pacing. Circulation 1990;82:108.
3. Lau CP, Butrous GS, Ward DE, Camm AJ. Comparison of exercise performance of six rate-adaptive ventricular cardiac pacemakers. Am J Cardiol 1989;63:833–838.
4. Sulke AN, Pipilis A, Henderson RA, Bucknall CA, Sowton E. Comparison of the normal sinus node with seven types of rate responsive pacemaker during everyday activity. Br Heart J 1990;64:25–31.

5. Lau CP, Mehta D, Toff WD, et al. Limitations of rate response of an activity sensing rate responsive pacemaker to different forms of activity. PACE 1988;10:141.
6. Mehta D, Lau CP, Ward DE, Camm AJ. Comparative evaluation of chronotropic responses of QT sensing and activity sensing rate responsive pacemakers. PACE 1988;11:1405–1412.
7. Candinas RA, Gloor HO, Amann FW, Schoenbeck M, Turina M. Activity-sensing rate responsive versus conventional fixed-rate pacing: a comparison of rate behavior and patient well-being during routine daily exercise. PACE 1991;14:204–213.
8. Callaghan F, Vollmann W, Livingston A, Boveja B, Abels D. The ventricular depolarization gradient: effects of exercise, pacing rate, epinephrine, and intrinsic heart rate control on the right ventricular evoked response. PACE 1989;12:1115–1130.
9. Callaghan F, Camerlo J, Tarjan P. The ventricular depolarization gradient: exercise performance of a closed-loop rate responsive pacemaker. PACE 1987;10:1212.
10. Singer I, Olash J, Brennan AF, Kupersmith J. Initial clinical experience with a rate responsive pacemaker. PACE 1989;12:1458–1464.
11. Paul V, Garratt C, Ward DE, Camm AJ. Closed loop control of rate adaptive pacing: clinical assessment of a system analyzing the ventricular depolarization gradient. PACE 1989; 12:1896–1902.
12. Singer I, Brennan AF, Steinhaus B, Maldonado C, Kupersmith J. Effects of stress and beta 1 blockade on the ventricular depolarization gradient of the rate modulating pacemaker. PACE 1991;14:460–469.
13. Lasaridis K, Paul VE, Katritsis D, Ward DE, Camm AJ. Influence of propranolol on the ventricular depolarization gradient. PACE 1991; 14:787–792.
14. Lau CP, Antoniou A, Ward DE, Camm AJ. Initial clinical experience with a minute ventilation sensing rate responsive pacemaker: improvements in exercise capacity and symptomatology. PACE 1988;11:1815.
15. Webb SC, Lewis LM, Morris-Thurgood JA, Palmer RG, Samderson JE. Respiratory-dependent pacing: a dual response from a single sensor. PACE 1988;11:730–735.
16. Lau CP, Ritchie D, Butrous GS, et al. Rate modulation by arm movements of the respiratory dependent rate responsive pacemaker. PACE 1988;11:744.
17. Lau CP, Ward DE, Camm AJ. Single chamber cardiac pacing with two forms of respiration-controlled rate responsive pacemakers. Chest 1989;95:352.
18. Heuer H, Koch T, Isbruch F, Gulker H. Pacemaker stimulation by a two sensor regulation. PACE 1987; 10:688.
19. Stangl K, Wirtzfeld A, Heinze A, Laule M, Seitz K, Gobl G. A new multisensor pacing system using stroke volume, respiratory rate, mixed venous oxygen saturation, and temperature, right atrial pressure, right ventricular pressure, and dP/dt. PACE 1988;11:712–724.
20. Sugiura T, Kimura M, Mizushina S, Yoshimura K, Harada Y. Cardiac pace-

maker regulated by respiratory rate and blood temperature. PACE 1988;1077–1084.

21. Sugiura T, Mizushina S, Kimura M, Fukui Y, Harada Y. A fuzzy approach to the rate control in an artificial cardiac pacemaker regulated by respiratory rate and temperature: a preliminary report. J Med Eng Tech 1991;15:107–110.

22. Alt E, Theres H, Heinz M, Matula M, Thilo R, Blomer H. A new rate-modulated pacing system optimized by combination of two sensors. PACE 1988;11:1119–1129.

23. Res JCJ, Boute W. A dual sensor in a rate responsive pacemaker: the QT interval and the T wave amplitude (abstr). Eur Heart J 1990;11:199.

24. Landman MAJ, Senden PJ, van Rooijen H, van Hemel WM. Initial clinical experience with rate adaptive cardiac pacing using two sensors simultaneously. PACE 1990;13:1615–1622.

25. Connelly DT, for The Topaz Study Group. Initial experience with a new single chamber, dual sensor rate responsive pacemaker. PACE 1992 (in press).

Chapter 14

Do We Really Need Automatic Pacemakers?

PHILIPPE RITTER, SERGE CAZEAU,

JACQUES MUGICA

Introduction

Modern cardiac pacemakers have become more and more sophisticated thanks to the incorporation of microprocessors. Extension of
RAM memory allows the introduction of new pacing functions as well
as extended diagnostic capabilities. However, simultaneous use of various functions may lead to misinterpretation of ECG tracings. Furthermore, programming requires the exact knowledge of all the functions
contained in the implanted pacemaker in order to provide the best hemodynamic and electrophysiologic status to the patient and to avoid
misfunctioning which may lead to complications.

Some pacemaker dysfunctions are avoided by a specific automatic
design. One example of this automatic function is the ventricular safety
pacing function. To avoid the effect of AV crosstalk (no ventricular pacing after atrial pacing because of ventricular sensing of the atrial spike
after the blanking period), ventricular safety pacing triggers ventricular
pacing after a period (around 100 ms) when the pacer detects an event
in the ventricle (of any origin) after the blanking period but within the
safety window. In other circumstances, one can imagine that the pacemaker might be able to recognize a given abnormality and might au-

New Perspectives in Cardiac Pacing, Vol. 3, edited by S. Serge Barold and Jacques Mugica,
Mount Kisco, NY, Futura Publishing Co., © 1993.

tomatically correct the programming settings for avoiding complications.

In our mind, automaticity implies the automatic reprogramming of the device to improve hemodynamics or electrophysiology by better reproducing the physiologic behavior of a given biologic parameter, or to improve the pacemaker function.

If the aim of automaticity is to improve the patient's status, manual control of the automatic function must remain available to adapt pacemaker function to every specific pathologic situation. On the other hand, if the aim of automaticity is to ensure the patient's safety, then we really need automatic pacemakers.

This discussion focuses on four examples to illustrate the importance of automatic safety functions: autocapture, autosensing, automatic protection against endless loop tachycardias, and fallback.

Autocapture

This system automatically adapts the pacing output to the physiologic and pathologic variations of pacing threshold. The goal is the reduction of current drain from the battery and the prevention of exit block in the ventricle. Autocapture was first developed by Telectronics-Cordis and introduced in the Prism device. The evoked QRS complex is measured after every ventricular pacing spike to determine efficacy of the stimulus.[1-3] The capture verification mechanism is triggered from time to time to adjust stimulus output. It is necessary to minimize the polarization voltage from pacing in order to sense cardiac depolarization just after the pacing spike from the same electrodes that pace the heart.[4] A triphasic waveform spike was designed to minimize the polarization artifact to allow accurate analysis of the evoked potential.[5,6] A positive precharge preceeds the conventional spike, which is followed by a positive postcharge to balance the residual negative charge. When the three phases of the output pulse are properly adjusted, the positive charge emitted during the precharge and the postcharge is approximately equal to the negative charge emitted during the negative pacing spike. Thus, the positive and negative charges canceled each other and the lead is charge-balanced. To adjust the duration of the positive precharge, a hardware feedback circuit delivers a pulse 120 ms after the stimulus, within the myocardial refractory period. Following completion of charge-balancing, the residual artifact is measured and averaged. A capture window is measured, which corresponds to the area integral of the first 24 ms of the evoked depolarization. The capture threshold is defined as being equal to one-third the amplitude of the capture window. The maximum allowable residual artifact is defined to be one-eighth of the amplitude of the capture window. If the residual artifact exceeds this value, charge-balancing is repeated in order to obtain an 8:1 signal-to-noise ratio. Then the automatic threshold searching algorithm accurately determines capture threshold. Upon loss of capture, a double duration pulse is triggered after 120 ms to avoid a ventricular pause and a 0.8 V safety margin is added to the capture threshold, and the pulse is again charge-balanced. Then the pacemaker will continuously verify ventricular capture. After every fourth pacemaker pulse, capture is checked. If capture is not detected, a back-up pulse is triggered. After three consecutive losses of capture, the whole process is repeated. So far, this system has been used only in the ventricle. However, the same technique could be used for automatic output regulation for atrial pacing.[7]

Autosensing

Control of sensitivity is of major importance, specially in dual chamber pacing. Oversensing of myopotentials or external interference may lead to pacemaker-mediated tachycardia or to pacemaker inhibition with syncope. Undersensing of atrial signals is frequent during exercise or during atrial tachycardias, resulting in VVI function. Autosensing was incorporated in the Intermedics Cosmos II DDD model and the Relay DDDR pulse generator. The objective of autosensing is to provide consistent sensing and prevent oversensing. The most sensitive setting must be programmed to use the automatic sensitivity program. The pulse generator achieves a steady state gradually by seeking the best minimum sensitivity. The device determines the sensing threshold automatically by measuring the lowest sensitivity that will sense the spontaneous signal. The pacemaker contains two sensing circuits set at two different sensitivity levels: an outer target and an inner target twice as sensitive as the outer target. The pacer measures the signal relative to these two levels, constantly readjusting the sensitivity levels such that the electrographic signal falls just below the outer target but well above the inner target. A sensing margin close to 100% is ensured. Unfortunately, the system is not designed to regain sensing if lost. Amplitude of the atrial signal can decrease during exercise. During undersensing by the Relay DDDR pacemaker, because autosensing does not correct the sensitivity level, the device functions in the DVI or DVIR mode without heart rate acceleration leading to dyspnea and fatigue on exertion. This behavior may theoretically lead to atrial arrhythmias, and we prefer not to use this feature. However, this system represents the first attempt of automatic adjustment of sensitivity.

Automatic Control of Endless Loop Tachycardias

Protection against retrograde conduction is better managed in modern dual chamber pacemakers than in the older-generation devices. Most of the devices are now well protected against endless loop tachycardias (ELT). However, this protection acts only when the rate of the suspected ELT is equal to the upper rate limit (URL), whereas 30–68.4% of the ELT episodes have a rate inferior to the upper rate limit.[8,9] The ELT rate depends on the duration of the AV interval and the retrograde VA conduction time. If the sum of these two intervals is longer than the upper rate interval (for ventricular pacing), the rate of the ELT will be less than the programmed upper rate. If the sum of these two intervals is shorter than the URL, the AV intervals are lengthened and the ELT rate is equal to the upper rate. In the Paragon II and Synchrony II (Siemens-Pacesetter) devices, the user must select a rate over which, after 10 or 127 ventricular beats, one P wave will not synchronize a ventricular stimulus to interrupt the ELT.

The best example of automaticity is provided by the Chorus II device (ELA Medical).[9] The concept of the protection against ELTs proposed by this model has already been described.[10,11] This algorithm is based on the stability of the VA retrograde conduction time (from the V paced to the retrograde P sensed). When the device meets the following criteria over eight ventricular beats, it will suspect the occurrence of an ELT episode: atrial sensing, ventricular pacing, with VP time less than 453 ms, and stability of the VP time within 16 to 31 ms. When these four criteria are fulfilled, the pacemaker will differentiate a normal sinus rhythm from an ELT. On the ninth beat, it modulates the AV delay (AVD) one time, but this process is automatic. If the stability of the VP ranged within 16 ms, the AVD modulation will shorten the AVD by 4 to 7 ms. If the stability of the VP time ranged within 31 ms, the AVD modulation will shorten the AVD by 63 ms. Furthermore, if the subsequent AVD shortening (accompanied by the same VV interval shortening) results in violation of the upper rate limit, then AVD modulation will not cause shortening but rather extension of the AVD. After modulation, if VA conduction time remains stable, the pacemaker identifies the rhythm as secondary to retrograde conduction. Then, after the next cycle, the postventricular atrial refractory period (PVARP) is extended to its maximum value (450 ms) in order to interrupt the ELT. If VP time does not remain within the VP stability range after AVD modulation, the pacemaker interprets the rhythm as sinus rhythm not influenced by AVD modulation. Sometimes, shortening of the VV interval induced by negative AVD modulation results in retrograde conduction block. In this situation, atrial pacing frequently occurs after the tachycardia. If so, the conclusion is that the rhythm was due to retrograde conduction, blocked after the AVD modulation, and this episode is registered by the pacemaker counter of ELT. When two consecutive ELT episodes occur, or when the number of ELTs per day exceeds a programmable value, then the device automatically reprograms the AVD value and, if necessary, the PVARP value.

In conclusion, this system is fully automatic and provides improved protection against ELTs as the algorithm is able to reprogram the device without intervention by the physician. However, the algorithm may not work in exceptional situations such as retrograde conduction times greater than 450 ms, or Wenckebach-like behavior of the retrograde conduction after negative AVD modulation. Despite these limitations, the success rate approaches 98%.[9]

Protection Against Atrial Arrhythmias

Occurrence of atrial tachycardia may lead to fast ventricular pacing with tachycardia-induced heart failure if the episode is prolonged. To avoid such a situation, fallback was designed to allow for a low ventricular pacing rate during episodes of atrial arrhythmias. In the Cosmos I (Intermedics), Quadra and Reflex DDD (Telectronics), and Chorus I and RM (Ela Medical), fallback is operating after the atrial rate exceeds the upper rate limit when the pacemaker is in the Wenckebach upper rate response. Then the ventricular pacing rate is decelerated until it reaches the fallback rate and AV synchrony is no longer maintained. The pacemaker functions in the VDI mode. This means that the pacing mode is VVT with the ability to sense atrial events. When the atrial tachycardia resumes, 1:1 AV synchrony returns. Although the overall efficacy of this response is satisfactory, acceleration of the ventricular rate prior to fallback initiation represents a disadvantage.

In the Telectronics pacemakers, one has to program the atrial rate of fallback onset and must be very careful in programming the 2:1 block rate higher than this atrial rate of fallback onset, otherwise the pacemaker never goes into the fallback mode. Then, the fallback onset ventricular rate must be programmed. We should keep in mind that Wenckebach operation induces a decrease in mean ventricular rate. As atrial rate accelerates, mean ventricular rate approaches the 2:1 AV block rate.

Consequently, if the fallback onset ventricular rate is equal to the URL, and once fallback is initiated, ventricular rate reaccelerates before decelerating again when reaching the fallback rate. In addition, if URL is programmed at a low value (110 or 100 bpm), fallback onset ventricular rate can be programmed at a higher value. Therefore, one must pay a lot of attention before programming this feature in theses devices.

In the Chorus I device, the number of ventricular cycles in the Wenckebach mode prior to fallback is programmable. If the physician programs 10 cycles, then the protection algorithm against endless-loop tachycardias will not work properly. Then the next step is 100 cycles, but intermittent atrial undersensing may sometimes cause the pacemaker to remain in the Wenckebach mode for a long time before going to fallback. In the Chorus RM, the first programmable setting is 50 cycles, which is a better compromise for optimizing pacemaker function. In this model, fallback causes pacing mode conversion from DDD to VVI, or from DDD to VVIR, or from DDDR to VVIR, depending on the selection programmed.

In all the devices decribed above, short total atrial refractory periods are required for optimal function as these pacemakers cannot sense atrial events in the postventricular atrial refractory period (PVARP).

The Quintech 931 and Harmony devices (Vitatron) provide an attempt to discriminate normal sinus acceleration from the onset of atrial arrhythmia. These pacemakers use a detection window (100 ms) below the programmed URL, in which the spontaneous atrial beats are counted. If the number of consecutive P waves sensed within this window is more than five and the atrial rate subsequently exceeds the URL, the pacemaker classifies the atrial rhythm as physiologic and responds in the Wenckebach mode. If fewer than five consecutive P waves have been counted at the moment the URL is exceeded, the atrial rhythm is defined as pathologic, PVARP is extended, URL is reduced, and the pacemaker response is in the block mode. An interesting fact is the ability of the device to sense atrial events in the PVARP after the absolute atrial refractory period. In addition, this feature may represent a good protection against endless loop tachycardias.

Atrial sensing within PVARP is of major importance for detecting fast atrial rates. The Chorus II device is able to sense atrial rates as fast as 425 bpm. Atrial events can be sensed 110 ms after the ventricular events and within PVARP. The device can differentiate normal sinus activity from premature atrial contractions (PAC). A window of atrial rate acceleration detection (WARAD) enables the pacemaker to make this differentiation. The WARAD is defined as a period that starts after an atrial event and lasts 75% (nominal value) of the preceding sinus interval. A normal sinus acitivity is defined as an atrial event outside the refractory periods and outside the WARAD. A PAC is defined as a sensed atrial event outside the refractory periods and within the WARAD. When a PAC is sensed, the device does not pace the ventricle and resets an atrial escape interval (AEI) equal to the WARAD value. At the end of the AEI, the device paces the atrium and the ventricle with a 31-ms AV delay, in order to minimize the ventricular escape interval and to optimize atrial sensing for this cycle. If a spontaneous atrial event is sensed during the AEI, an atrial arrhythmia suspicion phase is started for 30 seconds during which the URL is limited to 120 bpm (or less if URL is less than 120 bpm), and AV delay duration is 31 ms in order to optimize atrial sensing. If the atrial arrhythmia is sustained after 30 seconds, fallback operation is initiated. When the atrial rate decreases below 120 bpm, 1:1 AV association is reestablished.

This algorithm represents an interesting improvement of the fallback functioning. However, the differentiation between normal sinus acceleration and PACs is established on the WARAD value, which is an equivalent of the atrial event prematurity. The nominal value of 75% seems to be satisfactory for most patients; but in young patients, the 62.5% value is preferable as the percentage of cycle-to-cycle shortening of sinus intervals can be superior to 25% at exercise onset (for example, running up stairs). The user must be very cautious when programming the device.

If the WARAD value programming is inappropriate, fallback can be initiated at exercise onset.

The use of implantable sensors to judge the appropriateness of atrial rate is a new approach to the management of pacemaker-mediated tachycardias. Two devices have this capability: the Relay (Intermedics) and the DDDR-Meta (Telectronic).

In the Relay, a conditional ventricular tracking limit (CVTL) can be used to protect the patient against PMTs. This CVTL is set at 35 bpm above the lower rate and is not programmable. When the P-wave rate is 35 bpm above the lower rate in the absence of sensor-indicating exercise, the Relay will consider this rhythm as pathologic and will respond in a Wenckebach mode at the CVTL.[12] However, when the patient exercises, and when the sensor algorithm has indicated a heart rate acceleration superior to 20 bpm above the lower rate, the CVTL is no longer active. In the event of atrial tachycardia, sudden ventricular rate acceleration can occur after exercise onset until the patient returns to rest. On the other hand, if the patient's heart rate is close to the CVTL at rest, and at exercise onset, atrioventricular dissociation may occur, thus limiting exercise capacity.[13] A lower rate must thus be programmed at a high level if one wants to limit this problem.

In the DDDR-Meta, PVARP adapts according to sensor activity (but not to sinus rate), proportionally to the metabolic indicated rate (MIR). PVARP decreases until the maximum rate is reached where PVARP equals MIR minus the AV delay. The AV delay also shortens proportionally to MIR. In the DDDR mode, this pacemaker does not possess the ability to exhibit a Wenckebach upper rate response. When a P wave falls in the adapted PVARP, the next atrial spike is omitted and any P wave occurring before the next ventricular spike will not start an AV delay. The pacemaker temporarily works in the VVIR mode. To ensure that maximum stability of rate is maintained and that switching from VVIR to DDDR and back again is minimized, running documentation of atrial events is maintained by the atrial rate monitor (ARM). The ARM is updated for each P wave that is sensed, no matter what the current operational mode happens to be. The ARM is also updated whenever an atrial output occurs. If the PP interval is greater than the total atrial refractory period, the ARM will decrement (minimum = 0). If the PP interval is less than the total atrial refractory period, the ARM will increment (maximum = 3). At the time of each ventricular output (or when the R wave is sensed), the ARM is examined. If the count is at its minimum value of zero, the pacemaker will return to DDDR mode. Thus, in the presence of atrial arrhythmias, the pacemaker will continue to function in the VVIR mode as long as the PP interval is shorter than the adapted total atrial refractory period until slowing of the atrial rate no longer produces P waves within the adpated PVARP, whereupon AV synchrony is restored.

Once again, a propensity of developing AV dissociation during sinus rhythm can occur. Due to the long response time of the system, and if the patient starts to exercise, sinus rate may increase faster than the MIR. This leads to P waves falling within the relatively long PVARP with mode shifted to VVIR and AV dissociation.

These limitations cannot occur if the indication for DDDR pacing is appropriate, i.e., sinus chronotropic incompetence during exercise. AV synchrony will be maintained at exercise onset, as the heart rate acceleration will depend on the sensor-indicated rate. In the event of atrial arrhythmia, pacing mode conversion will operate properly.

In conclusion, do we really need automatic pacemakers? Yes, for safety reasons. Tools already exist but they are not all included in a single device. The autocapture system is not commercially available with the charge balancing system. The autosensing system cannot correct under-sensing automatically. The protection against endless loop tachycardias is smart but there are still few limitations in borderline situations. The fallback algorithms offer a satisfactory protection against sustained atrial arrhythmias but improvements are required for almost all the systems. Progress will probably come quickly as the computer-based pacemakers offer the ability to test new functions temporarily. Once the new function is validated, it can be implemented permanently in the implanted systems. Close cooperation between physicians and engineers will undoubtedly lead to new concepts and algorithms and bring us closer to a truly automatic pacemaker.

References

1. Boute W, Candelon B, Wittkampf FHM. Characterization of the endocardial evoked potentials. Clin Prog Electrophysiol Pacing 1986;4:47.
2. Nappholz TA, Whingham R, Hansen J, et al. Automatic detection of atrial and ventricular capture. Clin Prog Electrophysiol Pacing 1986;4:46.
3. Curtis AB, Vance F, Miller-Shifrin K. Characteristic variation in evoked potential amplitude with changes in pacing stimulus strength. Am J Cardiol 1990;66:416.

4. Curtis AB, Vance F, Shifrin K. A successful method for minimizing stimulus polarization artifact for accurate evaluation of intracardiac evoked potentials. PACE 1990;13:519.

5. Curtis AB, Vance F, Miller K. Automatic reduction of stimulus polarization artifact for accurate evaluation of ventricular evoked responses. PACE 1991;14:529.

6. Feld GK, Love CJ, Camerlo J, et al. A new pacemaker algorithm for continuous capture verification and automatic threshold determination: elimination of pacemaker afterpotential utilizing a triphasic charge-balancing system. PACE 1992;15:171.

7. Livingston AR, Callaghan FJ, Byrd CL, et al. Atrial capture detection with endocardial electrodes. PACE 1989;12:1896.

8. Limousin M, Bonnet JL. A new algorithm to solve endless loop tachycardia in DDD pacing: a multi-center study of 91 patients. PACE 1990;13:867.

9. Nitzsche R, Guenoun M, Lamaison D, et al. Endless loop tachycardias: description and first clinical results of a new fully automatic protection algorithm. PACE 1990;13:1711.

10. Lamaison D, Girodo S, Limousin M. A new algorithm for a high level of protection against pacemaker-mediated tachycardia. PACE 1988;11:1715.

11. Girodo S, Limousin M, Ritter P, et al. New algorithm for prevention and termination of pacemaker endless-loop tachycardia. In: Barold SS, Mugica J (eds.). New Perspectives in Cardiac Pacing, Futura Publishing Co., Mount Kisco, NY, 1988, p 405.

12. Lau CP, Li JPS, Cheng CH, et al. Sensor-initiated termination of pacemaker-mediated tachycardia in a DDDR pacemaker. Am Heart J 1991;121:595.

13. Lau CP, Tai YT, Fong PC, et al. The use of implantable sensors for the control of pacemaker-mediated tachycardias: a comparative evaluation between minute ventilation sensing and acceleration sensing dual chamber rate adaptive pacemakers. PACE 1992;15:34, 1992.

PART **III**

Selection of Pacing System and Follow-Up

Chapter 15

Considerations for the Selection of Rate-Adaptive Single Lead Atrial (AAIR) Pacing

JOHAN BRANDT, HANS SCHÜLLER

Introduction

The term "chronotropic incompetence" denotes an inability to adapt the heart rate adequately to the demands of exercise. There is currently no generally accepted strict definition of this phenomenon, but chronotropic incompetence has been reported to occur in 24% to 64% of patients with sinus node disease (SND) (Table 1). Chronotropic incompetence appears to increase in prevalence during follow-up of SND patients,[8,9] and clearly merits attention when selecting the optimal pacemaker system.

Arguments for Atrial Stimulation

Treatment-comparison studies in SND have demonstrated lower incidences of permanent atrial fibrillation,[10-13] congestive heart failure,[10-12] and possibly also systemic embolism[13,14] with atrial than with ventricular pacemaker treatment, and this appears to influence mortality during long-term follow-up.[11,12] The risk of the "pacemaker syndrome," i.e., symptoms and signs caused by inadequate timing of atrial and ventricular contractions, constitutes another drawback of ventricular pacing.[15] Furthermore, developments within the field of atrial leads have

New Perspectives in Cardiac Pacing, Vol. 3, edited by S. Serge Barold and Jacques Mugica, Mount Kisco, NY, Futura Publishing Co., © 1993.

TABLE 1

Prevalence of Chronotropic Incompetence in Sinus Node Disease

Reference	Definition	Prevalence
Abbott et al.[1]	Maximum HR less than 120/min	44%
Holden et al.[2]	(If maximum HR less than 120/min)	43%
Vallin, Edhag[3]	Maximum HR less than 135/min	52%
Johnston et al.[4]	Maximum HR less than 110/min	64%
Simonsen[5]	Maximum HR less than 125/min	40%
Prior et al.[6]	Maximum HR less than 85% of calculated	36%
Kallryd et al.[7]	Maximum HR less than 120	24%

HR = heart rate.

resulted in quite acceptable performance regarding mechanical stability and stimulation and sensing thresholds.[16–18] To withhold a pacing system providing atrioventricular (AV) synchrony from the patient with SND can therefore no longer be justified. Recently, ventricular inhibited pacing was stated to be an inappropriate treatment for SND in the British Pacing and Electrophysiology Group recommendations for pacemaker prescription.[19] However, the choice between single chamber atrial and dual chamber rate-adaptive pacing for the patient with SND and chronotropic incompetence has remained controversial.

Atrial Rate-Adaptive (AAIR) Pacing

Potential Problems

The main potential drawback of AAIR pacing is the possibility of inadequately slow AV conduction at high pacing rates, with long spike-Q intervals (Fig. 1). This may result in the occurrence of the "pacemaker syndrome" during exercise.[20–23] Clarke and Allen[20] observed this phenomenon in one patient and could subsequently reproduce it experimentally in two of ten cases. Den Dulk et al.[21] described this sequence of events in one case of dual AV nodal pathways; the clinical problem was solved when treatment with disopyramide was discontinued. Mabo,

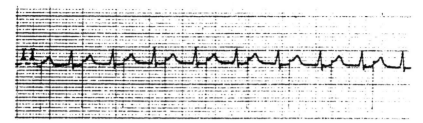

Figure 1. Rapid atrial pacing (rate 120 impulses/minute) resulting in a pro-longed spike-Q interval (320 ms). The atrial contractions occur during ventricular systole, when the AV valves are closed, with negative hemodynamic effects.

Pouillot, et al.[23] found inadequately prolonged PR intervals during exercise in 5 of 17 patients with AAIR pacing, and two of these had symptoms. In their study, as well as in other investigations of the AV conduction in this situation, drug treatment was an important factor. Edelstam et al.[24] showed that no important prolongation of the spike-Q interval occurred with an increased pacing rate during exercise with AAIR pacing except in patients on drugs with negative chronotropic effects. In a small similar study, Ruiter et al.[25] found approximately equal AV intervals at rest and maximum exercise without medication, but the AV intervals during exercise were considerably prolonged when beta-blocking drugs were given. This is in accordance with our findings in 42 patients with AAIR pacemakers: all showed enhancement of AV conduction during physical activity; the spike-Q intervals were significantly longer in patients treated by beta-blockers, whereas other antiarrhythmic drugs did not appear to have a significant negative effect on the AV conduction during exercise[26] (Fig. 2).

Another important consideration in patients with AAIR pacing is the adequate tuning of the rate increase and the choice of a suitable maximum pacing rate for the individual patient. Needless to say, significant atrioventricular conduction delay may be produced in any patient if a low level of exercise is accompanied by rapid atrial pacing ("atrial overpacing"). In our experience, a maximum pacing rate exceeding 130 impulses per minute is rarely motivated in these often elderly patients, and we aim at a pacing rate of approximately 90 per minute during normal walking.

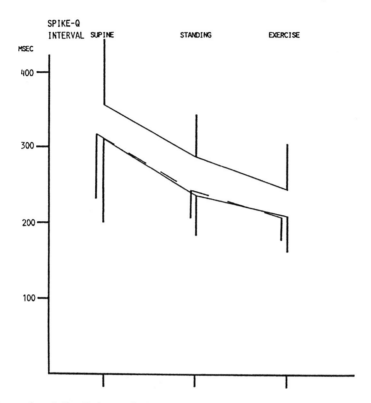

Figure 2. Spike-Q intervals (mean ± SD) at an atrial pacing rate of 120 impulses/minute in 42 patients with AAIR pacemakers. The spike-Q intervals were measured with the patients supine, standing, and immediately following exercise. Patients treated with antiarrhythmics other than beta blockers (n = 15; lower solid curve) showed spike-Q intervals not differing significantly from patients without antiarrhythmics (n = 20; broken curve). However, patients treated with beta blockers (n = 7; upper solid curve) had significantly longer spike-Q intervals during standing (p<0.02) and following exercise (p<0.05) than patients not on beta-blocking drugs (Student's *t*-test). (Used with permission of PACE.[26])

Atrial Fibrillation in Sinus Node Disease

The possibility of development of permanent atrial fibrillation must be considered in atrial pacing, as it renders the atria nonstimulatable. However, the yearly incidence of this arrhythmia in sinus node disease treated with atrial stimulation is low, approximately 1.4%.[13,27] The risk of permanent atrial fibrillation in these patients is significantly related to advanced age at pacemaker implantation, and it is very rare below 70 years of age.[27] Only a small minority of these patients show a slow ventricular rate and require reoperation to ventricular pacing.[27] There is experimental evidence that an increased atrial pacing rate may have an antitachyarrhythmic effect.[28] This raises the question whether AAIR stimulation may reduce the risk of atrial tachyarrhythmias compared to standard AAI pacing;[29] however, conclusive evidence thereof is lacking.

Atrioventricular Block in Sinus Node Disease

Another consideration is that of development of high grade AV block after atrial pacemaker implantation. In a recent long-term follow-up study of 213 patients, clinically significant AV block occurred in 1.8% of the patients per year.[27] This risk was considerably increased in the presence of complete bundle branch or bifascicular block; in the absence of such conduction disturbances, the yearly incidence was approximately 1.2%. This low incidence is in accordance with an earlier compilation of several other materials.[30]

Dual Chamber Rate-Adaptive (DDDR, DDIR) Pacing

Disadvantages of a Short Technical AV Delay

The main argument for the use of rate-adaptive dual chamber pacing systems in SND is that these do not rely upon the spontaneous AV conduction and that negative hemodynamic effects resulting from long spike-Q intervals during exercise are obviated. On the other hand, there is experimental evidence that AV sequential pacing may produce inferior hemodynamics compared to atrial stimulation, due to the unphysiologic contraction sequence of the ventricular myocardium.[31-35] The abnormal pattern of contraction resulting from right ventricular stimulation adversely effects left ventricular systolic function,[35-38] left ventricular diastolic properties,[35,39,40] and the overall cardiac pumping efficiency.[41,42] The impairment of systolic function has been demonstrated also during submaximal exercise.[35] The clinical relevance of these findings is presently uncertain. Nevertheless, it is obvious that whereas dual chamber stimulation will be of hemodynamic benefit during exercise to some patients, it is disadvantageous to others; this is schematically depicted in Figure 3.

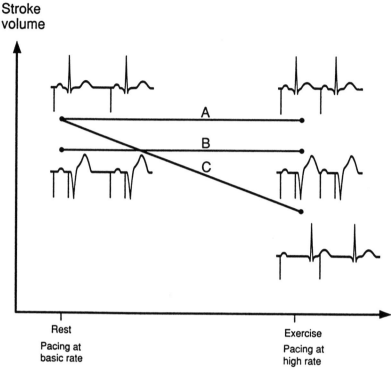

Figure 3. Schematic illustration of possible effects of atrial versus dual chamber rate-adaptive pacing during exercise. If AV conduction is normal (A), the physiologic activation sequence at rest and during exercise with increased pacing rate results in a higher stroke volume compared to AV sequential stimulation (B). This is due to the difference in ventricular activation pattern. However, AV sequential pacing is superior when impaired AV conduction during exercise with rapid atrial pacing results in an inappropriately long spike-Q interval, with a decreased stroke volume (C).

Disadvantages of a Long Technical AV Delay

It must be realized that not even a dual chamber system with normal technical function and no lead-related problems is a guarantee against occurrence of the "pacemaker syndrome."[15] The risk of this increases when a long technical AV delay is programmed (Fig. 4). Ongoing tech-

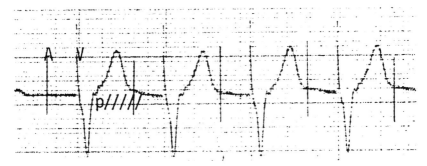

Figure 4. Dual-chamber pacing at a rate of 80 impulses/minute. The presence of retrogradely conducted P waves followed by atrial myocardial refractoriness precludes subsequent atrial capture, resulting in effective ventricular stimulation only.

nical refinements such as automatic adaptation of the AV delay to the stimulation rate will certainly prove valuable in this context.

Economic Aspects

A drawback of dual chamber systems is their cost.[43] At our institution, 96 patients have received AAIR pacemakers for sinus node disease with chronotropic incompetence since 1986. To date, a reoperation to a dual chamber system has been necessary in only two cases. The net hardware savings currently amount to approximately $167,000, compared to primary dual chamber rate-adaptive pacemaker implantation in all cases. Further, the difference in cost between atrial and dual chamber rate-adaptive pacing is likely to increase with time, due to the shorter life span and somewhat more complicated follow-up of dual chamber systems.

Conclusions

At present, rate-adaptive atrial pacing (AAIR) can be considered the first-line treatment for symptomatic sinus node disease with chronotropic incompetence. Patients with documented AV block, complete bundle branch block, or bifascicular block in addition to sinus node disease should receive a dual chamber rate-adaptive system (DDDR or DDIR) as the primary implant, as should patients in whom treatment with beta-blocking agents is deemed necessary.

References

1. Abbott JA, Hirschfeld DS, Kunkel FW, Scheinman MM. Graded exercise testing in patients with sinus node dysfunction. Am J Med 1977;62:330–338.
2. Holden W, McAnulty JH, Rahimtoola SH. Characterisation of heart rate response to exercise in the sick sinus syndrome. Br Heart J 1978;40:923–930.
3. Vallin HO, Edhag KO. Heart rate responses in patients with sinus node disease compared to controls: physiologic implications and diagnostic possibilities. Clin Cardiol 1980;3:391–398.
4. Johnston FA, Robinson JF, Fyfe T. Exercise testing in the diagnosis of sick sinus syndrome in the elderly: implications for treatment. PACE 1987;10: 831–838.
5. Simonsen E. Sinus node dysfunction (thesis, University of Odense) Odense. CAVI 1987:200–203.
6. Prior M, Masterson M, Blackburn G, Maloney J, Wilkoff B. Critical identification of patients with sinus node dysfunction for potential sensor-driven pacing (abstr). PACE 1988;11:512.
7. Kallryd A, Kruse I, Rydén L. Atrial inhibited pacing in the sick sinus node syndrome: clinical value and the demand for rate responsiveness. PACE 1989;12:954–961.
8. Gwinn N, Leman R, Zile M, Kratz J, Gillette J. Pacemaker patients become chronotropic incompetent with time (abstr). PACE 1990;13:535.
9. Vardas PE, Fitzpatrick A, Ingram A, Travill CM, Theodorakis G, Hubbard W, Sutton R. Natural history of sinus node chronotropy in paced patients. PACE 1991;14:155–160.
10. Rosenqvist M, Brandt J, Schüller H. Atrial versus ventricular pacing in sinus node disease: a treatment comparison study. Am Heart J 1986;111:292–297.
11. Rosenqvist M, Brandt J, Schüller H. Long-term pacing in sinus node disease: effects of stimulation mode on cardiovascular morbidity and mortality. Am Heart J 1988;116:16–22.
12. Santini M, Messina G, Porto MP. Sick sinus syndrome: single chamber pacing. In: Gomez FP (ed.). Cardiac Pacing, Electrophysiology, Tachyarrhythmias. Editorial Grouz, Madrid, 1985, pp 144–152.
13. Sutton R, Kenny R-A. The natural history of sick sinus syndrome. PACE 1986;9:1110–1114.
14. Sasaki S, Takeuchi A, Ohzeki M, Kishida H, Nishimoto T, Kakimoto S, Fukumoto H. Long-term follow-up of paced patients with sick sinus syndrome. In: Steinbach K, et al. (eds.). Proceedings of the VIIth World Symposium on Cardiac Pacing. Steinkopff Verlag, Darmstadt, 1983, pp 85–90.
15. Schüller H, Brandt J. The pacemaker syndrome: old and new causes. Clin Cardiol 1991;14:336–340.

16. Markewitz A, Hemmer W, Weinhold C. Complications in dual chamber pacing: a six-year experience. PACE 1986;9:1014–1018.

17. Parsonnet V, Hesselson AB, Harari DC. Long-term functional integrity of atrial leads. PACE 1991;14:517–521.

18. Wenke K, Markewitz A, Fülle P, Zipfel B. Langzeitergebnisse bei Verwendung zweier kohlenstoffbeschichteter Schraubelektroden im Vorhof. Herzschrittmacher 1989;9:93–98.

19. The British Pacing and Electrophysiology Group Working Party. Recommendations for pacemaker prescriptions for symptomatic bradycardia. Br Heart J 1991;66:185–191.

20. Clarke M, Allen A. Rate-responsive atrial pacing resulting in pacemaker syndrome (abstr). PACE 1987;10:1209.

21. den Dulk K, Lindemans FW, Brugada P, Smeets JLRM, Wellens HJJ. Pacemaker syndrome with AAI rate-variable pacing: importance of atrioventricular conduction properties, medication and pacemaker programmability. PACE 1988;11:1226–1233.

22. Pouillot C, Daubert C, Mabo P, Cazeau S, Paillard F, Le Breton H. The lack of adaptation in PR interval to heart rate: a frequent limitation for AAIR pacing (abstr). PACE 1990;13:504.

23. Mabo P, Pouillot C, Kermarrec A, Lelong B, Lebreton H, Daubert C. Lack of physiological adaptation of the atrioventricular interval to heart rate in patients chronically paced in the AAIR mode. PACE 1991;14:2133–2142.

24. Edelstam C, Nordlander R, Wallgren E, Rosenqvist M. AAIR pacing and exercise: what happens to AV conduction? (abstr). PACE 1990;13:1193.

25. Ruiter J, Burgersdijk C, Zeeders M, Kee D. Atrial Activitrax pacing. The atrioventricular interval during exercise (abstr). PACE 1987;10:1226.

26. Brandt J, Fahraeus T, Ogawa T, Schüller H. Practical aspects of rate-adaptive atrial (AAIR) pacing: clinical experiences in 44 patients. PACE 1991;14:1258–1264.

27. Brandt J. Permanent atrial pacing. Clinical studies. Thesis, University of Lund, Sweden, 1991 (obtainable from author).

28. Han J, Millet D, Chizzonitti B, Mae GK. Temporal dispersion of recovery of excitability in atrium and ventricle as a function of heart rate. Am Heart J 1966;71:481–487.

29. Kato R, Terasawa T, Gotoh T, Suzuki M. Antiarrhythmic efficacy of atrial demand (AAI) and rate responsive atrial pacing. In: Santini M, Pistolese M, Alliegro A (eds.). Proceedings of the International Symposium on Progress in Clinical Pacing. Excerpta Medica, Amsterdam, 1988, pp 15–24.

30. Rosenqvist M, Obel IWP. Atrial pacing and the risk for AV block. Is there a time for change in attitude? PACE 1989;12:97–101.

31. Gilmore JP, Sarnoff SJ, Mitchell JH, Linden RJ. Synchronicity of ventricular contraction: observations comparing haemodynamic effects of atrial and ventricular pacing. Br Heart J 1963;25:299–307.

32. Kosowsky BD, Scherlag BJ, Damato AN. Re-evaluation of the atrial contribution to ventricular function. Study using His bundle pacing. Am J Cardiol 1968;21:518–524.

33. Daggett WM, Bianco JA, Powell WJ Jr, Austen WG. Relative contributions of the atrial systole-ventricular systole interval and of patterns of ventricular activation to ventricular function during electrical pacing of the dog heart. Circ Res 1970;27:69–79.
34. Askenazi J, Alexander JH, Koenigsberg DI, Belic N, Lesch M. Alteration of left ventricular performance by left bundle branch block simulated with atrioventricular sequential pacing. Am J Cardiol 1984;53:99–104.
35. Rosenqvist M, Isaaz K, Botvinick EH, Dae MW, Cockrell J, Abbott JA, Schiller NB, Griffin JC. Relative importance of activation sequence compared to atrioventricular synchrony in left ventricular function. Am J Cardiol 1991;67:148–156.
36. Boerth RC, Covell JW. Mechanical performance and efficiency of the left ventricle during ventricular stimulation. Am J Physiol 1971:221:1686–1691.
37. Badke FR, Boinay P, Covell JW. Effects of ventricular pacing on regional left ventricular performance in the dog. Am J Physiol 1980;238:H858–H867.
38. Zhou J-T, Yu G-Y. Hemodynamic findings during sinus rhythm, atrial and AV sequential pacing compared to ventricular pacing in a dog model. PACE 1987;10:118–124.
39. Zile MR, Blaustein AS, Shimizu G, Gaasch WH. Right ventricular pacing reduces the rate of left ventricular relaxation and filling. J Am Coll Cardiol 1987;10:702–709.
40. Bedotto JB, Grayburn PA, Black WH, Raya TE, McBride W, Hsia HH, Eichhorn EJ. Alteration in left ventricular relaxation during atrioventricular pacing in humans. J Am Coll Cardiol 1990;15:658–664.
41. Koretsune Y, Kodama K, Nanto S, Ishikawa K, Taniura K, Mishima M, Inoue M, Abe H. The effect of pacing mode on external work and myocardial oxygen consumption. In: Steinbach K, et al. (eds.). Cardiac Pacing. Proceedings of the VIIth World Symposium on Cardiac Pacing. Steinkopff Verlag, Darmstadt, 1983, pp 181–186.
42. Baller D, Wolpers H-G, Zipfel J, Bretschneider H-J, Hellige G. Comparison of the effects of right atrial, right ventricular apex and atrioventricular sequential pacing on myocardial oxygen consumption and cardiac efficiency: a laboratory investigation. PACE 1988;11:394–403.
43. Eagle KA, Mulley AG, Singer DE, Schoenfeld D, Harthorne JW, Thibault GE. Single-chamber and dual-chamber cardiac pacemakers. A formal cost comparison. Ann Intern Med 1986;105:264–271.

Chapter 16

Single-Lead VDD Pacing

Giovanni Enrico Antonioli,

Lucia Ansani, Dario Barbieri,

Gabriele Guardigli,

Gianfranco Percoco, Tiziano Toselli

Introduction

The concept of an AV single lead for P-synchronous ventricular pacing, first developed more than 12 years ago to avoid the insertion of two leads, has now become a reality. In its present configuration, the AV lead represents the natural evolution of the original lead we first presented in 1979.[1,2] Since 1979, extensive clinical experience has shown that with available technology, reliable single-lead VDD pacing can be achieved successfully.[3-10] Indeed, this particular pacing mode was recently included in the Guidelines for Pacemaker Implantation promulgated by the American College of Cardiology/American Heart Association Task Force.[11]

Clinical Considerations

The development of the single-lead VDD system was based on physiologic, surgical, and practical considerations.

1. P-synchronous ventricular pacing (VDD or VAT) provides

New Perspectives in Cardiac Pacing, Vol. 3, edited by S. Serge Barold and Jacques Mugica, Mount Kisco, NY, Futura Publishing Co., © 1993.

the treatment of choice for patients suffering from AV block with normal sinoatrial function (SAF) because it preserves rate responsiveness and AV synchrony for maximum hemodynamic benefit.
2. Lead contact with the atrial wall is unnecessary in patients with complete heart block (CHB) and normal SAF (which remains unchanged over time) because atrial pacing is not required.
3. In the mid-1970s, we observed that floating unipolar electrodes in the mid-to-high right atrium consistently registered an atrial electrogram (EGM) showing important favorable characteristics for atrial sensing (Fig. 1). Our initial investigations involved 25 consecutive patients who underwent electrophysiologic study or pacemaker implantation. Atrial electrograms were recorded from 25 unmodified unipolar ventricular pacing leads with a surface area of 10–54 mm^2. Atrial recordings were obtained when the electrode tip was floating in the atrial blood pool before its insertion in the right ventricle. The electrode was directly connected to a standard high input impedance ECG recorder and electrograms were recorderd at high speed during several consecutive whole respiratory cycles, and then processed. Mean

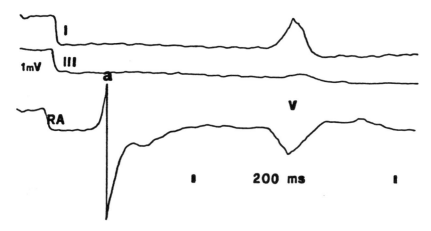

Figure 1. High-speed recording of the atrial electrogram from a floating unipolar tip-electrode. The atrial deflection is larger and sharper than the ventricular component.

TABLE *1*

Atrial Electrogram Characteristics Detected by 25 Unipolar Tip Electrodes Floating in the Mid-to-High Atrium Directly Connected to the High Impedance ECG Recorder

	Amplitude (mV)			dV/dt		Frequency Content (Hz)
	Mn	*Mx*	*t (ms)*	*Mn*	*Mx*	
Mean SD	1.11 ± 0.67	2.16 ± 1.07	7.64 ± 2.43	0.15 ± 0.09	0.29 ± 0.15	72.42 ± 24.25
Mn	0.50	0.90	4.00	0.05	0.12	41.66
Mx	3.00	4.80	13.00	0.43	0.69	125.00

Mean values and ranges of amplitude in mV, major intrinsic deflection duration (t) in ms, dV/dt, and frequency content.*

* Calculated with the simplified formula Hz = 1:2t.

Amplitude = 80% of peak-to-peak amplitude of the atrial signal; t = major intrinsic deflection duration; SD = standard deviation; Mn = minimum observed value; Mx = maximum observed value.

values and ranges of amplitude (mV), major intrinsic deflection duration (t), dV/dt, and frequency content (Hz), are summarized in Table 1. Frequency content of the signal, calculated with the simplified formula Hz = 1:2t and without complex signal analyzers, gives information about the center frequency of the bandpass amplifier that will be dedicated to detecting such a signal.[2] The different surface areas did not affect the atrial electrogram because of the high input impedance (higher than 2 megaohm) of the recorder.[12–15]

4. The necessity of two leads, one ventricular for pacing and the other atrial for sensing, proved to be the most important obstacle to the widespread utilization of the P-synchronous system, a mode already available in the early 1960s.[16] Today, the insertion of two leads in one vein is a routine procedure but, in the late 1970s, this approach was rarely used because of limited lead technology. Therefore, in the beginning, a single AV lead system capable of delivering P-synchronous ventricular pacing represented an attractive concept potentially applicable to the treatment of a large number of patients.

Lead Development

The above considerations generated the idea that P-synchronous ventricular pacing might be feasible with a single bipolar lead designed with a proximal unipolar electrode floating in the mid to high right atrium for atrial sensing and a distal unipolar electrode at the tip of the lead for ventricular pacing and sensing. Our first AV lead, designed with a coaxial structure, was similar to standard bipolar ventricular leads. Detection of atrial depolarization was achieved by a 60 mm^2 floating ring electrode mounted 12–18 cm from the tip. In our early experience with temporary and permanent VAT or VDT pacemaker implantations[1,2,17,18] a prior chest X-ray was necessary to determine the optimal distance between the ventricular and atrial electrodes.

In early designs, the unipolar ring atrial electrode was very sensitive to myopotentials, electromagnetic interference (EMI), and ventricular far-field signals. The evoked or spontaneous ventricular electrogram (EGM) registered by the floating atrial electrode demonstrated that the dV/dt of ventricular far-field signals is dramatically lower than that of the atrial signals. We compared the average amplitude, dV/dt, and the frequency content of the highest and fastest portion of each component (P and QRS) of the atrial electrogram in a series of 16 patients.[8] Maximum ventricular versus minimum atrial signal showed: 1.15 ± 0.35 mV vs. 1.72 ± 0.49 mV, 0.06 ± 0.02 dV/dt vs. 0.19 ± 0.09 dV/dt, 26.77 ± 10.11 Hz vs. 74.55 ± 23.82 Hz. All the differences were statistically significant (P<0.001). The characteristics of the ventricular EGM indicated that the far-field QRS signal was incapable of being detected by a properly designed atrial sensing circuit. Nevertheless, the single AV lead posed difficulties during implantation in terms of obtaining an optimal and stable position for both the atrial and the ventricular electrodes. The development of an active ventricular fixation lead with a 43 mm^2 atrial ring electrode 13 cm from the tip rendered positioning of the two electrodes easier and more reliable by minimizing lead dislodgement and atrial undersensing.

In 1982/1983 a single AV lead (as described above) connected to a Medtronic Enertrax 7100 pacemaker was implanted in three CHB patients for permanent VDD pacing.[19] One of these units still works perfectly after more than 9 years. One patient died of congestive heart failure 16 months after implantation; the VDD unit worked perfectly. The last unit was removed for battery exhaustion after 6 years of correct VDD functioning.[8,20] No ventricular synchronization (far-field atrial sensing) has occurred during long-term follow-up.

Development of Atrial Bipolar Configuration

The development of a bipolar configuration of atrial electrodes to eliminate EMI and myopotential oversensing was accomplished in the 1980s. In 1981, we showed that a bipolar configuration of the atrial electrodes greatly improved signal selectivity and we determined that the optimal spacing between the two poles of floating bipolar atrial lead ranged from 0.5 to 1 cm.[21,22]

In the early 1980s, two atrial dipole configurations were developed; one consisted of a double ring with a short, 5 mm (Fig. 2, type C), interelectrode distance,[21,22] and the other consisted of two hemirings forming an orthogonal dipole to the longitudinal axis of the lead, with 1 mm (Fig. 2, type D) interelectrode distance.[23,24] The former configuration has been substantially maintained in our updated model of a tripolar single AV lead with active ventricular fixation.

In the mid-to-late 1980s, two additional atrial bipolar electrode systems were developed, one with wide (30 mm, Fig. 2 type B) dipole spacing[10] and the other with two closely spaced, 7 mm (Fig. 2, type E) and diagonally positioned hemiring electrodes (diagonal atrial bipolar or

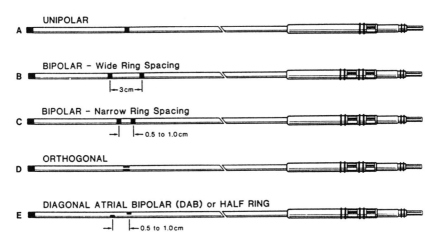

Figure 2. Five configurations of floating atrial sensing electrodes mounted on a ventricular pacing lead. See text for details.

DAB configuration).[4-7,9] At the same time, the availability of dedicated VDD pulse generators with specially designed atrial amplifiers capable of reliable detection of the atrial signal allowed extensive clinical application of single-lead VDD pacing. Figure 2 illustrates the five AV lead configurations that have been used for permanent single-lead P-synchronous ventricular pacing. Today, only the leads shown in Figure 2 B, C, and E remain commercially available. The main characteristics of atrial EGMs detected with these leads (with exception of type B) are included in Table 2.

Figure 3 shows examples of atrial EGMs detected by different electrode configurations. In our experience, the short longitudinal or diagonal dipole works best.[21,22,25,26] Figure 4 shows typical atrial EGMs in 34 patients in whom sharper atrial signals and better A/V ratios were recorded by 1-cm spacing compared to 3-cm spacing. Figure 5 depicts the efficacy of various single-lead systems in the detection of atrial activity. The A/V ratios detected with 1-cm spaced electrodes are better in all positions except the atrial floor, where the ratio is similar to the 3-cm spaced electrodes; on the other hand, all dipoles with spacing greater

TABLE 2

Atrial Electrogram Characteristics Detected by Four Different Floating Electrode Configurations (see Fig. 2). (Mean values within a whole respiratory cycle.)

Patient No.	Electrode Type	Amplitude (mV) ± SD	t (ms) ± SD	dV/dt ± SD	SI (Kohm) ± SD
39	A	1.87 ± 0.94	7.7 ± 2.6	0.23 ± 0.13	9.5 ± 2.2
14	B	3.45 ± 1.98	8.0 ± 1.7	0.42 ± 0.11	1.9 ± 0.5
20	C	3.57 ± 1.65	7.9 ± 1.9	0.43 ± 0.13	2.2 ± 0.4
41	D	2.06 ± 1.12	7.5 ± 1.6	0.37 ± 0.07	2.3 ± 0.7

A = unipolar; B = bipolar orthogonal; C = bipolar two rings (5 mm spaced); D = DAB (diagonal atrial bipolar); SI = sensing impedance at the atrial electrode-blood interface. See Table 1.

Sensing impedance (source-electrode) was measured with a variable resistor (from 100 to 0.5 Kohm) parallel connected to the recorder (half amplitude loading technique); the resistance value for which the signal amplitude was 50% of the one measured without parallel resistor was assumed to be the sensing impedance.[12-15]

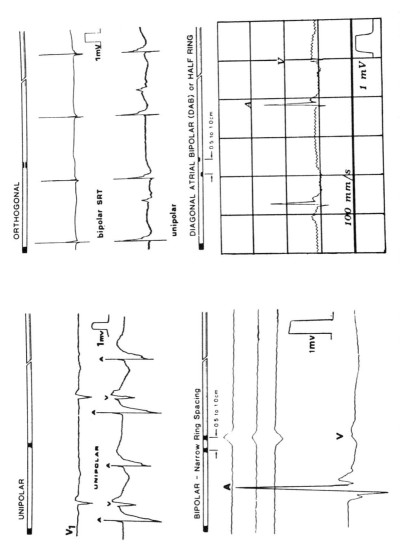

Figure 3. An example of atrial electrogram recorded from four different atrial electrode configurations (on AV single lead) floating in the mid-to-high right atrium.

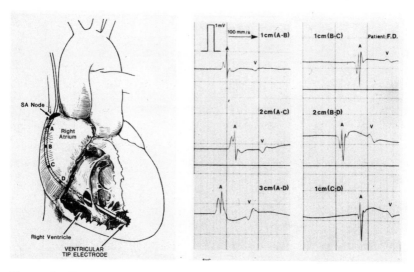

Figure 4. Representative acute atrial bipolar electrograms recorded by four 1-cm spaced electrodes (indicated as A, B, C, and D) mounted on an experimental multipolar AV lead.

than 1 cm yield unsatisfactory signal morphology. Therefore, a low atrial position should be avoided. A short dipole spacing is preferable, and when the lead is placed closer to the atrial wall, a better signal is obtained. Furthermore, placement of the atrial dipole in the mid-to-high atrium helps reject the ventricular far-field signal because the atrial electrodes are further away from the ventricular myocardium.[25] Also, the Fast Fourier analysis of atrial EGM shows the best frequency range for sensing is provided by a short dipole floating in the mid-to-high right atrium.[26]

Factors Influencing Atrial Signal Detection

Many conditions can affect the characteristics of the atrial EGMs detected by a floating electrode:[25–28]

1. spacing between electrodes;
2. distance from myocardial wall: attenuation and biological filtering;
3. dipole orientation;

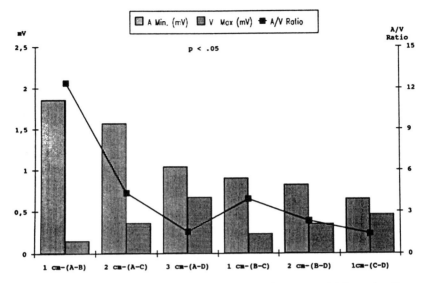

Figure 5. Signal amplitudes (histograms, left scale, mV) and A/V ratios (line, right scale) as measured from different dipole spacings with the experimental multipolar electrode-lead indicated in Figure 4. The differences between atrial and ventricular signal amplitudes and between calculated A/V ratios were statistically significant (P<0.05).

4. electrode size: if too large, it will cause field potential averaging; if too small, it will show a source impedance higher than that required to chronically maintain at the optimal value of 100 the ratio between true pacemaker input impedance and source-electrode impedance;

5. interference patterns: distortion of the depolarization field because the two electrodes are at different relative distances from the myocardium or because boundary effects of myocardium tissues;

6. differential gain: the gain of the atrial differential amplifier must be sufficiently high to maintain the best discriminatory function;

7. phase imbalance: if the dipole is too widely spaced or the electrode surface area is too large, the two electrodes can sense interfering signals having identical or near-identical morphology and amplitude but different phase. This phase difference, i.e., the time of arrival of the signal at the sensing

electrodes, can result, by the differential process, in an adequate atrial signal capable of triggering a ventricular output in the VDD mode;

8. aging of cardiac muscle: development of interfiber collagen.

In addition, the floating condition itself induces morphology and amplitude variations of the signal, during deep breathing, coughing, change in the posture, etc.

Patient Selection

The ideal candidates for the single-lead VDD pacing are patients suffering from advanced or complete AV blocks (CHB) and uncompromised SAF. In many patients, mild sinus node dysfunction does not preclude a substantial increase in atrial rate according to physiologic requirements.

Retrograde VA conduction occurs in the 30–40% of CHB patients with partial or complete heart block.[29] Thus, in the presence of sinus bradycardia with a cycle length longer than the programmed lower rate interval of a VDD pulse generator, escape ventricular pacing (VVI mode) can induce retrograde VA conduction and endless loop tachycardia. Therefore, extreme sinus bradycardia is a contraindication to VDD pacing. Unsynchronized ventricular pacing after intermittent sinus bradycardia can be avoided by programming the lower rate to a value less than the minimum sinus rate determined with Holter recordings.[30] Although the recently published ACC/AHA Guidelines for Pacemaker Implantation[11] indicated that retrograde VA conduction constituted a contraindication to VDD pacing, we believe that retrograde VA conduction should not be a deterrent to single-lead VDD pacing provided the patients are carefully selected and the pulse generator appropriately programmed. Both right and left atrial dimensions should be carefully evaluated by 2D echocardiography. For single AV lead pacing, atrial chamber diameters should not be larger than the accepted maximum values.[31] In our center, we accept maximum values of 4 × 3 cm and 3 × 3 cm, respectively, for left and right atrial diameters measured in the apical four-chamber view. Evaluation of atrial size permits identification of patients at risk for arrhythmias, a situation where DDD or other pacing modes would be more appropriate.[32,33] Patients with paroxysmal supraventricular tachyarrhythmias and persistent sinus bradycardia or sinus arrest should not receive a VDD pacemaker.

Chronotropic atrial function with respect to the patient's age should also be assessed. Exercise tests and 24-hour dynamic ECG recordings yield important information about the variations of the sinus rates in daily life.

Implant Procedures

If all the above conditions are met, a VDD single-lead pacing system can be implanted. During the procedure, careful handling and positioning of the lead is of the utmost importance.

1. After having fixed the ventricular tip in the selected position, the lead should be manipulated in order to produce an atrial dipole as close as possible to the medium high atrial wall, as shown in Figure 6. An acceptable atrial signal (amplitude ≥ 0.5 mV) during maneuvers such as deep breathing and coughing should be consistently registered. Evaluation of the atrial EGM during arm and shoulder movements is also important.

2. Constant P-wave synchronization during all the implant maneuvers is extremely important because amplitude and morphology of the atrial signal during daily activity is influenced by a variety of factors. As all measurements are carried out in the supine position, the lowest acceptable P-wave amplitude should be the one measured during deep inspiration. In this respect, some recent studies[34,35] have shown that morphological variations of the P-wave in any given patient are not accompanied by significant changes in the frequency content. Obviously, the lowest acceptable amplitude of the atrial signal must be decided according to the programmability range of the pacemaker to be implanted.

3. Since the atrial electrode floats in the blood stream, anatomico-histologic changes do not affect the detected signal, as seen with contact electrodes over time. Chronic measurements made from single AV leads during reintervention or by telemetry do not show significant variations of the EGM characteristics, even several years after implantation. Characteristics of atrial signals measured between 3 months and 6 years after the implant in six of our patients who required a reintervention, confirmed (by direct measurement) the absence of chronic signal attenuation. At pacemaker removal,

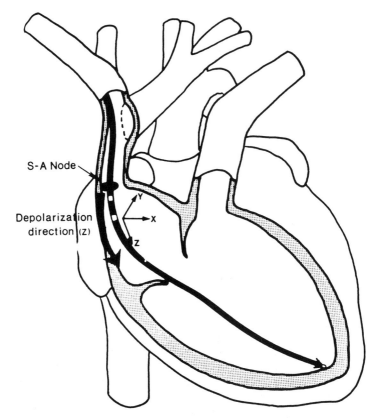

Figure 6. Diagram illustrating the correct position of a single lead with a short atrial dipole.

all six cases showed atrial signal amplitudes capable of driving a specifically designed VDD pacemaker with morphologies similar to those transmitted by telemetry.

Pacemaker Programming

Programming of single-lead VDD and conventional VDD systems is similar and basically simpler and less critical than a VVIR system.

The following parameters have to be carefully programmed:

1. **Atrial sensitivity.** Atrial sensitivity should be programmed at sufficiently high values to assure synchronization on the minimum atrial signal detected at the time of implantation (for example, a minimum P-wave amplitude of 1 mV requires a programmed sensitivity of at least 0.5 mV). The pulse generator should possess a wide range of atrial sensitivity settings to compensate for loss of atrial sensing due to dipole sliding to both higher (superior vena cava) or lower (atrial floor) positions and to allow discrimination between antegrade and retrograde P waves.[36,37]

   The availability of a programmable bandwidth of the atrial amplifier (ABW) is very helpful for two reasons: (a) Interfering myopotentials, not sufficiently rejected by the pacemaker circuit, can be drastically attenuated by a programming of the atrial bandwidth in the low frequency range (20–110 Hz); and (b) retrograde P waves with the same amplitude as but lower frequency content than the antegrade ones can be ignored by the atrial amplifier if the ABW is programmed in the high frequency range (40–200 Hz). This avoids the need of programming the atrial refractory period to a long value, to maintain an adequate upper tracking rate.[35,36]

2. **Postventricular atrial refractory period (PVARP).** PVARP should be programmed to contain retrograde P waves. If specific algorithms to prevent endless loop tachycardia are not available, the PVARP extension will limit the upper rate, possibly affecting the 1:1 atrial tracking during exercise.

3. **AV delay.** Since in the VDD pacing mode the pacemaker only senses atrial activity, the AV delay must be programmed to take into account the delay in detecting atrial depolarization (20–40 ms). Since a single-lead VDD system with dynamic AV delay is not yet available, the AV delay must be programmed according to the hemodynamically most effective value found by means of Doppler echocardiography and exercise testing.[38]

4. **Lower rate.** The lower rate must be programmed at a value lower than the minimum sinus rate detected in 24-hour Holter ECG to prevent asynchronous (VVI) ventricular pacing and retrograde VA conduction.

Clinical Experience

Two multicenter studies of two different single-lead VDD systems have demonstrated satisfactory performance.

In the first trial, our improved atrial unipolar single lead (Fig. 2, type A) was implanted in more than 250 patients between October 1985 and March 1989.[8] The lead was connected to the CPI ULTRA II 910 VDD pacemaker, chosen for its widely programmable options (see Table 3). Our contribution to this trial included 98 patients, 72 of which are still in follow-up. The single AV lead was introduced through the right cephalic vein in 85 patients and through the right subclavian vein in 13 patients.

TABLE 3

Timing and Sensing Characteristics of Atrial Circuit of Three Different VDD Pacemakers Available for Permanent Pacing in the Last Years

Parameters	Ultra II[1]	Phymos[2]	Twinal-30[3]
BR (bpm)	30–90 (1 bpm/step)	40–120 (16 steps)	30–120 (1 bpm/step)
UR (bpm)	100–180 (10 bpm/step)	ARP + AVD	65–150 (27 steps)
AVD (ms)	60–130 (10 ms/step)	50–225 (25 ms/step)	60–300 (20 ms/step)
ARP (ms)	175–475 (25 ms/step)	250–400 (50 ms/step)	100–600 (20 ms/step)
AS (mV)	0.25–0.50–0.75 1.0–1.5–2.5–4.0	0.1–0.2	0.1–0.2–0.3–0.4–0.5–0.6 0.7–0.8–1.0–1.2–1.4 2.0–2.5–2.8–4.0–5.6
ABW (Hz)	na	na	Lo (20–110) Hi (40–200)

BR = basic rate: UR = upper rate; ARP = atrial refractory period; AVD = AV delay; AS = atrial sensitivity; ABW = atrial bandwidth; na = not available; Lo = Low frequency range; Hi = high frequency range.

[1] Cardiac Pacemaker Inc., St. Paul, Mn.

[2] MEDICO Italia SRL, Rubano, Italy.

[3] LEM Biomedica SRL, Florence, Italy/Cardiac Control Systems Inc, Palm Coast, FL.

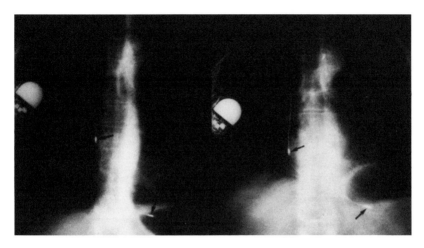

Figure 7. Frontal plane chest X-ray showing a single AV lead during held inspiration (left) and held expiration (right). Arrows indicate the atrial and ventricular electrodes.

Figure 7 shows the chest X-ray of one of the patients. In our series, at implantation, the mean maximum and minimum values of atrial EGM characteristics measured within a whole respiratory cycle were 2.64 ± 1.05 mV and 1.65 ± 0.38 mV amplitude, 0.31 ± 0.12 and 0.18 ± 0.09 dV/dt. The follow-up protocol included serial Holter recordings (Fig. 8), telemetric evaluation of the atrial signal, and serial stress tests before discharge, after 30 and 90 days and, when possible, every 6 months. Atrial channel oversensing phenomena, checked by means of isometric exercise and superior limb movements involving the pectoral muscles, were negligible. Three months after the implant, two patients underwent reoperation. At that time, minimum/maximum atrial amplitude values were not different from those measured at the implant: 1.8/3.5 vs. 1.8/3.6 and 1.1/2.6 vs. 1.1/2.6 mV, respectively. During a mean follow-up of 36 months, 5 patients required conversion to the VVI mode due to complete loss of sensing (2 patients, 1 and 3 years after the implant), or chronic atrial fibrillation (3 patients, 24, 30, and 33 months after the implant). Sixty-seven patients out of 72 (93%) are actually being paced in VDD mode. In the whole population, a high quality atrial signal could be recorded by serial telemetric analysis (Fig. 9). AV synchrony was also

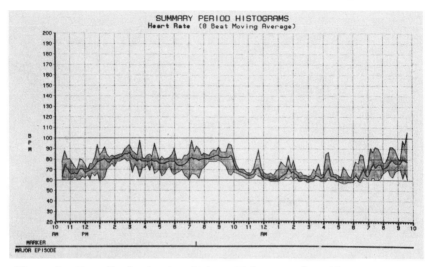

Figure 8. Rate distribution in a 24-hour Holter recording. Heart rate ranges between 58 (lower line) and 105 bpm (top line); sinus tracking is preserved also at low frequency values, a lower rate limit of 50 bpm being programmed.

maintained during exercise. Serial 24-hour Holter ECG recordings performed in all patients confirmed these data. Occasional loss of atrial synchronization was recorded with Holter monitoring, involving only four to five beats. In the worst cases, loss of synchronization was observed in less than 3% of the total observation period, which is less than 40 minutes in the 24-hour recording. None of the patients developed pacemaker-mediated tachycardias that could not be prevented by proper reprogramming.

In the second trial, a new coaxial tripolar single AV lead manufactured by LEM Biomedica (Florence, Italy) in both tined and retractable screw-in ventricular tip versions, was implanted in 514 patients in 30 Italian centers since November 1988.[7,39] The lead, with a diagonal atrial bipolar (DAB) configuration (Fig. 2, type E), was connected to a dedicated pacemaker LEM/CCS Twinal-30 (LEM Biomedica, Florence, Italy/Cardiac Control Systems, Inc, Palm Coast, Florida) with extensive programmability (see Table 3). Figure 10 shows a chest X-ray of a patient with one of these systems. In this trial, the implantation procedures were similar to those of our original experience. At implantation, the mean

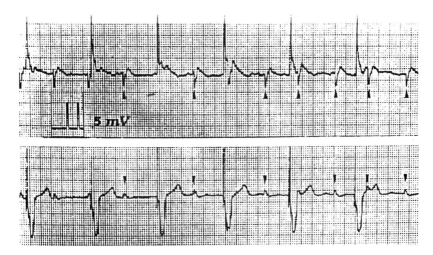

Figure 9. The upper strip is a telemetric recording of a chronic endoatrial electrogram; the lower strip is the corresponding surface ECG. During telemetry, the implanted pulse generator is temporarily converted to the VVI mode and provides reference 5 mV marker signals on the surface ECG. The atrial electrogram ranges between 2.5 and 3.5 mV.

amplitude of the atrial signal was 2.0 (0.4–6.8) mV and the mean programmed atrial sensitivity was 0.4 mV (0.1– 1.5).

A follow-up protocol common to all the participating centers was adopted, including telemetric evaluations of atrial EGM, provocative tests for myopotential interferences, Holter recordings, and exercise stress tests. During a mean follow-up of 15.2 months,[7,39] all of the investigators reported excellent function of the single-lead VDD systems. Interference by myopotentials was detected only occasionally (causing ventricular output inhibition in three cases, ventricular synchronization in one case); occasional loss of atrial sensing was observed in 11 patients (2.1%) during Holter monitoring, and was corrected by reprogramming of atrial sensitivity. Provocative oversensing phenomena were negligible. Twenty patients died of unrelated causes (3 of stroke, 5 of advanced heart failure, 12 of extracardiac pathology). One patient was lost to follow-up but his unit worked perfectly at the last evaluation. Four hundred ninety-three patients are still being followed. Twenty-seven patients (5.5%) required conversion to the VVI mode because of complete loss

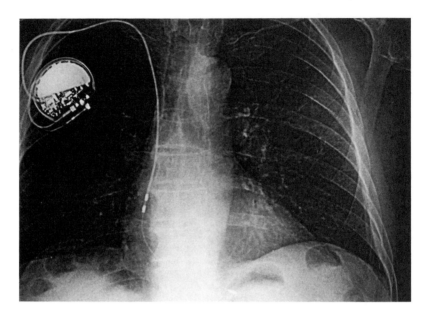

Figure 10.   Frontal plane chest X-ray showing an implanted DAB (diagonal atrial bipolar configuration) single-lead (LEM Biomedica, SRL-Italy/Cardiac Control Systems, Inc-USA) VDD pacemaker.

of sensing (15 patients), chronic atrial fibrillation (11 patients), or development of an extreme sinus bradycardia (1 patient). In five patients, the system had to be replaced. Four hundred sixty-one patients (93.5%) remain paced in the VDD mode. Corresponding results were obtained with a similar system in the US in patients with CHB and normal SAF.[4–6,9,40]

Conclusion

The success of single-lead VDD pacing depends on using special pulse generators dedicated to this mode of pacing and special implantation techniques to detect an appropriate atrial electrogram. The atrial dipole should be positioned in the middle-high atrium to detect the best atrial signal while active ventricular fixation greatly simplifies the implantation procedure. At implantation, a variety of maneuvers should be performed, including deep respiration, coughing, arm and shoulder movements, changes in positions, etc. to check the correct position of the atrial dipole and fluctuations of the atrial signal. Proper programming of atrial sensitivity, lower rate, PVARP, and AV delay are essential.

The reported experience over an 11-year period with different single AV lead configurations, from the first VDT pacemaker implantation in 1980 to the last VDD device in 1992, has been satisfactory. The single AV lead system provides excellent AV synchrony, consistently observed during daily activities and physical exercise with a remarkably low incidence of atrial undersensing, interference, lead dislodgement, pacemaker syndrome, and endless loop tachycardia.

Further improvements in lead technology will undoubtedly occur in the future. In this respect, we recently successfully used in nine patients a new tripolar single AV lead (connected to a dedicated LEM/CCS Twinal-30 pacemaker) with 5 mm spaced full rings atrial dipole (Fig. 2,

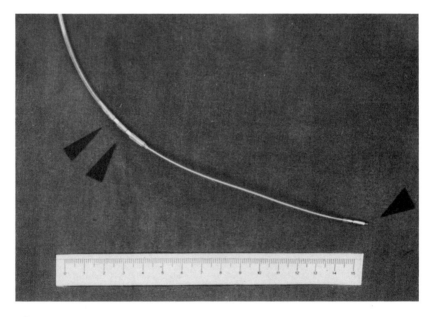

Figure 11. Tripolar single AV leads. Arrowheads indicate the two 5-mm spaced atrial ring electrodes and the ventricular retractable screw-in tip.

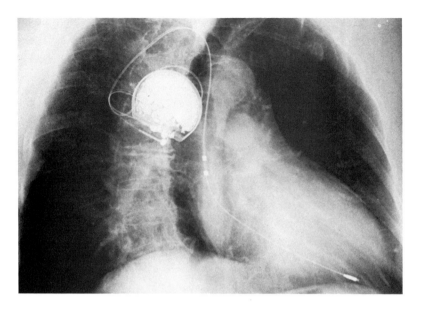

Figure 12.   Lateral chest X-ray showing single AV lead (with narrow-spaced AV ring electrodes connected to a LEM Biomedica, SRL-Italy/Cardiac Control Systems, Inc-USA VDD pacemaker.

type C) with an active retractable screw-in ventricular tip (Figs. 11 and 12).

The future of VDD single lead pacing appears bright. A new VDDR single-lead system (Intermedics, Inc, Angleton, Texas) recently presented at Cardiostim '92[41] represents the "natural" evolution of the systems we described herein. The dipole of the new system is a 7-mm diagonal atrial bipolar (Fig. 2, type E) electrode and the characteristics of the atrial sensing amplifier resemble those of the VDD pacemaker presently used. The availability of a VVIR mode, replacing the VDD if sinus function defaults, represents an advantage but also a potential drawback. The advantage relates to the maintenance of ventricular rate modulation in patients who develop chronic atrial fibrillation or atrial chronotropic incompetences after implantation. The drawback is closely related to the above advantage, i.e., the availability of rate responsiveness in terms of the VVIR mode may result in less careful evaluation of SAF so that the patient may not derive the full benefit of AV synchrony in a VDD/VVIR device.

References

1. Antonioli GE, Grassi G, Baggioni GF, et al. A simple P-sensing ventricle stimulating lead driving a VAT generator. In: Meere C (ed.). Cardiac Pacing, chap 34/9, PaceSymp Montreal, Canada, 1979.
2. Antonioli GE, Grassi G, Baggioni GF, et al. A simple new method for atrial triggered pacemaker. Preliminary clinical trials. G Ital Cardiol 1980;10:679.
3. Cornacchia D, Fabbri M, Maresta A, et al. Clinical evaluation of VDD pacing with a unipolar single-pass lead. PACE 1989;12:604.
4. Furman S, Gross J, Andrews C, Ritacco R. Atrial synchronous pacing with a single pass lead (abstr). PACE 1989;12:677.
5. Varriale P, Pilla AG, Tekriwal M. Single-lead VDD pacing system. PACE 1990;13:757.
6. Longo E, Catrini V. Experience and implantation techniques with a new single-pass lead VDD pacing system. PACE 1990;13:927.
7. Percoco GF, Ansani L, Barbieri D, et al. A new single lead VDD pacing system. PACE 1990;13(II):1906.
8. Antonioli GE, Ansani L, Baggioni GF, et al. Single-lead VDD pacing: Long term experience. In: Santini M, Pistolese M, Alliegro A (eds.). Progress in Clinical Pacing 1990, p 431, Excerpta Medica, Amsterdam, 1990.
9. Furman S, Gross J, Andrews C, Ritacco R. Single pass lead atrial synchronous pacing (abstr). PACE 1991;14(II):693.
10. Curzio G. A multicenter evaluation of a single-pass lead VDD pacing system. PACE 1991;14:434.
11. Dreifus LS, Fisch C, Griffin JC, et al. Guidelines for implantation of cardiac pacemaker and antiarrhythmia devices. ACC/AHA Task Force Report. JACC 1991;18:1.
12. Furman S, Hurzeler P, De Caprio V. Cardiac pacing and pacemakers III. Sensing the cardiac electrogram. Am Heart J 1977;93(6):794.
13. Barold SS, Ong LS, Heinle RA. Matching characteristics of pulse generator and electrode. A clinician's concept of input and source impedance and their effect on demand function. In: Meere C (ed.). Cardiac Pacing, Montreal, Pacesymp, 34-3, 1979.
14. Antonioli GE, Baggioni GF, Grassi G. Variations of endocavitary ECG parameters as a function of electrode area and pacer input impedance. Trends updating. In: C Meere (ed.): Cardiac Pacing, Montreal, Pacesymp, 34-1, 1979.
15. Bornzin G, Stokes K. The electrode-biointerface sensing. In: Barold SS (ed.). Modern Cardiac Pacing, Futura Publishing Co, Mount Kisco, New York, 1985.
16. Nathan DA, Samet P, Center S, Wu CY. Long-term correction of complete

heart block. Clinical and physiologic studies of a new type implantable synchronous pacer. Progr Cardiovasc Dis 1964;6:538.

17. Antonioli GE, Grassi G, Baggioni GF, et al. VAT and VDT system using a single bipolar catheter. 1st Asian-Pacific Symp Cardiac Pacing, Jerusalem, June 16–19, 1980. PACE 1980;3:362.

18. Antonioli GE, Grassi G, Marzaloni M, Sermasi S. A new implantable VDT pacemaker using a single, double-electrode catheter. In: Feruglio GA (ed.). Cardiac Pacing, p 1093 (Europacing Florence 1981), Piccin, Padova, 1982.

19. Antonioli GE. Single pass lead: What is the future? In: Perez Gomez F (ed.). Cardiac Pacing, p 986, Torremolinos 1985, Editorial Grouz, Madrid, 1985.

20. Sermasi S, Marzaloni M, Antonioli GE. Reliability of single-lead for permanent VDD pacing. Euro-Pace 1989, May 28–31, Stockholm, Sweden, PACE 1989;12(II):1165.

21. Antonioli GE, Sermasi S, Marzaloni M, et al. A comparison study of intra-atrial electrograms (IAE) from different types of floating atrial electrode (abstr). PACE 1983;6:9.

22. Sermasi S, Marzaloni M, Rusconi L, et al. Analysis of atrial electrograms derived from different floating atrial electrodes. In: Aubert AE, Hector H (eds.). Pacemaker Leads, p 27, Elsevier BV, Amsterdam, 1985.

23. Goldreyer BN, Olive AL, Leslie J, et al. A new orthogonal lead for P-synchronous pacing. PACE 1981;4:638.

24. Olive AL, Goldreyer BN, Brueske RE, Amundson DC. A new single lead for atrial sensing and ventricular pacing. In Feruglio GA (ed.). Cardiac Pacing, p 1101 (Europacing Florence 1981), Piccin, Padova, 1983.

25. Antonioli GE, Brownlee RR, Audoglio R. Science, theory and clinical considerations related to sensing atrial depolarization in single-lead VDD pacing. In: Antonioli GE, Aubert AE, Hector H (eds.). Pacemaker Leads 1991, p 115, Elsevier BV, Amsterdam, 1991.

26. Barbieri D, Ansani L, Guardigli G, et al. High-resolution and frequency content analysis of floating endo-atrial signals at different dipole lengths. In: Antonioli GE, Aubert AE, Hector H (eds.). Pacemaker Leads 1991, p 135, Elsevier BV, Amsterdam, 1991.

27. Myers GH, Kresh YM, Parsonnet V. Characteristics of intracardiac electrogram. PACE 1978;1:90.

28. Brownlee RR. Toward optimizing the detection of atrial depolarization with floating bipolar electrodes. PACE 1989;12:431.

29. Furman S. Sensing and timing the cardiac electrogram. In: Furman S, Hayes D, Holmes D (eds.). A Practice of Cardiac Pacing, 2nd edition, Futura Publishing Co, Mount Kisco, New York, 1989.

30. Barold SS, Mugica J. Stimuler ou détecter l'oreillette sauf contre-indication. Règle d' or de la stimulation cardiaque des années 90. Stimucoeur 1992;20:129.

31. Feigenbaum H. Echocardiography. Fourth edition, Lea & Febiger, Philadelphia, 1986.

32. Barold SS. The DDI mode of cardiac pacing. PACE 1987;9:480.

33. Sutton R. Pacing in atrial arrhythmias. PACE 1990;13:1823.

34. Aubert AE, Hector H, De Geest H. Single lead electrogram analysis. In: Antonioli GE, Aubert AE, Hector H (eds.). Pacemaker Leads 1991, p 89, Elsevier BV, Amsterdam, 1991.

35. Cornacchia D, Fabbri M, Maresta A, et al. Real-time morphology and spectrum analysis of atrial signal sensed by floating bipole in chronic single-lead VDD pacing. In: Antonioli GE, Aubert AE, Hector H (eds.). Pacemaker Leads 1991, p 143, Elsevier BV, Amsterdam, 1991.

36. Klementowicz PT, Furman S. Selective atrial sensing in dual chambers pacemakers eliminates endless-loop tachycardia. JACC 1986;7:590.

37. Rognoni G, Occhetta E, Perucca A, et al. A new approach to the prevention of endless-loop tachycardia in DDD and VDD pacing. PACE 1991;14:1828.

38. Mehta D, Gilmour S, Ward DE, Camm AJ. Optimal atrioventricular delay at rest and during exercise in patients with dual chamber pacemakers: A noninvasive assessment by continuous wave Doppler. Br Heart J 1989;61: 161.

39. Percoco GF, Ansani L, Barbieri D, et al. Single lead VDD pacing: The Italian experience with a short atrial dipole. In: Antonioli GE, Aubert AE, Hector H (eds.). Pacemaker Leads 1991, p 207, Elsevier BV, Amsterdam, 1991.

40. Furman S, Gross J, Andrews C. Single-lead VDD pacing. In: Antonioli GE, Aubert AE, Hector H (eds.). Pacemaker Leads 1991, p 183, Elsevier BV, Amsterdam, 1991.

41. Lau CP, Tai YT, Li J, et al. Clinical experience with the first single lead VDDR pacing system. Eur JCPE 1992;2(Suppl 1A):18.

Chapter 17

Adverse Effects and Limitations of Rate-Adaptive Pacing

ELENA B. SGARBOSSA, SERGIO L. PINSKI,

ELIZABETH CHING, JAMES D. MALONEY

Introduction

The development of appropriate sensors for rate-adaptive cardiac pacing has presented an exciting challenge to the pacemaker community.[1-3] Several sensors have already been incorporated into approved pulse generators, while others remain under clinical investigation. An ideal sensor would faithfully emulate the normal sinus node by employing a reliable indicator of metabolic needs as the input parameter. The reliability of a sensor depends both on the parameter being sensed and on the measurement technique.[4] Typically, assessment of the performance of new sensors has been based almost exclusively on formal exercise testing; at times this has led to suboptimal results, since the demands of other activities have not been considered. Although significant advances have been made, the goal of an "ideal" sensor has not yet been achieved; therefore, the search for the most "physiologic" sensor (including the combination of two or more sensors in the same unit[5]) is still ongoing.

The present review addresses adverse effects and limitations of rate-adaptive cardiac pacing. For the purposes of the discussion, adverse effects have been classified into three categories (Table 1): (1) adverse effects depending on the sensor; (2) adverse effects peculiar to a specific pacing

New Perspectives in Cardiac Pacing, Vol. 3, edited by S. Serge Barold and Jacques Mugica, Mount Kisco, NY, Futura Publishing Co., © 1993.

TABLE *1*

Classification of Limitations and Adverse Effects with Rate-Responsive Systems

Sensor-Related
  Inappropriate increases in pacing rate
  Lack of achievement or maintenance of an appropriate pacing rate

Technical and Hardware-Related

Pacing Mode-Related and Programming-Related
  VVIR mode
  AAIR mode
  Dual-chamber modes

Patient-Related
  Children
  Elderly
  Patients with congestive heart failure
  Patients with myocardial ischemia
  Patients with cardiac arrhythmias
  Patients undergoing diagnostic and therapeutic procedures

mode; and (3) adverse effects depending on patient characteristics. We understand that the classification is somewhat artificial, because some of the adverse effects depend upon the interaction of more than one factor. However, the classification provides a useful framework for the discussion of the limitations of rate-adaptive pacing. Sensors clinically available in the United States are covered more extensively. Regarding investigational sensors, emphasis is placed on those more widely discussed in the literature and on those with which we have personal experience.

Sensor–Related Adverse Effects

There is agreement regarding the properties that an ideal sensor should meet. The sensor should be *sensitive* to the patient's needs (detecting exercise as well as postural changes or other stresses); *specific* (it should not respond to environmental factors or to changes not related with increased metabolic needs); *accurate* (its response should be proportional to the metabolic requirements); and *rapid* enough to start its response.[6] Imperfect performance of some of these tasks may lead to either inappropriate increases in pacing rate or to lack of achievement or maintenance of an appropriate pacing rate.

Inappropriate Increases in Pacing Rate

Sensor-mediated tachycardias occur when the sensor-determined rate is higher than the requirement of the physiologic condition.[7] Apart from rare technical failures or inappropriate programming, such tachycardias are a reflection of the imperfect specificity and proportionality of the sensor to discriminate noise from the physiologic changes which it is supposed to detect.

Sensing of physical activity has been the most extensively used variable in clinical practice (single chamber: Medtronic Activitrax/Legend, Siemens Pacesetter Sensolog/Solus, CPI Excel, Biotronik Ergos; Intermedics Dash; dual chamber: Medtronic Synergist/Elite, Siemens Pacesetter Synchrony, Intermedics Relay). Their algorithms for detection of vibration peaks allow activity-sensing systems to generate a fast speed of response and to achieve maximal rates rapidly. As these sensors respond to motion, not to actual body need, they are not very specific. Vibrations from sources other than skeletal muscles may result in stimulation of the sensor and consequent increases in pacing rate. Nonphysiologic rate increases are common in situations with high levels of vibration, such as riding an automobile on a bumpy road,[8] public transportation, flights,[9,10] or dental drilling.[11] Almost any deformity of the pacemaker can generate signals of sufficient amplitude to cause an increase in the pacing rate.[8,12] For example, the rate often increases when patients lie on their pacemaker while in bed. Through programming of a higher activity threshold, most of these inappropriate increases in rate can be prevented.

A special type of tachycardia with activity sensors involves a positive feedback loop and, therefore, a tendency to self-perpetuate.[13] In the presence of pacemaker pocket stimulation (e.g., due to a "flipped" unipolar generator) the sensor may be activated. This leads to an increase in pacing rate, and the acceleration in rate then increases pocket vibration. Lowering the pacing output and/or pacemaker reversal inside the pocket may be necessary to interrupt the feedback.[7] Likewise, an activity-sensing pacemaker implanted in a retromammary position can be activated by the cardiac impulse itself and induce a positive feedback.[14] The loop can be avoided by reprogramming the pacemaker to a lower response threshold.

Newer activity-sensing systems, which consist of a non–piezoelectric sensor (CPI Excel)[15] or have a different spacial arrangement of the piezoelectric sensor (Intermedics Dash/Relay), measure changes in velocity of motion and therefore behave as "accelerometers." Since these sensors sense acceleration rather than vibration, they do not need to be in direct contact with body tissues and thus are included into the pacemaker circuitry. Accelerometers seem to be more specific than conventional activity sensors. The problem of rate augmentation caused by direct pressure on the pacemaker or environmental vibration is significantly reduced.[16]

Several pacemakers have central venous temperature sensors (Intermedics Nova MR and Circadia, Biotronik Thermos, Cook Kelvin). This sensor utilizes a pacing electrode with a thermistor close to the tip, and responds to the increases in blood temperature resulting from the heat generated by muscular activity. Although relatively specific, temperature-sensing pacemakers can be "deceived" by increases in mixed venous temperature secondary to enviromental factors (e.g., hot bath) or by factors that are only partly related to the metabolic needs (e.g., fever, eating).[17] In those cases, the temperature sensor will "erroneously" increase the pacing rate. These episodes of tachycardia are transient, but a self-perpetuated loop has been described in the presence of diaphragmatic stimulation. Diaphragmatic muscular contraction increases blood temperature, which in turn leads to sustained upper rate limit pacing. Lowering of the pacing output to eliminate diaphragmatic pacing will interrupt the positive feedback loop.[18]

Central venous temperature frequently falls with the inititation of exercise.[17–19] Pacemaker algorithms identify this initial drop and respond with an initial rate increase to a preprogrammed interim rate (Kelvin, Thermos) or to 85 beats per minute (Nova). Depending on the level of activity and the programming, this interim rate may or may not be appropriate. A temperature dip (with subsequent pacing at the interim rate) has been also observed in the setting of treadmill testing when patients were told that exercise would start, but the treadmill failed to turn on.[17] The dip is probably secondary to redistribution of cold blood from peripheral circulation to the central core, induced by autonomic influence in anticipation to exercise. Emotion and nervousness have been described as sources of abnormal acceleration in heart rate in patients with temperature-controlled pacemakers, especially when sensitive rate-responsive settings are programmed.[19] The exact mechanism of this response is unknown, but involuntary muscle tensing could be involved. For example, one of our patients with a Kelvin pacemaker showed an inappropriate paced rate of 120 bpm in anticipation to a tilt-table test.

A respiratory rate-sensing pacemaker (Biotec Biorate) has been shown to improve exercise performance,[20] but its specificity is less than perfect. The system will increase the pacing rate not only during exercise, but also during hyperventilation and coughing.[21] In the present devices, there is a rate cutoff at 60 breaths/min to prevent the pacemaker from responding to psychogenic hyperventilation. However, in patients with tachypnea due to heart failure, a potential positive feedback may occur, with a sustained rapid paced rate.

Another cause of abnormal augmentation in heart rate with respiratory rate pacemakers is swinging of an arm. The response is maximal with the arm ipsilateral to the auxiliary lead and can be attenuated by swinging both arms.[22,23] By careful programming, in some patients this characteristic can be advantageously used to obtain a "dual sensing" device. However, an inappropriate rate response can still occur if the subject swings only one arm[6] (Fig. 1).

Minute ventilation (Telectronics Meta 1202 and 1250) correlates better with sinus rate during exercise than the respiratory rate, and it also varies with emotional stress and fever.[21] The rate-adaptiveness provided by this sensor is, in general, workload-related. Swinging of the arms can induce some increase in the pacing rate. Minute ventilation pacemakers are less affected by hyperventilation than respiratory rate pacemakers, since hyperventilation induces more changes in the respiratory rate than in the minute ventilation.[24] During artificial mechanical ventilation, the rate is linearly related to both tidal volume and respiratory rate.[25] Overall, this sensor is one of the most specific available, and so inappropriate rapid pacing rates are uncommon.

A pacemaker (Medtronic Deltatrax) that detects changes in right ventricular pressure or maximum positive right ventricular dP/dt, reflecting, in part, right ventricular contractility, is being clinically tested. The sensor consists of a piezoelectric crystal that is part of the unipolar right ventricular lead. Experience with the system is limited,[26,27] but inappropriate increments in pacing rate have not been reported. A potential problem with the dP/dt sensor is that an increase in pacing rate may induce an increment in the inotropic state of the myocardium

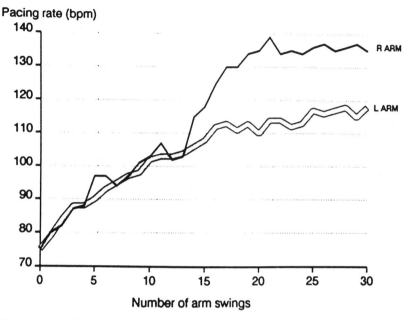

Figure 1.   Effect of swinging arm movement in a patient with a Biorate pace-maker with the tip of the auxiliary lead in the right second intercostal space. The arm swinging was performed during apnea. A higher pacing rate was achieved when the arm on the side of the auxiliary lead was swung (from reference 6, with permission).

(Treppe effect). This may translate into a further increase in the right ventricular dP/dt, creating a positive feedback loop. However, it has been suggested that the magnitude of this Treppe effect is small.[28]

Two other intracardiac parameters—the right ventricle stroke volume[29] and the right ventricular pre-ejection interval[30]—can be derived from measurements of impedance changes in the right ventricle. A pace-maker (CPI Precept 1100 and 1200) can be programmed to respond to either parameter. Measuring the stroke volume will allow the pacing rate to increase in response to augmented venous return during exercise. The pre-ejection interval is more specific, since it responds to adrenergic-mediated increases in contractility and thus is not affected by the pre-load.[30] In patients without structural heart disease, right- and left-sided measurements correlate fairly well.[31,32] However, this might not be true in patients with structural heart disease affecting predominantly one ventricle. An inappropriate increase in heart rate in one of our patients with coronary artery disease and severe left ventricular dysfunction with a DDDR pacemaker programmed to respond to the pre-ejection interval could have been the result of different responses of the ventricles to the adrenergic stimulation (Fig. 2). Rarely, the preejection interval sensor may induce inappropriate increases in pacing rate when assuming the upright posture.[33]

The QT-sensing system (Vitatron TX/Quintech/Rhythmix) is sensitive to adrenergic stimulation and is therefore able to respond to psychologic stress. The response to emotional stress, however, may at times be too pronounced.[34,35] There are also reports of undesirable increases in the paced rate while patients are dreaming.[36] Oscillations (e.g., transient inappropriate increases and decreases in the pacing rate, often occurring during exercise) were relatively frequent with the early models, but less common with the software in more recent versions of the QT-sensing pacemaker.

The QT sensor is also susceptible to a self-perpetuating positive feedback loop tachycardia. Shortening of the QT interval during exercise or stress will induce an increase in the pacing rate, which will then further shorten the QT. Newer versions of this pacemaker minimize the possible occurrence of this loop by providing a nonlinear slope adjustment algorithm: a higher slope is utilized at slow pacing rates and a smaller slope at high rates to prevent inappropriate rate acceleration.[37]

Lack of Achievement or Maintenance of an Appropriate Pacing Rate

The sensitivity of a sensor to emotional, vasodilatory, postural stresses, to exercise, and to diurnal rhythm changes is crucial for the achievement of a physiologically adequate increase in the pacing rate. Likewise, the speed of the sensor (e.g., the activation and deactivation times) will also be critical to the achievement and maintenance of the required increases in pacing rates. The response should be also accurate: the magnitude of the changes should be proportional to the need.

Because of their algorithm designed to detect high frequency vibration peaks, activity-sensing pacemakers do not respond to physiologic changes that are associated with minimal (e.g., Valsalva maneuver or

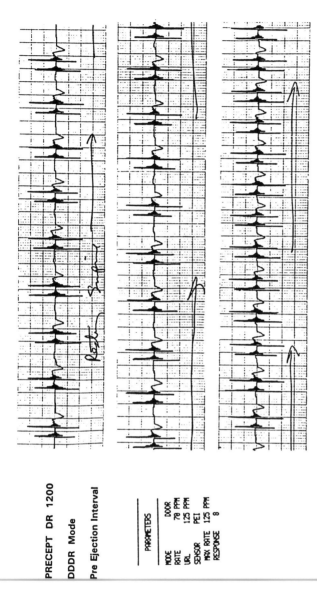

Figure 2. Inappropriate increase in heart rate induced by a DDDR pacemaker responding to the right ventricular pre-ejection interval. The patient had coronary artery disease, severe left ventricular dysfunction, complete AV block, and chronotropic incompetence. Two years after implant, he developed crescendo angina and acute pulmonary edema. Electrocardiographic strips, coincident with attacks of angina and exacerbation of heart failure, showed pacing at increasingly rapid rates. Most likely, a deleterious positive feedback loop was operative. An initial increase in rate precipitated angina and ischemia-induced left ventricular dysfunction. The reactive sympathetic discharge shortened the pre-ejection interval in the normally functioning right ventricle and triggered further increases in the paced rates. This exacerbated ischemia and failure in the left ventricle. Angina and heart failure did not recur after the reprograming the pacemaker to the DDD mode (continuous strip).

handgrip), or no (e.g., emotional stress, fever) body movement.[38] For example, it has been observed that the rate response to movement of the arm on the contralateral side of the implanted activity sensor is less than that to movement of the ipsilateral arm. Walking up stairs produces a paradoxical lesser response than descending the same staircase because the "heel strike" rate is lesser when ascending, although the metabolic needs are reversed.[39] Likewise, pacing rate is faster when walking downhill than uphill.[40] Some patients have learned to partly correct these disadvantages: they accelerate their heart rate in anticipation of physical effort by tapping on the generator before climbing stairs or starting exercise.

With early models of activity-sensing pacemakers, the pacing rate decreased abruptly after the termination of exercise as a result of the sudden cessation of body movement.[41] This pattern of recovery (short and unrelated to the level of exertion), differs from the normal physiologic response, in which the heart rate decreases exponentially at a rate related to previous exercise load and duration and to the level of cardiovascular fitness.[42] When patients were allowed to compare in a blinded fashion between an abrupt or a rate-modulated decay of the pacing rate, most of them preferred the latter.[43] Current models (Legend, Elite, Synchrony) provide for programmability of a recovery or deceleration time[44-46] (Fig. 3). This feature represents an improvement over previous units, but does not completely mimick the physiologic rate decay (see Fig. 8).

Central venous temperature follows closely the muscular activity, but its rate-responsiveness is slow. A brief burst of activity may be completed before temperature increases and a consequent cardiac rate response takes place; consequently, the "physiologic" tachycardia will

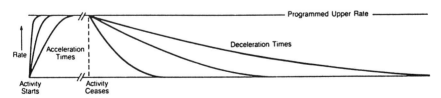

Figure 3. Deceleration time is the time required to achieve 90% of the difference between the maximum (or steady-state) sensor-derived pacing rate and the programmed lower rate limit.

occur after the end of the activity.[1] Moreover, this response is unpredictable because the initiation of exercise in a patient who is already warmed up by previous exercise does not cause a fall in central temperature. On the other hand, activities accompanied by fast heat dissipation (e.g., swimming) may blunt the rate response.

As a result of the slow responsiveness of its sensor, patients with minute ventilation pacemakers can also fail to achieve an appropriate rate after a sudden increase in the metabolic requirements. Talking while exercising can significantly attenuate the response of this sensor. This is more likely due to a disorganized breathing pattern during talking, which leads to a reduction on sensed minute ventilation.[24] Programming of minute ventilation pacemakers currently requires an exercise test after which the system automatically calculates the optimal slope value. It should be noted that during supine exercise respiratory movements are less marked than those in the upright position. If the initial exercise test is performed in the supine position, then the slope chosen by the pacemaker may be too smooth for regular upright exercise.[47]

The stroke volume sensing system has the theoretical advantages of good proportionality during exercise and a fast response. Some shortcomings of the system should be noted. In normal subjects, there is a transient decrease in stroke volume when standing[48,49] due to redistribution of about 700 mL of blood towards the legs. This is compensated for by a sympathetic-mediated increase in heart rate. However, the stroke volume pacemaker will not only fail to adapt its rate response to this postural change, but it might actually decrease the pacing rate (Fig. 4), potentially leading to symptomatic orthostatic hypotension. This is more likely to occur in patients with cardiac disease paced in the VVIR mode than with dual chamber rate-adaptive modes.[50,51]

Similar to what is true for minute ventilation sensor systems, setting the rate response or the response slope in systems based on stroke volume measurements while the patient exercises in supine position may not bring the ideal rate responsiveness and slope when exercising in upright position. To avoid these idiosyncrasies, these pacemakers should always be programmed in the upright position.[52]

The response of the QT interval sensing pacemaker during exercise is, in general, proportional to the workload. Although a failure of the QT interval to shorten during exercise despite a normal catecholamine response has been reported,[53] it is probably a rare event. With early devices, a delayed response accompanied by postexercise tachycardia was

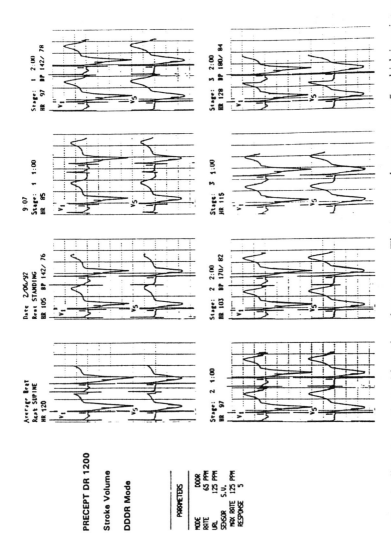

Figure 4. Treadmill test in a patient with stroke volume sensor. The response slope was set at 5, which is an intermediate value for this device (range: 1 to 8). As the sensor detects volume variations, the paced rate is high in supine position and decreases as soon as the patient stands. It continues to slow down while the blood volume is redistributing, even after the initiation of exercise (stage 1). The rest pacing rate range is only reached again during the stage 3 of the test.

common.[54] The current software with nonlinear slope adjustment partially circumvents this problem.[37,55] A shortcoming of the system can result in an inappropriate fall in the pacing rate when most needed; with very short QT intervals at high pacing rates, the T wave could fall before the sensing window (within the pacemaker refractory period) and determine an abrupt loss of rate adaptiveness.[56]

One of the limitations of QT sensing devices is that the QT interval can be measured in paced beats only, since the amplitude of T waves that follow spontaneous depolarizations is usually too low to be sensed. This is not a problem in pacer-dependent patients, but in patients with an intrinsic rate higher than the paced rate, the rate responsive mechanism remains inhibited with a consequent poor rate response to exercise. This situation was observed in patients with the initial TX1 model. A practical solution was to program the lower rate limit above of the patient intrinsic heart rate at rest, allowing the measurement of the evoked QT interval. The costs of this approach were increased battery drainage and the loss of the normal activation and contraction patterns. Subsequent versions of this pacemaker are able to "track" the stimulus-T interval by intermittently effecting an overdrive capture,[6] and therefore function in the rate responsive mode even when the intrinsic rate is higher than the programmed lower rate.

The heart rate/stimulus-T interval relationship can vary significantly in the same subject from one occasion to another. Frequent reprogramming, guided by the results of stress tests and Holter monitoring, was necessary to ensure maintenance of an adequate rate-responsiveness in patients with QT interval-sensing pacemakers.[57] The latest version (Vitatron Rhythmix), however, incorporates a built-in real-time Holter monitor and automatic slope-adjustment capability. The pacing rate/QT relationship is automatically measured daily both at the resting rate (e.g., during sleep) and each time the upper rate limit is reached in order to correct for long-term changes in this relationship.[37] An additional feature helps to achieve an optimal rate response. If the upper rate limit is not reached during an 8-day period, the pacemaker then automatically increases the slope by one step.[37]

Through the incorporation of two or more different sensors in the same pacemaker most instances of inappropriate pacing rates could be, in theory, avoided. Useful combinations would include a sensor with a fast response (e.g., activity) with a slower-responding but more workload-related parameter. Several of these combinations have been proposed. A pacemaker responding to both activity and the QT interval has been shown to provide a more physiologic response to exercise than either sensor alone.[58] Potential problems with combinations of sensors can be envisioned. It will be necessary to associate the multiple sensors in one lead; in theory, right ventricular parameters (oxygen saturation, central venous temperature, dP/dT) could be measured from the same lead. Another drawback of sensor combinations will be the need for complex algorithms to discriminate between possible contradictory inputs from the different sensors.[59]

Technical and Hardware Factors

Unfortunately, programmers from diverse manufacturers are different and demand operator familiarity with their particular specifications. Attempts at programming incompatible features cause most programmers to display a warning, automatically resetting a feasible combination of parameters. However, certain devices may accept the incompatible programmed features, leading to practical problems. In the Medtronic Activitrax models, the physician could choose a rate-response setting (slope) able to truncate the sensor-driven pacing rate below the programmed upper rate limit. Thus, even when the patient might attain high levels of activity, the generator would not neccessarily reach the programmed upper rate. The newer Legend, instead, allows the achievement of the upper rate limit regardless of the rate-response settings. The Siemens Pacesetter Synchrony II would allow the operator to "program" all the features related with the sensor, even if the sensor feature is "OFF." Programming eccentricities are known to occur with several different rate-responsive pacemakers.[60]

Additional problems may arise with sensors that require especially designed leads. Use of a conventional unipolar or bipolar pacing lead is a highly desirable feature. The requirement of a special lead might make the choice of a rate-adaptive system more difficult when replacing a generator. One of the main advantages of activity-sensing systems is that they fit almost any preexistent lead configuration. Only AAIR pacing in an unipolar configuration is not recommended, since far-field sensing may occur. Avoidance of QRS complex sensing by programming a long refractory period is not possible in some models (Activitrax 8403), whereas a decrement in the sensitivity may lead to loss of P-wave sensing.

The Meta pacemaker requires only a conventional bipolar lead. However, the subthreshold pulses (20 Hz) emitted by the device to measure transthoracic impedance interfere with ECG monitoring machines, which provide pacemaker enhancement artifacts, such as transtelephonic monitoring devices. The interference can be avoided by the application of a magnet over the generator (which turns it temporarily to the nonresponsive mode), repositioning the ECG electrodes in the low abdominal wall, or utilizing transmitters in which the pacemaker enhancement artifact can be turned off.[61] Interference with the detection of pacemaker spikes and with the interpretation of the underlying cardiac rhythm on a regular ECG during stress test was observed in our hospital (Fig. 5).

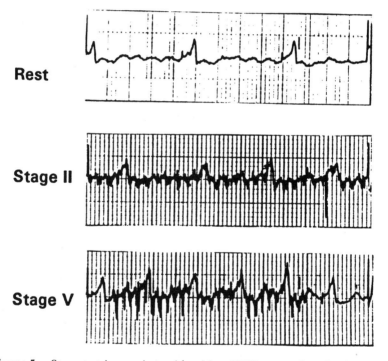

Figure 5. Stress test in a patient with a Meta VVIR pacemaker. During exercise, the low amplitude pulses are readily obvious on the ECG, making difficult the detection of spikes and of the underlying rhythm, in this case atrial fibrillation.

On rare occasions, the same low amplitude pulses have been the cause of oversensing[62,63] and activation of the noise-reversion mode.[64]

The respiratory rate pacemaker senses thoracic impedance by a two-electrode configuration between the pacemaker generator and the tip of an auxiliary lead, which is tunneled subcutaneously 8 to 10 cm from the pocket to a site on the thorax. Complications reported with this auxiliary lead include displacement, sensing failure, and skin erosion[23] (Fig. 6).

The functioning of specially designed intracardiac electrodes can be

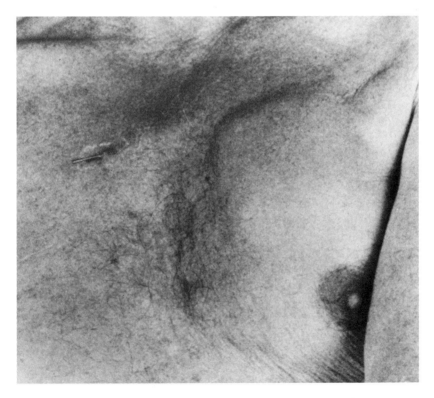

Figure 6. Erosion of the auxiliary lead in a patient with a Biorate pacemaker (from reference 6, with permission).

affected by the engulfment of the electrode within the cardiac trabeculae or by fibrin coating. For example, deposits of fibrin on the optoelectronic sensor, which measures central venous oxygen saturation (Medtronic Oxytrax), diminish the transparency of the system.[65] In animals, there is an exponential fall in sensitivity of the optical sensor early after implantation, which reaches a plateau within 3 months and can eventually lead to sensor failure.[66] A system using two different wavelengths has been proposed as a means to provide long-term stability of the measuring ability of the optoelectronic sensor, but it has not been tested clinically yet.[66] The dP/dt sensing pacemaker also requires a specially designed lead (Medtronic 6220S), which has the pressure sensor located 28 mm proximal to the tip. A stylet cannot be advanced beyond that point. This, in theory, could make implant difficult, but in the early experience with this lead, no implant attempts had to be abandoned.[26,27]

The QT sensing system does not require a special lead but is only available in an unipolar configuration. It is, therefore, subject to limitations common to unipolar leads. Myopotential interference is relatively common, but generally can be managed by decreasing the pacemaker sensitivity.[67] In order to avoid local skeletal muscle stimulation from the indifferent electrode, the generator cannot be placed deeply into the skeletal muscle. Thus, patients with little subcutaneous tissue or in young women in whom the cosmetic result is important are not ideal candidates for QT-sensing pacemakers. Furthermore, sensing of endocardial T wave can deteriorate with time. The use of an electrode with a small area (<12 mm^2), porous surface structure (preferably carbon), and atraumatic fixation significantly improves T-wave sensing.[68]

A limitation common to sensors that measure intracardiac parameters is their requirement of a ventricular lead, which eliminates their use in single chamber rate-adaptive atrial pacemakers. This situation is not likely to become a major concern in the United States, where atrial pacemakers are seldom utilized,[69] but could limit its use elsewhere.

The delivery of an alternate current or pulsed constant carrier signal is a common feature in all sensor systems that measure impedance. Since the carrier is continuous, it produces considerable battery drain. New techniques of measurement that tend to minimize this disadvantage are now in study. With bipolar leads, for example, the trailing edge voltage of the pulse generator can be used to measure end-diastolic and end-systolic volumes and thus calculate the stroke volume.[70]

Mode-Related and Programming-Related

There is a wide range of possibilities among which the physician can choose at the time of programming a rate-adaptive pacemaker. This diversity, at times, makes difficult the selection of the best combination of features for a particular patient. Several exercise tests, Holter monitors, transtelephonic transmissions, prolonged telemetry sessions, and adjustments in medication (all carrying a considerable resource and financial cost) may be required before the patient feels confortable.[71] Thus, it is imperative for the operator to be aware of the multiple problems that may arise during the follow-up. At the time of pacemaker implant and initial programming, clinical characteristics of the patient including age (heart rate reserve decreases with age,[72]) presence of congestive heart failure,[73] activity level, AV conduction disease, bundle branch block, chronotropic competence, and concomitant noncardiac diseases must be evaluated in order to provide the most physiologic pacing mode at rest as well as during exercise. Perhaps the most important physician task is to carefully study the technical manual of each device in order to prevent avoidable mistakes. Here we present some common problems related with the pacing mode or with suboptimal programming.

VVIR Mode

The exact incidence of pacemaker syndrome with VVIR pacemakers is unknown.[74] The behavior of ventriculoatrial (VA) conduction in an individual patient may be capricious, and thus the occurrence of pacemaker syndrome is difficult to predict. In some patients, retrograde conduction may be present only during a limited range of ventricular pacing rates, and the VVIR mode increases the probability that this detrimental rate range will be attained at least intermittently. Also, the VVIR mode maximizes the duration of pacing and thus the duration of the pacemaker syndrome when present. At the same pacing rate, VA conduction is more likely to be present during exercise than at rest.[75] On the other hand, in patients in whom ventriculoatrial conduction is present only at lower rates, the VVIR exercise response may take the patient outside this range and avoid continuous ventriculoatrial conduction.

There are few reports of pacemaker syndrome during exercise in patients with VVIR pacemakers. A patient had to stop a stress test after

19 seconds because of dizziness, and a simultaneous 40 mm Hg fall in the blood pressure was recorded with an intraarterial catheter.[76] The mechanism of pacemaker syndrome was probably loss of AV synchrony at sensor-driven pacing rates. In two patients with sinus node dysfunction, marked exertional dyspnea was associated with ventriculoatrial conduction, cannon A waves in the pulmonary wedge capillary pressure, and ventilation-perfusion mismatching.[77] Symptoms disappeared by pacing in the AAIR mode. In our experience, pacemaker syndrome with VVIR pacemakers is uncommon, but this could be related to our preferential selection of patients with chronic atrial fibrillation and/or AV junctional ablation for this pacing modality. We agree that the VVIR mode should be avoided when VA conduction is present, and it is definitely contraindicated when symptoms are produced by temporary ventricular pacing at the time of initial pacemaker implantation.[78]

AAIR Mode

The potential development of AV conduction disturbances is the main limitation of atrial pacing. When patients are appropriately selected, the incidence of high degree AV block in patients paced in the AAIR mode is low.[79,80] More frequent is the appearence of an inappropriate response of the PR interval during exercise, which, when marked, can lead patients with sick sinus syndrome to a form of pacemaker syndrome when paced in the AAIR mode.[81,82] Normally, a progressive shortening of the cycle length is accompanied by shortening of the PR interval, allowing an abbreviation of the diastolic interval. The relationship between the PR and the spontaneous heart rate follows a sigmoidal rather than a linear curve.[83] However, in some patients with baseline first degree AV block[81] or in those treated with beta blockers or other antiarrhythmic drugs,[84] the AV interval (atrial spike-QRS) does not shorten with faster atrial paced rates and can even paradoxically prolong. As a result, the atrial spike can fall on the next mechanical ventricular systole, leading to an atrial contraction against closed AV valves and to a form of pacemaker syndrome (Fig. 7).

The incidence of this abnormal regulation of the AV interval depends on the characteristics of the populations analyzed (presence of congestive heart failure, use of antiarrhythmic drugs, etc).[73] For example, a normal behavior of the spike-V interval at exercise has been reported in patients

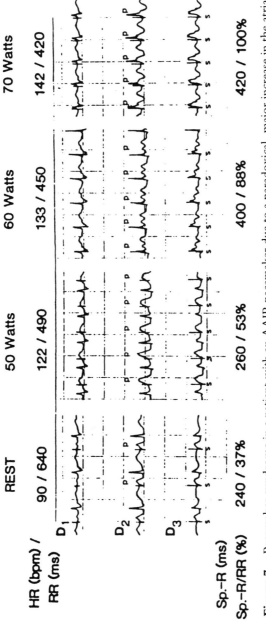

Figure 7. Pacemaker syndrome in a patient with an AAIR pacemaker due to a paradoxical, major increase in the atrial stimulus–R wave interval during exercise. At peak exercise, the P waves fall within the R wave of the preceding cycle (from reference 84, with permission).

with normal AV interval at rest and Wenckebach point below 120 beats per minute.[85]

The use of unipolar electrode configurations in this pacing modality has been reported to be associated with sensing of far-field QRS complexes.[81] Thus, programming of bipolar configuration is usually recommended for atrial pacemakers.

Dual Chamber Rate Adaptiveness

One of the main concerns with dual chamber rate-adaptive systems is the excessive current drain that they induce. Pacing both the atrium and the ventricle at rates grater than 70 beats per minute for much of the day would deplete lithium power sources within a few years. Manufacturers find it difficult to reliably predict generator replacement time indicators for these systems, but the incorporation of real-time telemetry aids the physician in following the progress of power source depletion.

In patients with dual chamber rate-adaptive systems who have only mild degrees of chronotropic incompetence, the potential for competition between intrinsic and sensor-driven atrial depolarizations exists, even with atrial sensing modes such as DDDR and DDIR (Fig. 8). This could eventually lead to atrial fibrillation. Dual chamber rate-adaptive pacemakers allow sensor-driven atrial pacing during the PVARP. A high sensor-driven atrial pacing rate can be programmed, while the tracking rate can be limited by programming a long atrial refractory period. These settings will avoid tracking of nonphysiologic tachycardias and at the same time provide adequate rate response during exercise. Some DDDR systems allow the direct programming of the maximum tracking rate lower than the maximum sensor-driven rate. This programming can result in a maximum sensor-driven pacing interval shorter than the total atrial refractory period. At high sensor-driven rates, the atrial sensing window may disappear, causing the pacemaker to actually operate in the DVIR mode. The addition of rate adaptiveness, based on chronotropic incompetence evident only during strenous exercise, can therefore be not only superfluous but also detrimental for patients who do not engage in such strenuous activity during everyday life.

The presence of some degree of chronotropic response will also make the ECG interpretation problematic.[86] In theory, when independent maximum tracking and sensor-driven rates are programmed, no intrinsic

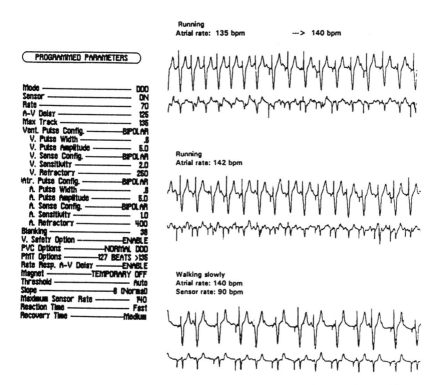

Figure 8.   Patient with a DDDR pacemaker implanted after a catheter ablation of the AV junction for an ectopic atrial tachycardia. A long PVARP (400 ms) was programmed to avoid tracking of the atrial tachycardia whereas the maximum sensor indicated rate of 140 bpm would allow chronotropic response during exercise. However, as the patient showed intrinsic chronotropic response during this test, sinus P waves falling in the PVARP were not tracked, although pseudotracking can be observed preceding the 3rd and 6th QRS complexes (middle strip); and the 2nd, 5th, 8th and 11th QRS complexes (bottom strip). The device started behaving as DVIR, with atrial competitive pacing and loss of AV synchrony. This was exacerbated after finishing exercise. Repeated atrial competition could trigger atrial fibrillation. Note also the abrupt decay in the pacing rate after exercise finished.

P wave will be tracked after the maximum tracking rate is exceeded. However, if the sensor-indicated and sinus rates are similar, a P wave sensed during the atrial sensing window will inhibit the next atrial spike and will result in apparent P-wave tracking at the sensor-driven rate ("pseudotracking") (Fig. 8), that is, above the maximum tracking rate.[87] Furthermore, if adaptive shortening of the AV delay was also enabled, the resultant cycle length variation on the ECG is very likely to be mistakenly diagnosed as pacemaker malfunction. A similar electrocardiographic appearance can also be seen in the DDIR mode (see Fig. 13). Atrial activity falling within the atrial sensing window will appear as tracked by the ventricular spike, although the pacemaker is actually incapable of atrial tracking. For both DDDR and DDIR modes, the maximum tracking rate is programmed to a single value, but it behaves as if it were variable and equal to the sensor-driven rate when the sensor-driven rate exceeds the programmed maximum tracking rate.[87]

DDDR Mode

In DDDR systems, the sensor can be used not only to provide rate-adaptive pacing but also to regulate other parameters, such as the AV delay, the upper rate limit Wenckebach behavior ("sensor-driven rate smoothing"), and the total atrial refractory period. Regulation of the duration of the atrial refractory period by a sensor can prevent pacemaker-mediated tachycardias. With the Meta DDDR pacemaker, a relatively long atrial refractory period at rest will exclude retrogradely conducted P waves, while a sensor-induced shortening of the atrial refractory period during exercise will facilitate atrial sensing as the upper rate is approached. A potential disadvantage of this method is its increased requirement on the speed and the response of the sensor.[13] The sinus cycle length at the onset of exercise decreases rapidly. A sensor with a delay of 20 seconds in response to exercise will result in the inability of the TARP to shorten fast enough to track the normal sinus activity. This will result in transient AV dissociation. In consequence, the clinical usefulness of a long TARP which prevents PMTs, will be limited during bursts of exercise by a slowly reacting sensor. In order to avoid this behavior, a shorter initial TARP has to be programmed at rest, to accommodate for this sudden sinus rate "jump." Sensor-derived information can be used advantageously to avoid tracking of inappropriate tachyarrhythmias.[88] The pacemaker could judge the appropriateness of

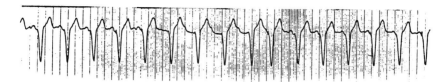

Figure 9.   Meta 1250 DDDR. Automatic switching to VVIR after detection of atrial fibrillation (6th complex QRS). Once the device has identified two normal P waves (8th and 9th complex QRS), it returns to the DDDR mode.

a high atrial rate by comparing it with the sensor-indicated rate. When these two rates are in discrepancy, the pacemaker may prevent tracking the inappropriate atrial rate by either switching to a nontracking mode as VVIR,[88,89] or by restricting its response temporarily to a tolerable lower level (conditional ventricular tracking limit.[88,90] Although in general useful, these capabilities can at times lead to an inappropriate loss of atrioventricular synchrony.

Automatic mode switching is provided in the Meta 1250 DDDR.[88,89] When a P wave is detected inside the PVARP, the mode switches from DDD(R) to VDIR mode (ventricular pacing, atrial and ventricular sensing) (Fig. 9). This will impede the tracking of pathologic atrial tachycardias or pacemaker-mediated tachycardia. To allow the restoration of AV synchrony in case the mode switching is the result of retrograde conduction, the algorithm also provides a 240 ms extension of the pacing cycle after eight ventricular paced beats (Fig. 10). The drawback of this mechanism is that patients with frequent ventricular premature beats with VA conduction or frequent premature atrial beats will have recurrent instances of mode switching throughout the day. The same will happen when sinus tachycardia is not accompanied by a comparable sensor activation. This is more likely if a long PVARP and conservative sensor parameters are programmed (Figs. 10 and 11). This inappropriate mode switching could lead to bothersome symptoms or to pacemaker syndrome.[89] Rate-responsive asynchronous ventricular pacing mode can instead be observed if noise (e.g., myopotentials[88]) is detected in the atrium channel. It should be noted that VVI pacing is also the end-of-life behavior of the system. In one of our patients with persisting ventricular pacing, the diagnosis of premature battery depletion was easily made by the absence of the intermittent 240 ms extension in the pacing cycle and by the fixed rate of 63.5 bpm, which did not increase with exertion.

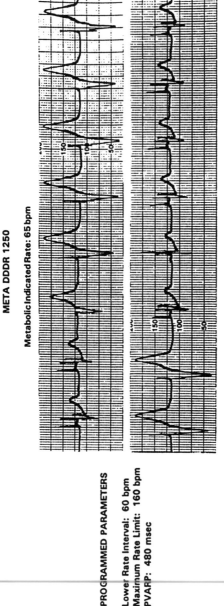

Figure 10. Patient with frequent PVCs, with VA conduction. Detection of a P wave within the PVARP triggers the mode switching to VVIR. Once eight consecutive P waves have been counted by the device, the VA interval will be extended by 240 ms. This will allow the next spontaneous P wave to fall after the PVARP, or an atrial paced event will take place. (Continuous strips). Patients with frequent PVCs may have prolonged episodes of AV asynchrony due to this inappropriate mode switching.

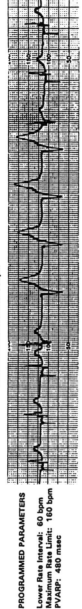
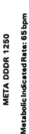

META DDDR 1250

Metabolic Indicated Rate: 65 bpm

PROGRAMMED PARAMETERS

Lower Rate Interval: 60 bpm
Maximum Rate Limit: 160 bpm
PVARP: 480 msec

Figure 11.   Same patient as in Figure 10. A PVC with retrograde P wave induces the switching to VVI(R) mode. After the fourth paced ventricular beat, another PVC allows restoration of synchronized AV pacing. The reason for this behavior is the absence of retrograde P wave conduction in this particular PVC (note the different T wave following the PVC).

In other pacemakers (Relay, Circadia), the information received by the sensor regarding physical activity can be used to judge the appropriateness of a high sensed atrial rate, modulating the pacemaker's response. If the sensor input is below a specified level, indicating lack of exercise, the device can track sensed atrial events only to a tolerable low limit—the conditional ventricular tracking limit (CVTL). Wenckebach-type behavior ensues at the CVTL until the sensor input increases, indicating that exercise is occurring, or until the sensed atrial rate decreases. If the sensor input indicates exercise, the DDDR pacemaker can track up to the programmed maximum rate.[90]

When setting the CVTL option, however, the patient's characteristics must be taken into account. Currently, the CVTL is only programmable "ON" or "OFF" and is set automatically at 35 beats/min above the programmed lower rate. At faster heart rates, if the sensor is not activated, the P wave will not be tracked. When using this feature, some patients may need to have their lower rate programmed faster than

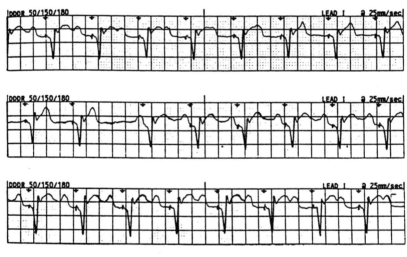

Figure 12. Inappropriate triggering of the CVTL response in a patient with an Intermedics Relay, DDDR mode. Strips were obtained at rest, with the lower rate limit programmed at 50 to permit checking of atrial sensing. Wenckebach behavior is seen as the intrinsic atrial rate is 85 bpm. The CVTL does not allow the pacemaker to track higher rates, if the sensor is not activated. This patient is 18 years old and his lower rate limit was set at 82 bpm with circadian response "on," and the inappropriate response showed above was not observed during long-term monitoring.

the indispensable. Otherwise, relatively high resting intrinsic heart rates (e.g., 85 bpm) may be inconveniently followed by Wenckebach behavior (Fig. 12).

DDIR Mode

The DDIR pacing mode may be particularly useful in patients with sinus node dysfunction and frequent paroxysmal atrial tachyarrhythmias. As long as the intrinsic rate is below the sensor-indicated rate, normal AV synchrony is maintained.[91] However, if the resting sinus rate is above the lower rate limit, or if the intrinsic chronotropic response is faster than the sensor-indicated one, AV dissociation occurs. The resulting ir-

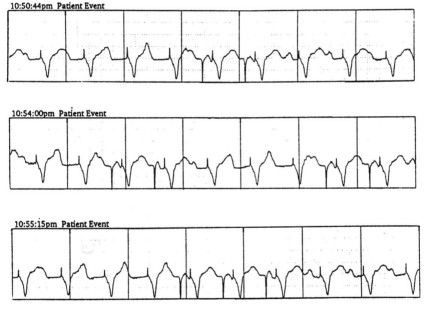

Figure 13. Holter recording during symptomatic episodes in a patient with a dual chamber pacemaker programmed in the DDIR mode. The spontaneous sinus rate was higher than the sensor-indicated rate. This led to intermittent AV asynchrony, since in this pacing mode intrinsic P waves are sensed but not tracked. The asynchrony was unpleasantly perceived by the patient. This manifestation of "pacemaker syndrome" required the reprogramming of the device to the DDDR mode.

regularity of the AV and PV intervals may be unpleasantly perceived by the patient (Fig. 13). The ECG interpretation of DDIR pacing may be very complex, especially if the physician is not fully acquainted with the modality. Pacemaker malfunctions may be readily misdiagnosed (Figs. 14 and 15).

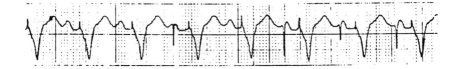

(PROGRAMMED PARAMETERS)

Mode	DDI
Sensor	ON
Rate	80
A-V Delay	175
Vent. Pulse Config.	BIPOLAR
V. Pulse Width	.6
V. Pulse Amplitude	2.5
V. Sense Config.	BIPOLAR
V. Sensitivity	4.0
V. Refractory	275
Atr. Pulse Config.	BIPOLAR
A. Pulse Width	.6
A. Pulse Amplitude	3.0
A. Sense Config.	BIPOLAR
A. Sensitivity	.75
A. Refractory	300
Blanking	38
V. Safety Option	ENABLE
Rate Resp. A-V Delay	ENABLE
Magnet	TEMPORARY OFF
Threshold	Auto
Slope	12
Maximum Sensor Rate	150
Reaction Time	Fast
Recovery Time	Medium

Figure 14. Interpretation of the DDIR mode function can be difficult. This strip was taken from a patient who was referred for presumptive malfunction of his pacemaker, after analysis of the surface ECG. However, the device is functioning as expected for a DDIR mode, showing some apparently tracked P waves.

10:33:11pm

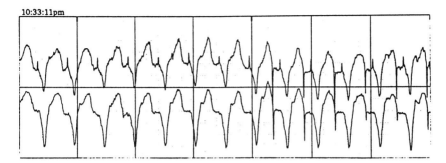

Figure 15. Pseudotracking in DDIR pacemaker. DDDR pacing mode might be inferred from this strip, that in this case would have a relatively long programmed AV delay since the P waves fall in the T waves. However, on the second half of the strip, starting of the atrial pacing cannot be attributed to faster sensor-driven rate, since the VV interval has not shortened. Atrial undersensing could rather be misdiagnosed from the first atrial spike occurrence. But the programmed pacing mode is DDIR. The P waves are only pseudotracked, falling into the atrial sensing window.

Patient-Related Factors

Several factors capable of influencing a particular sensor system are related to the specific characteristics of the patients.

Children

The selection of rate-responsive pacemaker systems for infants and small children is still limited. Activity-sensing pacemakers are at the present time the only ones compatible with epicardial pacing. In older children, activity-sensing pacemakers implanted in the infraclavicular area have worked adequately,[92] but their response when implanted in the abdomen is largely unknown. Similarly, minute ventilation pacemakers have provided physiologic rate-adaptiveness in children older than 6 years of age.[93] However, younger children are not suitable candidates because the system cannot recognize respiratory rates above 60 breaths per minute.

Thus far, temperature-sensing leads may be too large for implanting in small children. None of the leads that measure intracardiac parameters are available with an active fixation mechanism, an important feature when using transvenous pacing in the presence of congenital cardiac malformations or postoperative changes in anatomy.

Elderly Patients

Aging leads to several modifications in the normal physiology of healthy subjects. Furthermore, superimposed cardiac, pulmonary, or muscle-skeletal diseases are frequent and require additional consideration at time of programming a rate-adaptive pacing system. Elderly patients exercise mainly with short bursts of physical activity;[94] for many of them, walking upstairs or floor scrubbing will be the most strenuous activity.[95] Therefore, they are less likely to get benefit from sensors with long reaction times, such as minute ventilation or central venous temperature. Activity-sensing pacemakers seem to be more adequate for this pattern of activity.

There is scarce experience with sensors that measure intracardiac parameters in very elderly subjects. Many changes in the hemodynamic profile accompanying exercise in this population have been described. These include alterations in both active and passive viscoelastic properties of the left ventricle, cardiac dilatation, and lesser response to β-adrenergic stimulation,[96] all of which may interfere with an optimal rate adaptiveness. For example, changes in central venous temperature are more pronounced in elderly subjects, probably due to reduced heat dissipation since the blood flow to the skin during exercise is markedly reduced. This could lead to an exaggerated rate response by a temperature-sensing system.

Patients with Congestive Heart Failure

The presence of heart failure interferes with normal rate-adaptive pacing. Decreased exercise tolerance is a hallmark of heart failure.[97] Patients with heart failure will often cease to exercise before slow-acting sensors can be activated. For example, central venous temperature may show the expected decrease with the initiation of exercise. However, this is frequently followed by a markedly slower rise: right ventricular temperature often does not return to baseline until the patient has stopped

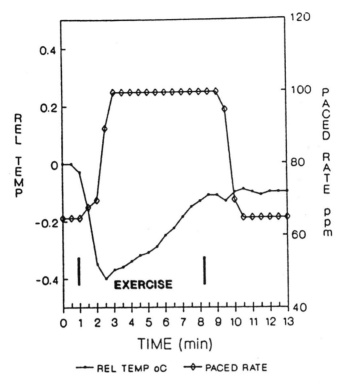

Figure 16. Treadmill test in a patient with congestive heart failure and a temperature sensor system (Kelvin Cook 500). After the initial drop in the temperature, the pacemaker increased the pacing rate to the interim rate (100 bpm). However, as exercise continued, temperature did not increase above the initial baseline temperature. Thus, appropriate rate response was not achieved.

exercise. Thus, the pacing rate proportioned by a temperature-sensing system may be inappropriately delayed or absent[17] (Fig. 16).

There are few data available regarding the behavior of dP/dt, stroke volume, and preejection interval sensors in patients with ventricular dysfunction, congestive heart failure, or cor pulmonale. These conditions themselves and the drugs used in their treatment (positive inotropes, diuretics, vasodilators) can be expected to modify the response of the sensors. Further research into this area is needed.

Patients with Myocardial Ischemia

Heart rate is one of the main determinants of myocardial oxygen consumption. Therefore, rate-adaptive pacing can trigger episodes of cardiac ischemia in susceptible individuals. At any heart rate, myocardial oxygen consumption (and the ischemic potential) is lower with atrial than with AV sequential pacing; also, it may be lower with AV sequential than with ventricular pacing.[98] Although not contraindicated, rate-adaptive pacemakers must be used with great caution in patients with active coronary artery disease. Specifically, the patient's ischemic threshold must be taken into account when programming the upper rate limit and other settings of rate-adaptive pacemakers.[99] Angina is not a satisfactory safety marker for patients with coronary artery disease and rate-adaptive pacemakers. The detrimental effects of ischemia on ventricular function precede the development of angina; in some patients ischemia can be essentially silent. Noninvasive evaluation of ventricular function at different pacing rates should be undertaken in all patients to determine the highest permissible rate.[100] In properly selected patients with coronary artery disease, rate-adaptive pacing can actually improve exercise tolerance.[101]

Parameters determined by a right ventricular pressure sensor can vary during myocardial ischemia. As dP/dt is increased by preload and afterload, eventual cardiac ischemia may raise the right ventricular pressure and dictate a rise in pacing rate, aggravating the ischemia. Similarly, in patients with a respiration sensor, QT interval or PEI sensors, hyperventilation or catecholamine release due to chest discomfort could trigger an increase in pacing rate.

On the other hand, drugs used in the management of angina pectoris can also interfere with the normal functioning of specific sensors. Acute beta blockade markedly attenuates the response to exercise driven by the QT rate-responsive system, and the rate response cannot be restored by increasing the slope or by altering the T-wave sensitivity or T-wave sensing window. Atenolol administered as treatment of hypertension on a chronic basis, however, did not interfere significantly with the QT driven pacing rate.[57] In humans with dP/dt sensing pacemakers, pharmacologic vasodilatation with nitrates increased dP/dt and the resulting pacing rate.[26] On the contrary, vasodilators may reduce the stroke volume and the pacing rate mediated by stroke volume sensor-driven systems.[102] Drug-induced vasodilatation may reduce the central venous temperature by 0.24°C,[6] leading to an erroneous interpretation of beginning exercise by a temperature-sensor system. The effects of these phenomena require further evaluation.

Patients with Cardiac Arrhythmias

Patients with cardiac arrhythmias may have particular problems with rate-responsive pacemakers. Many ventricular tachyarrhyhtmias are rate-dependent (e.g., can be triggered by a high paced rate). Different mechanisms might be operative, including heterogeneous shortening of myocardial refractory periods, provocation of myocardial ischemia, and precipitation of "triggered" arrhythmias. Figure 17 depicts the initiation of a sustained ventricular tachycardia in a patient with a rate-responsive pacemaker during a treadmill exercise test. To avoid this complication, a relatively low maximal rate should be programmed in patients prone to the development of ventricular tachyarrhythmias.

Drugs that modify the relationship between the heart rate and the QT interval (class I and class III) are likely to disrupt the rate response of QT sensor systems. The effects of beta blockers on QT pacemakers were described above. Finally, as explained in a prior section, extreme prolongation of the AV interval induced by antiarrhythmic drugs can induce pacemaker syndrome during exercise in patients with AAIR pacemakers.[84]

Implantable defibrillators are being increasingly used in patients with ventricular arrhythmias, many of whom also require chronic rate-responsive pacing. The need to avoid double-counting (e.g., sensing of both the pacemaker pulse and the resulting QRS complex by the defibrillator) by meticulous intraoperative testing should be emphasized. Double-counting of a fixed rate of 70 bpm is not likely to trigger a defibrillator discharge, as the cutoff rates are usually programmed above 150 bpm; however, a sensor-driven rate of 100 bpm will certainly result in a defibrillator shock if double-counting exists. Minute ventilation pacemakers have been successfully implanted in patients with defibrillators; the low-amplitude pulses used for measuring transthoracic impedance have not triggered shocks.[103]

Special Procedures

In a similar way to what is recommended for standard pacing systems, devices with rate-adaptive capabilities should be tested before and

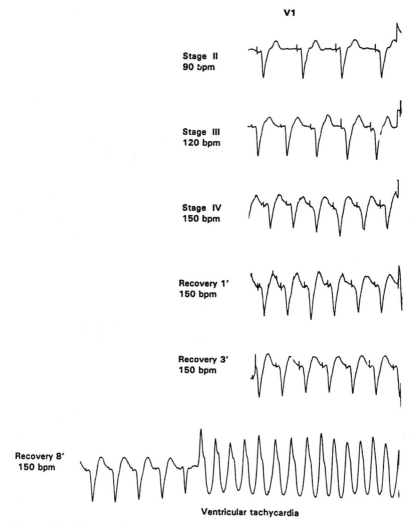

Figure 17. Treadmill test in a patient with coronary artery disease and left ventricular dysfunction with a Meta VVIR pacemaker. The programmed maximum rate was 150 bpm. The test was stopped as a result of the development of severe dyspnea (stage IV). However, due to sustained tachypnea, the sensor-driven rate remained at its maximum value during the recovery, contributing to the initiation of rapid sustained ventricular tachycardia which had not occurred before.

after certain procedures. These include surgery (with electrocautery or cardioplegia; the latter is especially important for temperature-sensing systems), radiofrequency ablation, external cardioversion or defibrillation, magnetic resonance imaging, radiation therapy sessions, lithotripsy, and any procedure that involves electrical current in contact with body tissues. Probably the safest option is to turn the rate-responsiveness feature "off" during these maneuvers. In patients who do not show spontaneous cardiac rhythm, the pacemaker should be temporarily reprogrammed to an asynchronous mode if possible.

References

1. Furman S. Rate-modulated pacing. Circulation 1990;82:1081–1094.
2. Tyers GFO. Current status of sensor-modulated rate-adaptive cardiac pacing. J Am Coll Cardiol 1990;15:412–418.
3. Alt E, Heinz M, Theres H, Matula M. Function and selection of sensors for optimum rate-modulated pacing. In: Barold SS, Mugica J (eds.). New perspectives in cardiac pacing. 2. Futura Publishing, Mount Kisco, NY, 1991, pp 163–202.
4. Rossi P. Rate-responsive pacing: biosensor reliability and physiological sensitivity. PACE 1987;10:454–466.
5. Landman MAJ, Senden PJ, van Rooijen H, van Hemel NM. Initial clinical experience with rate adaptive cardiac pacing using two sensors simultaneously. PACE 1990;13:1615–1622.
6. Lau CP, Camm AJ. Rate-responsive pacing: technical and clinical aspects. In: El-Sheriff N, Samet P (eds.). Cardiac Pacing and Electrophysiology. W.B. Saunders Co., Philadelphia, 1991, 524–544.
7. Lau CP, Tai YT, Fong PC, Cheng CH, Chung FLW. Pacemaker mediated tachycardias in single chamber rate responsive pacing. PACE 1990;13:1575–1579.
8. Stangl K, Wirtzfeld A, Lochschmidt O, Basler B, Mittnacht A. Physical movement sensitive pacing: comparison of two "activity"-triggered pacing system. PACE 1989;12:102–110.
9. Toff WD, Leeks C, Joy M, et al. The effect of aircraft vibration on the function of an activity-sensing pacemaker (abstr). PACE 1987;10:423.
10. Gordon RS, O'Dell KB, Low RB, Blumen U. Activity-sensing pesmanent internal pacemaker dysfunction during helicopter aeromedical transport. Ann Emerg Med 1990;19:1260–1263.
11. Rahn R, Zegelman M, Kreuzer J. The influence of dental treatment on the Activitrax (abstr). PACE 1988;11:852.
12. Wilkoff B, Shimokochi D, Schaal S. Pacing rate increase due to application of steady external pressure on an activity sensing pacemaker (abstr). PACE 1987;10:4–23.

13. Lau CP. Sensors and pacemakers mediated tachycardias. PACE 1991;14: 495–498.
14. Ahmed R, Gibbs S, Ingram A, Chan SL, Sutton R. Pacemaker-mediated tachycardia with left retrommamary implantation of VVIR (activity-sensing) pacemakers. Eur J Cardiac Pacing Electrophysiol 1992;2:144–147.
15. Millerhagen J, Bacharach D, Wollins J, Maile K. An accelerometer-based adaptive-rate pacing system. PACE 1990;13:1079–1218.
16. Lau CP, Tai YT, Fong PC, et al. Clinical experience with an activity sensing DDDR pacemaker using an accelerometer sensor. PACE 1992;15:334–343.
17. Sellers TD, Fearnot NE, Smith HJ, Di Lorenzo DM, Knight JA, Schmaltz MJ. Right ventricular blood temperature profiles for rate responsive pacing. PACE 1987;10:467–479.
18. Volosin KJ, O'Connor WH, Fabiszewski R, Waxman HL. Pacemaker-mediated tachycardia from a single chamber temperature sensitive pacemaker. PACE 1989;12:1596–1599.
19. Zegelman M, Winter UJ, Alt E, et al. Effect of different body-exercise modes on the rate response of the temperature-controlled pacemaker Nova MR. Thorac Cardiovasc Surg 1990;38:181–185.
20. Rossi P, Rognoni G, Occhetta E, et al. Respiration-dependent ventricular pacing compared with fixed ventricular and atrial-ventricular synchronous pacing: aerobic and hemodynamic variables. J Am Coll Cardiol 1985;646–652.
21. Mond HG, Kertes PJ. Respiratory rate. In: Rate responsive cardiac pacing. Telectronics and Cordis Pacing Systems, 1988, pp 37–40.
22. Lau CP, Ritchie D, Butrous GS, et al. Rate modulation by arm movements of the respiratory dependent rate responsive pacemaker. PACE 1988;11: 744–752.
23. Santomauro M, Fazio S, Ferraro S, et al. Follow-up of a respiratory rate modulated pacemaker. PACE 1992;15:17–21.
24. Lau CP, Antoniou A, Ward DE, Camm AJ. Reliability of minute ventilation as a parameter for rate responsive pacing. PACE 1989;12:321–330.
25. Lau CP, Lee CP, Wong CK, Cheng CH, Leung WH. Rate responsive pacing with a minute ventilation sensing pacemaker during pregnancy and delivery. PACE 1990;13:158–163.
26. Bennett T, Sharma A, Sutton R, Camm JA, Erickson M, Beck R. Development of a rate adaptive pacemaker based on the maximum rate-of-rise of right ventricular pressure (RV dP/dt max). PACE 1992;15:219–234.
27. Ovsyshcher I, Guetta V, Bondy C, Porath A. First derivative of right ventricular pressure, dP/dt, as a sensor for a rate adaptive VVI pacemaker: initial experience. PACE 1992;15:211–218.
28. Sharma AD, Yee R, Bennett T, et al. The effects of ventricular pacing on right ventricular maximum positive dP/dt: implications for a rate-responsive pacing system based on this parameter (abstr). PACE 1987;10:1228.
29. Wortel HJJ, Ruiter JH, De Boer HGA, Heemels JP, Van Mechelen R. Impedance measurements in the human right ventricle using a new pacing system. PACE 1991;14:1336–1342.

30. Chirife R. Physiological principles of a new method for rate responsive pacing using the pre-ejection interval. PACE 1988;11:1545–1554.
31. Sperry RE, Burns CA, Rogera RR, Ellenbogen KA, Nixon JV, Wood M. Can pre-ejection interval determined by right ventricular impedance predict changes in left ventricular pre-ejection period? (abstr) J Am Coll Cardiol 1992;19:65A.
32. Burns CA, Sperry R, Rogers R, Nixon V, Ellenbogen KA. Can impedance based pacemakers accurately determine changes in left ventricular stroke volume? (abstr) J Am Coll Cardiol 1992;19:149A.
33. Ruiter JH, Heemels JP, Kee D, van Mechelen R. Adaptive rate pacing controlled by the right ventricular preejection interval: clinical experience with a physiological pacing system. PACE 1992;15:886–894.
34. Dodinot B, Godenir JP, De Sousa M. Is the evoked QT principle a reliable rate-responsive sensor? (abstr) PACE 1987;10:419.
35. Hedman A, Hjmemdahl P, Nordlander R, Aström H. Effects of mental and physic stress on central haemodynamics and cardiac sympathetic nerve activity during QT interval-sensing rate-responsive and fixed-rate ventricular inhibited pacing. Eur Heart J 1990;11:903–915.
36. Maisch B, Langenfeld H. Rate adaptive pacing-clinical experience with three different pacing systems. PACE 1986;9:997–1004.
37. Boute W, Gebhardt U, Begemann MJS. Introduction of an automatic QT interval driven rate responsive pacemaker. PACE 1988;11:1804–1814.
38. Lau CP, Mehta D, Toff WD, Stott RJ, Ward DE, Camm AJ. Limitations of rate-response of an activity-sensing rate-responsive pacemaker to different forms of activity. PACE 1988;11:141–150.
39. Soberman J, McAlister H, Klementowicz P, Andrews C, Furman S. Paradoxical response in activity-sensing pacemakers (abstr). PACE 1988;11:507.
40. Candinas RA, Gloor HO, Ammann FW, Schoenbeck M, Turina M. Activity-sensing rate responsive versus conventional fixed-rate pacing: a comparison of rate behavior and patient well-being during routine daily exercise. PACE 1991;14:204–213.
41. Lindemans FW, Rankin IR, Murtaugh R, et al. Clinical experience with an activity-sensing pacemaker. PACE 1986;9:978–986.
42. Hammond HK, Froelicher VF. Normal and abnormal heart rate responses to exercise. Prog Cardiosvasc Dis 1985;17:271–296.
43. Lau CP, Wong CK, Cheng CH, Leung WH. Importance of heart rate modulation on the cardiac hemodynamics during postexercise recovery. PACE 1990;13:1277–1285.
44. Legend 8416/8417/8418. Technical Manual. Medtronic Inc., Minneapolis, MN, 1989.
45. Elite. Technical Manual. Medtronic Inc., Minneapolis, MN, 1990.
46. Synchrony II 2022 and 2023. Technical Manual. Pacesetter-Siemens, Sylmar, CA, 1991.
47. Zegelman M, Beyersdorf F, Kreuzer J, Cieslinski G. Rate responsive pacemakers: assessment after two years. PACE 1986;9:1005–1009.

48. Salo RW, Pederson BD, Olive AL, Lincoln WC, Wallner TG. Continuous ventricular volume assessment for diagnosis and pacemaker control. PACE 1984;7:1267–1272.
49. Wortel HJJ, Ruiter JH, De Boer HGA, Heemels JP, Van Mechelen R. Impedance measurements in the human right ventricle using a new pacing system. PACE 1991;14:1336–1342.
50. Hoeschen RJ, Reimold SC, Lee RT, Plappert TJ, Lamas GA. The effect of posture on the response to atrioventricular synchronous pacing in patients with underlying cardiovascular disease. PACE 1991;14:756–759.
51. Leitch JW, Arnold JM, Klein GJ, Yee R, Riff K. Should a VVIR pacemaker increase the heart rate with standing? PACE 1992;15:288–294.
52. Precept, Technical Manual. CPI Inc., St Paul, MN, 1990.
53. Fyfe T, Robinson JF. Failure of Quintech TX pacemaker caused by loss of stimulus-T interval shortening during exercise. Br Heart J 1986;56:391.
54. Mehta DM, Lau CP, Ward DE, et al. Comparative evaluation of chronotropic responses of QT sensing and activity sensing rate responsive pacemakers. PACE 1988;11:1404–1412.
55. Baig MW, Green A, Wade G, Kovanci E, Constable PDL, Perrins EJ. A randomized double-blind, cross-over study of the linear and nonlinear algorithms for the QT sensing rate adaptive pacemaker. PACE 1990;13:1802–1808.
56. Bowes RJ, Schofield PM, Slaven Y, Southern S, Bennett DH. Programming the TX T-wave sensing rate responsive pacemaker. In: Belhassen B, Feldman S, Copperman Y (eds.). Cardiac Pacing and Electrophysiology. Proceedings of the VIIIth World Symposium on Cardiac Pacing and Electrophysiology. Ketrpress Entreprises, 1987, pp 95.
57. Fananapazir L, Rademaker M, Bennett DH. Reliability of the evoked response in determining the paced ventricular rate and performance of the QT or rate responsive (TX) pacemaker. PACE 1985;8:701–714.
58. Rickards AF. initial experience with a new single chamber, dual sensor rate responsive pacemaker (abstr). Eur J Cardiac Pacing Electrophysiol 1992;2:A23.
59. Landman MAJ, Senden PJ, Buys EM. Sensor cross checking in a dual sensor pacemaker during activity artifacts and emotional stress (abstr). Eur J Cardiac Pacing Electrophysiol 1992;2:A23.
60. Leman RB, McVenes RD, Kratz JM, Gilette PC. Programming eccentricities of an activity sensing pacemaker. PACE 1990;13:3–6.
61. Meta MV. Clinical study summary data. Telectronics Pacing Systems, Englewood, CO, 1988.
62. Wilson J, Lattner S. Apparent undersensing due to oversensing of low amplitude pulses in a thoracic impedance sensing, rate responsive pacemaker. PACE 1988;11:1479–1481.
63. Ortega DF, Salazar AI. Oversensing in AAIR, respiration-controlled pacemaker: possible role of impedance-detection carrier pulses (abstr). Eur J Cardiac Pacing Electrophysiol 1992;2:A63.
64. Forbath P, Hart J, Besser W, et al. Interference reversion resulting from

transthoracic impedance measurement in a minute ventilation, rate-modulating pulse generator (abstr). PACE 1989;12:640.

65. Wirtzfeld A, Heinze R, Stanzl K, Hoekstein K, Alt E, Liess HD. Regulation of pacing rate by variations of mixed venous oxygen saturation. PACE 1984;7:1257–1262.

66. Seifert GP, Moore AA, Graves KL, Lahtinen SP. In vivo and in vitro studies of a chronic oxygen saturation sensor. PACE 1991;14:1514–1527.

67. Lau CP, Linker NJ, Butrous GS, Ward DE, Camm AJ. Myopotential interference in unipolar rate responsive pacemakers. PACE 1989;12:1324–1330.

68. Boute W, Derrien Y, Wittkamok FHM. Reliability of evoked endocardial T wave sensing in 1500 pacemaker patients. PACE 1986;9:948–953.

69. Bernstein AD, Parsonnet V. Survey of cardiac pacing in the United States in 1989. Am J Cardiol 1992;69:331–338.

70. Chirife R. A new sensor for right ventricular volumes using the trailing edge voltage of a pulse generator output. PACE 1991;14:659.

71. Sulke N, Dritsas A, Chalnbers J. Is accurate rate response programming neccessary? PACE 1990;13:1031–1044.

72. Hayes DL, Von Feldt L, Higano ST. Standardized informal exercise testing for programming rate adaptive pacemakers. PACE 1991;14:1772–1776.

73. Luceri RM, Brownstein SL, Vardeman L, Goldstein S. PR interval behavior during exercise: implications for physiological pacemakers. PACE 1990;13:1719–1723.

74. Buckingham TA, Woodruff RC, Pennington DG, Redd RM, Janosik DL, Labovitz AJ, Graves R, Kennedy HL. Effect of ventricular function on the exercise hemodynamics of variable rate pacing. J Am Coll Cardiol 1988;11:1269–1277.

75. Cazeau S, Daubert C, Mabo P, et al. Dynamic electrophysiology of ventriculoatrial conduction: implications for DDD and DDDR pacing. PACE 1990;13:1646–1655.

76. Wish M, Cohen A, Swartz J, Fletcher R. Pacemaker syndrome due to a rate-responsive ventricular pacemaker. J Electrophysiol 1988;2:504–507.

77. Fujiki A, Tani M, Mizumaki K, Asanoi H, Sasayama S. Pacemaker syndrome evaluated by cardiopulmonary exercise testing. PACE 1990;13:1236–1241.

78. Dreifus LS, Fisch C, Griffin JC, Gillette PC, Mason JW, Parsonnet V. Guidelines for implantation of cardiac pacemakers and antiarrhythmia devices. A report of the American College of Cardiology/American Heart Association Task Force on assessment of diagnostic and therapeutic cardiovascular procedures (Committee on Pacemaker Implantation). J Am Coll Cardiol 1991;18:1–13.

79. Brandt, Fahraeus T, Schuller H. Rate-adaptive atrial pacing (AAIR): clinical aspects. In: Barold SS, Mugica J (eds.). New Perspectives in Cardiac Pacing. 2. Futura Publishing, Mount Kisco, NY, 1991, pp 303–312.

80. Rosenqvist M, Obel IWP. Atrial pacing and the risk for AV block: is there a time for a change in attitude? PACE 1989;12:97–101.

81. den Dulk K, Lindemans FW, Brugada P, Smeets JL, Wellens HJ. Pacemaker syndrome with AAI rate variable pacing: importance of atrioventricular conduction properties, medication, and pacemaker programmability. PACE 1988;11:1226–1233.
82. Schüller H, Brandt J. The pacemaker syndrome: old and new causes. Clin Cardiol 1991;14:336–340.
83. Barbieri D, Percoco GF, Toselli T, Guardigli G, Ansani L, Antonioli GE. AV delay and exercise stress test: behavior in normal subjects. PACE 1990;13:1724–1727.
84. Mabo P, Pouillot C, Kermarrec A, Lelong B, Lebreton H, Daubert C. Lack of physiological adaptation of the atrioventricular interval to heart rate in patients chronically paced in the AAIR mode. PACE 1991;14:2133–2142.
85. Brandt J, Fahraeus T, Ogawa T, Schüller H. Practical aspects of rate adaptive atrial (AAIR) pacing: clinical experiences in 44 patients. PACE 1991;14:1258–1264.
86. Hayes DL, Higano ST, Eisinger G. Electrocardiographic manifestations of a dual-chamber, rate-modulated (DDDR) pacemaker. PACE 1989;12:555–562.
87. Higano ST, Hayes DL. P wave tracking above the maximum tracking rate in a DDDR pacemaker. PACE 1989;12:1044–1048.
88. Lau CP, Tai YT, Fong PC, Li JPS, Chung FLW, Song S. The use of implantable sensors for the control of pacemaker mediated tachycardias: a comparative evaluation between minute ventilation sensing and acceleration sensing dual chamber rate adaptive pacemakers. PACE 1992;15:34–44.
89. Vanerio G, Patel S, Ching E, et al. Early clinical experience with a minute ventilation sensor DDDR pacemaker. PACE 1991;14:1815–1820.
90. Lee MT, Adkins A, Woodson D, Vandegriff J. A new feature for control of inappropriate high rate tracking in DDDR pacemakers. PACE 1990;13:1852–1855.
91. Vanerio G, Maloney JD, Pinski SL, et al. DDIR versus VVIR pacing in patients with paroxysmal atrial tachyarrhythmias. PACE 1991;14:1630–1638.
92. Zeigler VL, Gilette PC, Kratz J. Is activity sensored pacing in children and young adults a feasible option? PACE 1990;13:2104–2107.
93. Yabek SM, Wernly J, Chick TW, Bermann Jr W, McWilliams B. Rate-adaptive cardiac pacing in children using a minute ventilation biosensor. PACE 1990;13:2108–2112.
94. Schuchert A, Kuck KH, Bleifeld W. Effects of body constitution and age on maximum pacing rate of activity-modulated rate responsive pacemakers. PACE 1991;14:1467–1472.
95. Chung FLW, Lau CP, Wong CK, Tai YT, Fong PC, Sorrell A. Activity-initiated rate adaptive cardiac pacing in patients over 75 years old (abstr). PACE 1991;14:655.
96. Rodeheffer RJ, Gerstenblith G, Becker LC, Fleg JL, Weisfeldt ML, Lakata EG. Exercise cardiac output is maintain with advancing age in healthy

human subjects: cardiac dilatation and increased stroke volume compensate for a diminished heart rate. Circulation 1984;69:203–213.

97. Liang CS, Steward DK, LeJemtel TH, et al. Characteristics of peak aerobic capacity in symptomatic and asymptomatic subjects with left ventricular dysfunction. Am J Cardiol 1992:69:1207–1211.

98. Baller D, Wolpers HG, Zipfel J, Bretschneider HJ, Hellige G. Comparison of the effects of right atrial, right ventricular apex, and atrioventricular sequential pacing on myocardial consumption and cardiac efficiency: a laboratory investigation. PACE 1988;11;394–403.

99. de Cock CC, Visser F Stokker LO, et al. Efficacy and safety of rate responsive pacing in patients with coronary artery disease and angina pectoris. PACE 1989;12:1405.

100. Shefer A, Rozenman Y, David YB, Flugelman MY, Gotsman MS, Lewis BS. Left ventricular function during physiological cardiac pacing: relation to rate, pacing mode, and underlying cardiac disease. PACE 1987;10:315–325.

101. de Cock CC, Visser FC, Stokkel L, Roos JP. Rate-responsive pacing after myocardial infarction and angina pectoris (abstr). PACE 1990;13:1192.

102. McKay RG, Spears R, Aroesty JM, et al. Instantaneous measurement of left and right ventricular stroke volume and pressure-volume relationships with an impedance catheter. Circulation 1984;69:703–710.

103. Ilvento J, Wilkoff B, Dorian P, Vidaillet H, Fee J. Favorable interaction between implantable cardioverter-defibrillators and impedance based rate responsive pacemakers (abstr). PACE 1991;14:629.

104. McGuinn WP, Wilkoff BL, Maloney JD, et al. Treatment of autonomically mediated syncope with rapid AV sequential pacing on demand (abstr). J Am Coll Cardiol 1991;17:271A.

Chapter 18

The Follow-Up of Dual Chamber Rate-Adaptive Pacemakers

CHU-PAK LAU

Introduction

Dual chamber rate-adaptive (DDDR) pacemakers are currently the most sophisticated pacemakers in use. While there are still a number of controversial areas with the use of DDDR pacing,[1] more information is now available on the programming of a DDDR pacemaker and the role of the sensor in defining the rate response, the atrioventricular interval (AVI), the postventricular atrial refractory period (PVARP), and the management of pacemaker-mediated tachycardias. The follow-up and programming of such pacemakers, therefore, involve not only the rate-adaptive sensor(s) and the conventional DDD functions, but also the interactions between the sensor(s) and DDD parameters made possible in the DDDR pacing mode. A systematic approach is recommended that should include clinical evaluation, pacemaker programming, and the management of special DDDR-related problems and complications (Table 1).

Clinical Assessment

Symptom assessment is the most important aspect of follow-up of patients with rate-adaptive pacemakers. Adverse symptoms of palpita-

New Perspectives in Cardiac Pacing, Vol. 3, edited by S. Serge Barold and Jacques Mugica, Mount Kisco, NY, Futura Publishing Co., © 1993.

TABLE *1*
Follow-Up of Patients with DDDR Pacemakers

Types	*Details*
Clinical	Symptoms (e.g., palpitations, breathlessness, angina). Quality of life and well-being. Hemodynamics and exercise capacity.
Programming	
DDD	LRI and URI
	AVI
	PVARP
	A and V sensing and pacing function
	Crosstalk
	PMT response
Sensor	Matching rate response to workload
	Speed of onset and recovery from an exercise
DDD/Sensor	Sensor-determined LRI and URI
Interactions	Sensor-determined AVI and PVARP
	PMT response using the sensor
Special Problems	Complications of implantation
	Patients undergoing general anesthesia
	Sensor-mediated tachycardias
	Pacemaker syndrome
	Atrial arrhythmias induction
	Technical problems

A = atrial; AVI = atrioventricular interval; LRI = lower rate interval; PMT = pacemaker-mediated tachycardias; PVARP = postventricular atrial refractory period; URI = upper rate interval; V = ventricular.

tion may suggest an inappropriately fast sensor-determined rate, and if this occurs during sleep in a patient with an activity-sensing pacemaker, the possibility of the sensor being activated by the patient lying directly on the pacemaker should be considered.[2] Palpitations can also complicate excessive arm swinging in patients with respiratory-sensing pacemakers.[3,4] Some patients may temporarily experience palpitations when their fixed-rate pacemakers are upgraded, and a gentle rate-adaptive function initially is advisable. In patients with ischemic heart disease, worsening of angina pectoris can be a problem, but this usually resolves with judicious adjustment of the upper rate.[5]

There is now good evidence that rate-adaptive pacing is superior to

VVI pacing, not only in enhancing cardiac hemodynamics during exercise, but also on clinical grounds. Symptoms of shortness of breath on exercise and energy during daily activities are likely to improve,[6] as well as some improvement in the formal quality of life.[6,7] Although the improvement in measures of quality of life with the addition of AV synchrony to VVIR pacing may not be statistically significant,[8] there is little doubt that hemodynamics at rest and at low levels of exercise are significantly better.[9–12] Most patients prefer dual chamber pacing over VVIR pacing,[8] and symptomatic improvement may occur only after several weeks.[6] Hemodynamic and exercise tolerance can be formally tested with either treadmill or cycle ergometry, and a protocol with gradually increasing workload may be more appropriate for the usual pacemaker recipients.[13,14] A significant proportion of elderly patients may not be able to perform these exercises.[15] The distance covered by these patients during a standard 12-minute walking test is a reproducible and simple means of assessing the benefits of rate-adaptive pacemakers during daily activities.[15] A learning effect occurs between the first and second 12-minute walking tests, but thereafter, this effect is small.

Programming

At the time of pacemaker implantation, most DDDR pacemakers will be in the DDD mode. The activation of the DDDR mode involves matching the sensor level to the workload and programming of the speed of onset and recovery from an exercise. By using submaximal exercise protocols, the DDDR mode can be activated as soon as the patient is ambulant after implantation. However, in the author's experience, reprogramming of initial sensor setting is often necessary on long-term follow-up when the patients' conditions improve and become more active. A reassessment of the rate-adaptive function can be carried out at 6–8 weeks post implantation together with the assessment of sensing and pacing functions.

Programming of DDD Functions

Standard protocols for programming DDD functions have been published.[16] In addition to conventional DDD parameters, the importance of a judiciously adjusted AVI is increasingly recognized. The AVI varies in different patients and during different physiologic conditions. The optimal AVI can be determined in an individual patient with non-invasive assessment such as echo- or Doppler-guided cardiac output measurements.[17–20] In normal individuals, the PR interval also shortens on exercise,[21] which can be imitated in some DDDR pacemakers that automatically decrease the AVI with rate (or with a sensor). This is reported to enhance exercise duration, maximum oxygen uptake and carbon dioxide production,[22] and an elevation of the anerobic threshold.[22] A non-physiologic AVI not only adversely affects cardiac hemodynamics but also results in a reduced sense of well being.[23]

In patients with sinus node disease treated with dual chamber pacemakers, the resting AVI should be programmed to allow maximum intrinsic conduction. Using a radionuclide ventriculogram, Rosenqvist et al.[24] showed that AAI pacing results in better cardiac output, left ventricular ejection fraction, and preserved normal septal motion than DDD pacing. In a small group of patients, Harper et al.[25] also demonstrate improved peak oxygen uptake and oxygen pulse during exercise during intrinsic conductions than during P wave synchronous ventricular pacing.

In programming the AVI, it is also important to consider the conduction delay to the left atrium and ventricle induced from the corresponding right-sided atrial or ventricular pacing.[26] Left ventricular mechanical contraction is delayed if it is activated through right ventricular pacing compared to intrinsic conduction. An "optimal" AVI for the right heart will be too short for the left heart if the right ventricle is paced. By similar reasoning, the interatrial conduction time will also vary, depending on whether the right atrium is sensed or paced. These factors should be taken into account in programming the AVI.

Programming of the Sensor(s)

Matching Sensor Level to Workload

In a closed-loop rate-adaptive pacing system, the change in sensor level during exercise leads to a rate change, which in turn induces a physiologic change in the opposite direction. Thus, a negative feedback loop on the sensor is established. An example is the sensing of central venous oxygen saturation. Exercise with a fixed heart rate causes a fall in the oxygen saturation, which is detected by an oxygen sensor. The resultant rate change improves the cardiac output, causing an increase in oxygen saturation. Thus, the system is highly physiologic and automatically "sets" the optimal pacing rate. Theoretically, the need for sensor programming will be minimal.

Most rate-adaptive pacemakers utilize an open loop logic: the change in pacing rate does not have any effect on the sensor level responsible for the change. Thus, a physician has to ascribe a clinically determined rate-response/workload relationship, the so-called "slope" of rate response. A variety of exercise protocols and monitoring methods have been designed to standardize and simplify the optimization of the rate-responsive slope.

Exercise Methods: Treadmill exercise is one of the most widely employed exercise methods. Conventional exercise protocols are targeted to getting exercise data at the maximally achieved workload and are suitable for defining ischemia and for testing of the more athletic individuals. Since pacemaker recipients are usually elderly, it is important to obtain heart rates for submaximal exercise intensities. Alt[13] and Wilkoff et al.[14] proposed the use of a more gradual exercise protocol in assessing the degree of chronotropic incompetence and rate adaptation. The Chronotropic Assessment Exercise Protocol is a 2-minute stage protocol with gradual increase in the treadmill speed and grade.[14] Predicted heart rate at any stage of exercise can be derived from the age, resting heart rate, and functional capacity (maximum exercise capacity).

Cycle ergometry has also been used to program rate-adaptive pacemakers. This obviates the influence of the patient's body weight, and workloads can be accurately assessed. However, the rate response is significantly lower during cycle ergometry than during treadmill exercise for an equivalent workload.[28] As a full treadmill protocol may be time consuming or cannot be performed by some patients, brief treadmill exercise, e.g., lasting for 2–3 minutes at different speeds and grades, may be used to assess the accuracy of programming.[29] Brief exercise tests can also be used to estimate the speed of rate response.

The most common muscular exercise performed by pacemaker recipients is walking, and a walking test is a convenient stress test for programming rate-adaptive function and can be carried out by almost all pacemaker recipients. A rate of 90–100 bpm is usually ascribed as the approximate pacing rate achieved.[15,29] This clinical practice is supported by the heart rates attained by 195 normal subjects during "casual" and "brisk" walk.[30] Despite variability in the resting heart rates, most normal subjects attained a rate of 85–100 bpm and 100–110 bpm during casual and brisk walk, respectively.

Autoprogrammability: To simplify programming, some rate-adaptive pacemakers automatically infer from the sensor level derived from a given workload to a physician-ascribed pacing rate. In one type of activity sensing pacemaker (Sensolog and Synchrony models, Siemens Ltd.), sensor data are collected during casual and brisk walking and the rate-adaptive parameters can be inferred from published graphs to achieve the desired heart rate response.[31-33] As the algorithm employed for activity sensing in this pacemaker involves an integration of activity signals, the rate-responsive parameters as programmed by treadmill exercise tend to result in a higher rate for ordinary walking and are also highly dependent on the footwear worn by the patient.[31-32,34]

Another approach to achieve rate-adaptive parameters for ordinary exercise is utilized in an accelerometer-based activity-sensing pacemaker (Relay or Dash, Intermedics Inc., Freeport, TX).[35] Acceleration data are collected over a 3-minute exercise test (e.g., causal walking) and it is automatically coupled to a programmable rate response, the so-called "tailored to patient." The rate-adaptive slope has a triphasic relation to workload (Fig. 1), with a flat intermediate portion to represent ordinary exercise and more aggressive curves for low and high levels of exercise. The flat intermediate slope will result in a relatively stable rate response during daily activities once the "tailored to patient" function is activated with an ordinary walking exercise. In addition, the rate responses during ordinary workloads are only minimally affected by a change in slope because of substantial overlap of the rate-responsive curves for the ordinary workload response (Fig. 1). Therefore, to ensure that the maximum pacing rate can be attained in the more athletic patients, a formal exercise test still needs to be carried out to examine the rate-response characteristics at the higher workload.

In a minute ventilation sensing pacemaker (META-DDDR, Telectronics Pacing Systems, Englewood, CO), the impedance-derived minute ventilation level is reflected by the so-called rate responsive factor (RRF) derived from telemetry.[36] The rate-adaptive parameter can be de-

Relay : Effect of △Slope

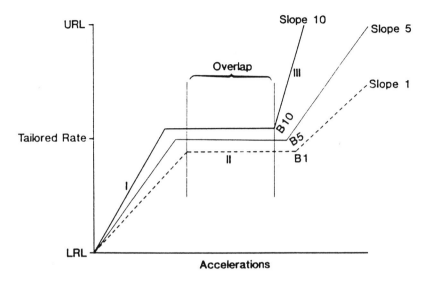

Figure 1. Triphasic rate-responsive curves of an accelerometer-based activity-sensing DDDR pacemaker. Phase I and III represent low and high levels of accelerations, respectively, and are related to a steeper slope of rate change. Phase II represents ordinary activities at which the change in rate is small. The transition between phase II and III is termed the breakpoint, which remains relatively constant at different slope values. Thus, there is substantial overlap in rate changes during the ordinary level of acceleration despite the use of a different slope. B_1, B_5, and B_{10} = breakpoints at slope 1, 5, 10, respectively; LRL = lower rate limit; URL = upper rate limit. Reproduced with permission from Futura Publishing Co.[35]

rived by performing an exercise test in the VVI but minute ventilation sensing mode to derive the minimum RRF value at peak exercise. Using this RRF to set the rate-responsive slope, the maximum pacing rate will be reached at an equivalent peak exercise load. Alternatively, the rate-responsive slope can be set using submaximal exercise tests to achieve a desired heart rate response.

Monitoring Function: The rate response during exercise can be monitored electrocardiographically during treadmill or cycle ergometry,

HISTOGRAMS

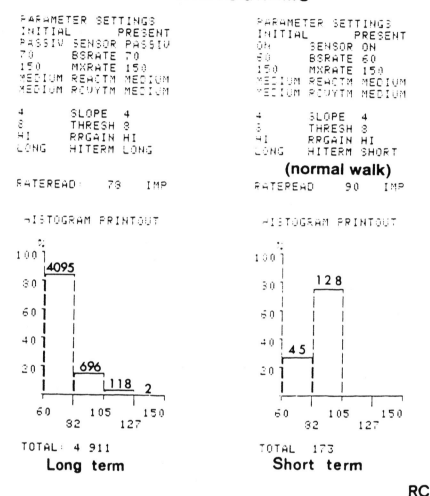

Figure 2.   Rate histograms of a patient with Sensolog 703. The number on top of each histogram bin (which was shown only on the programmer screen but is labeled here to give an idea of the size of each bin) represents the number of times that a pacing rate occurred within the bin range. The long-term histogram represents sampling over an 18–48 hour period and the short-term histogram was made in this example during normal walking for 2 minutes. Reproduced with permission from Futura Publishing Co.[31]

or by telemetry if informal exercise is carried out. To simplify programming, some pacemakers have built-in rate-monitoring software. The pacing rate for exercise can be allocated as percentages or counts into different rate ranges, the so-called rate histograms (Fig. 2).[31] This is useful to see the "spread" of rate response for an activity, although it cannot show the time sequence of rate response. Another approach is the use of rate profiles, which are like a built-in Holter (Fig. 3).[35] The rate response for an activity can be profiled over a programmable period of time. In addition, it is also possible to calculate the rate response at different rate-adaptive slopes with the recorded sensor data without the need for repeating the exercise (Fig. 3).

Holter monitoring is often used to program rate-adaptive pacemakers. While very useful to detect rate-adaptive sensor malfunction,

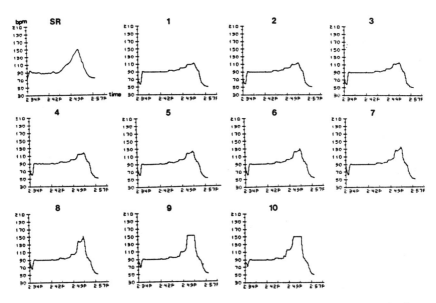

Figure 3.   Utility of calculated rate profile for optimizing rate response in the accelerometer-based activity-sensing pacemaker. This patient had normal sinus response during graded treadmill exercise (top left). The corresponding sensor-determined rate at different slopes (1–10) can be obtained for this exercise using the calculated rate profile software. In this patient, a slope value of 7 or 8 shows the best approximation to the sinus response. SR = sinus rate. Reproduced with permission from Futura Publishing Co.[35]

there are few data on how to use Holter-derived parameters to optimize rate response,[37] and analysis tends to be tedious and time consuming.

Onset and Termination of Rate Response

At the onset of exercise, the normal heart rate increases almost immediately without significant delay, with over half of the heart rate changes occurring within the first minute of exercise.[38,39] Thus, an appropriate speed of rate response is important, especially in patients who exercise only for brief periods of time. Compared with normals, the activity-sensing pacemakers have the best speed of onset of rate response,[29] which is now available as a programmable option. In patients with atrial rate-adaptive pacemakers, sudden rate increase may result in functional AVI prolongation so that an atrial contraction may take place simultaneously with the previous ventricular contraction and results in pacemaker syndrome.[40] This is a special situation when the addition of ventricular pacing is important to avoid adverse hemodynamic consequences of rate-adaptive atrial pacing.

The rate of decay of pacing rate after recovery may also be important. A physiologic rate of decay[41] may contribute to earlier recovery of hemodynamics and lower lactate accumulation after exercise. An appropriate pattern of decrease of pacing rate is especially important in patients who have achieved a high rate at peak exercise. The rate decay pattern is now programmable in a number of rate-adaptive pacemakers. In some sensors, such as the sensing of minute ventilation central venous temperature, oxygen saturation, and stroke volume, the decay of sensor value after exercise is related to previous workloads and can be used to modulate the pacing rate recovery after exercise.

The Maximum and Minimum Sensor-Indicated Rates

Apart from rate-responsive slopes, a minimum and maximum rate has to be ascribed. Unlike the case of VVI pacing in which an average rate has to be programmed, the baseline rate becomes less important in rate-adaptive pacemakers as a higher rate can be achieved by sensor-driven pacing during exercise. A lower pacing rate at sleep is physiologically attractive[42] and can be battery conserving.

The patient's age, activity, and the presence of ischemic heart disease should be taken into account in choosing the maximum sensor-driven rate. In general, a higher upper rate may be of benefit in the young patients and in children. In a review of nine studies on physiologic pacemakers, Nordlander et al.[43] found that the percentage of improvement in maximal exercise capacity was linearly related to the maximum rate achieved. However, Holter recordings of patients with complete heart block treated with VDD pacemakers show that the usual pacemaker recipients (mean age 68–70 years) achieved a rate of 150 bpm in less than 0.5% of the time in the day.[44] During 12-minute walking tests, there is no objective difference between an upper rate of 125 and 150 bpm on the distance covered.[15] Thus, it seems that an upper rate of 125–150 bpm can be chosen for most patients. In patients with angina pectoris, it is worthwhile to perform an exercise test to see if the programmed upper rate can improve exercise capacity without unduly aggravating anginal symptoms.

The value of the lower and upper rates can also significantly affect submaximal rate response. The "slopes" of rate response usually vary according the lower and upper rates programmed, and this should be considered in programming rate-adaptive settings (Table 2).

TABLE *2*

Effect of Lower Rate Programming in 12 Patients with DDDR Pacemakers (4 Minute Ventilation Sensing, 8 Activity Sensing)*

	Stages of Exercise				Peak Exercise
Lower Rate	*1*	*2*	*3*	*4*	
80	102	106	112	110	137
70	96	103	110	101	130
60	87	97	103	113	127
50	86	91	110	111	125

* The pacing rate (bpm) attained during submaximal exercise stages (1 and 2) were significantly affected by the programmed lower rate, although the maximum rate achieved at the end of exercise was not affected. The upper rate in all patients was 150 bpm.

Interactions Between DDD and Sensors

In current DDDR pacemakers, sensor(s) are used to determine and vary conventional DDD intervals and to control pacemaker-mediated tachycardias.

The Lower and Upper Rates

The programmed lower rates in a DDDR pacemaker are identical for P-wave sensing and for sensor-driven pacing. However, a sensor may be used to determine a separate lower rate during sleep.[35,45] In some DDDR pacemakers, a 24-hour clock is incorporated to act as a "sensor" to reduce the resting rate during sleep. The sleeping hours can be confirmed to be a resting period by the persistent lack of activity registered by the sensor (Fig. 4). Other examples include the use of diurnal fluctuation in temperature to change the resting rate at day and night time, so that the lower rate may become a spontaneously varying parameter. The occurrence of an activity during the "sleep rate" will be detected by the sensor, and rate response will occur at the programmed lower rate.

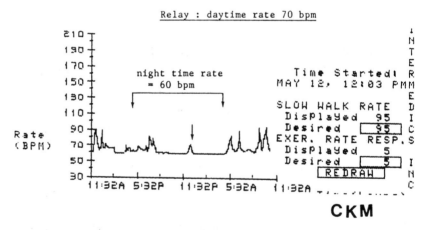

Figure 4. Diurnal changes of the lower rate according to the time of the day in an accelerometer-based activity-sensing DDDR pacemaker. A recorded rate profile obtained by telemetry is shown. An activity during sleep (arrow) resulted in rate response despite a lowered minimum rate.

In some DDDR pacemakers (Synchrony, Siemens Ltd.), a separate upper rate can be programmed for P-wave sensing and sensor-driven pacemakers. For the following discussion, the upper rate interval (URI) refers to the minimum P-wave tracking interval before pacemaker Wenckebach or 2:1 tracking of P wave occurs, and the sensor upper rate interval (SURI) for the minimum interval allowed for sensor-driven pacing. The SURI is shorter or equal to URI. Depending on the interactions between sinus rate (SR) and sensor-indicated rate (SIR), the following conditions may occur during exercise[46-48]:

1. Within the URI, when SR is faster than SIR, P-wave tracking will occur.
2. Within the URI, when SIR is faster than SR, atrial pacing will occur.
3. In most DDD pacemakers, a PP interval shorter than the URI will be tracked in a Wenckebach-like manner (Fig. 5A). However, a sudden rate drop will be avoided in a DDDR pacemaker because the sensor will determine the escape interval, so that "sensor-smoothing" of upper rate behavior will occur (Fig. 5B). If the SIRI is also shorter than URI, the P wave will be apparently tracked above the programmed upper rate (Fig. 5C).
4. Within the SURI, but shorter than the URI, SIR faster than SR will result in atrial pacing. It is possible in some pacemakers that atrial pacing will occur within the PVARP, which is programmed in conjunction with the URI as one of the DDD parameters (Fig. 5D).

Sensor-Determined AVI and PVARP

These parameters are determined by the sensor in a minute ventilation sensing DDDR pacemaker (META-DDDR). In this pacemaker, both the sensor-defined and P-wave tracking lower and upper rates are identical. The change in minute ventilation level is used to determine the SIRI.

In the DDDR mode, the AVI shortens during exercise according to the minute ventilation sensor.[49-51] The AVI equals to the sum of either 80 ms ("short") or 100 ms ("long") plus $\frac{1}{16}$ of SIRI. This interval always shortens as rate increases.

The programmed value of PVARP base is the PVARP in effect at

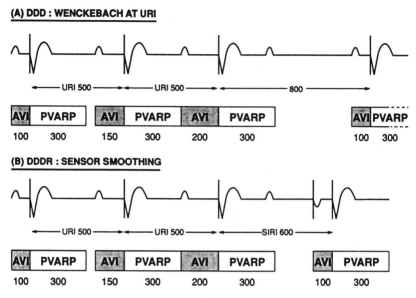

Figure 5. Upper rate behavior in a pacemaker with separately programmable upper rates for P wave tracking and for the sensor. The following intervals are programmed: atrioventricular interval (AVI) = 100 ms; postventricular atrial refractory period (PVARP) = 300 ms; sensor-determined upper rate interval = 350 ms; sensor-indicated rate interval (SIRI) = decreasing from 600 to 350 ms during exercise; upper rate interval for P wave tracking (URI) = 500 ms; and a PP interval of 450 ms is assumed. (A) Wenckebach P wave tracking as PP interval is shorter than URI in the DDD mode. (B) The same situation as in A, but in the DDDR mode and with the SIRI 600 ms. The fourth P wave is not tracked. However, instead of an extension of cycle length to 800 ms in A, the sensor set the lower escape interval to 600 ms, thus resulting in "sensor smoothing." Continued.

the lower rate limit (Fig. 6A). Thus, an atrial tracking interval (ATI) occurs after the PVARP at the lower rate limit if the sum of PVARP and AVI is shorter than the LRI. In the DDDR mode, the PVARP at the upper rate limit interval (which is also the minimum SIRI) is, in general, equal to the difference between the URI and the AVI. If a relatively "long" PVARP base is programmed, the PVARP will shorten (in a slope of 1 in 16) until the minimum value at the maximum rate limit. The ATI will disappear at the maximum rate. AV sequential pacing will always occur at the maximum rate as PP intervals shorter than the

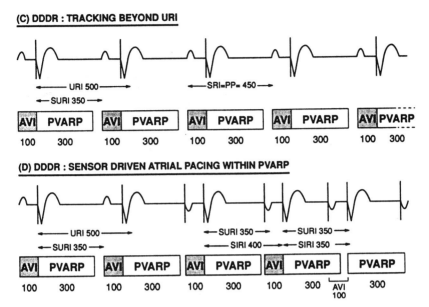

Figure 5. (C) The same condition as in B, but with the SIRI just equal to the PP interval of 450 ms. Although this PP interval is shorter than the URI, it is within the SURI and thus the P wave will be apparently tracked beyond the upper rate. In practice, as the P-wave sensing window is short, intermittent P-wave sensing and atrial pacing will occur as the P-wave rate and sensor-indicated rate may not exactly match. (D) Atrial pacing within the PVARP. The patient is undergoing exercise resulting in sensor activation and atrial overdrive pacing (third complex). As the SIRI shortens to 350 ms, atrial pacing will occur within the PVARP as the SURI is programmed independent of the PVARP.

URI will always fall within the PVARP and will not initiate ventricular pacing.

In situations where a relatively "short" PVARP base and low upper rate are programmed (Fig. 6B), the PVARP does not necessarily shorten as the rate increases as the upper rate would not be compromised by the short PVARP. A short ATI will be present at the upper rate limit which will allow tracking of intrinsic P wave if the SR is higher than the SIR (Fig. 6B). The ventricular response will, however, be determined by the programmed upper rate. The pattern of upper rate behavior is also affected by the automatic mode switching algorithm (see below).

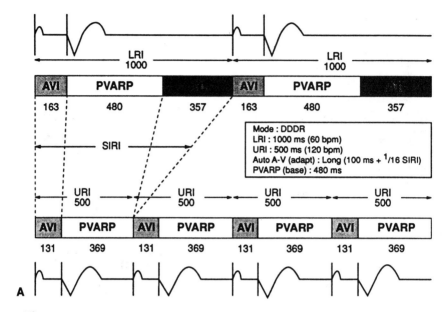

Figure 6. Schematic representation of the adaptation of the AV interval and PVARP in the META-DDDR at different PVARP base during exercise. The LRI and URI are 1000 and 500 ms, respectively, with the "long" auto AV adapt programmed. (A) PVARP = 480 ms. At rest, the LRI equals the sum of AVI, PVARP, and an atrial tracking interval (ATI). At peak exercise, the ATI disappears and both the AVI and PVARP shorten so that the URI equals to the sum of AVI and PVARP. Continued.

Sensor and Pacemaker-Mediated Tachycardias[52]

Several interactions between the implanted sensors and pacemaker-mediated tachycardias are possible in a DDDR pacemaker.

Sensor-Initiated Termination: Endless-loop tachycardias in dual chamber pacemakers can be terminated by pacemaker reprogramming to a nonatrial tracking mode, magnet application, chest wall stimulation, chest thumping, or the induction of myopotential oversensing.[53] In the DDDR pacemaker, the sensor can be used to terminate magnet-unresponsive endless-loop tachycardia.[54] For example, tapping an activity sensing pacemaker that employs a piezoelectric sensor results in AV se-

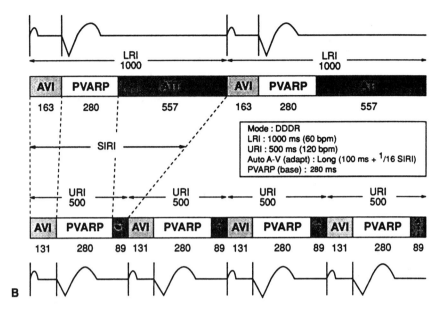

Figure 6. (B) PVARP = 280 ms. At rest, the LRI still equals to the sum of AVI, PVARP, and ATI, although the ATI is much longer. At peak exercise, AVI still shortens according to the sensor-indicated rate interval (SIRI). However, PVARP does not shorten as the sum of PVARP and AV interval at peak exercise is still shorter than the programmed URI. Thus, a short ATI persists at the upper rate limit. Reproduced with permission from Futura Publishing Co.[50]

quential pacing at an increasing rate and thus terminates the endless-loop tachycardia by overdrive pacing. The other potential sensor that can be easily initiated by either the patient or the physician is impedance-based respiratory sensing pacemaker,[3,4] which can be activated by hyperventilation or arm swinging. The use of implantable sensors thus offers the potential for sensor-initiated overdrive termination of endless-loop tachycardias during emergency situations.

Amelioration of the Consequences of Pacemaker-Mediated Tachycardias: One of the consequences of pacemaker-mediated tachycardia is rapid ventricular stimulation. The use of an implantable sensor in a DDDR pacemaker may allow the pacemaker to judge the

AF RESPONSE

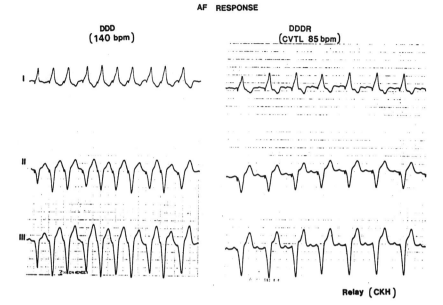

Figure 7. Ventricular responses in a patient with the Relay pacemaker during spontaneous atrial flutter (AF). The upper rate was 150 bpm and the atrial sensitivity was at 0.8 mV. Irregular ventricular tracking at 140 bpm occurred in the DDD mode. The rate was regularized and reduced to 85 bpm when DDDR mode was programmed such that the conditional ventricular tracking response (CVTL) was activated. Reproduced with permission from Futura Publishing Inc.[35]

appropriateness of a high atrial rate and to restrict the pacemaker response temporarily to a tolerably lower level—the conditional ventricular tracking limit (CVTL).[35,55] When the sensor indicates exercise, the system can ignore the CVTL and accelerates to the maximum programmed tracking rate (Fig. 7).

Sensor Prevention of Pacemaker-Mediated Tachycardias:
As discussed earlier, a sensor can be used to determine the AVI and PVARP at rest and during exercise.[49-51] At rest, with the sensor registering absence of exercise, the total atrial refractory period (TARP) can be kept long, thus excluding retrogradely conducting P waves or atrial tachycardias that will fall within the TARP and will not lead to ventricular pacing. On exercise with the sensor indicating the need for a rate re-

sponse, the TARP can be shortened by the sensor and allows an approach to the upper rate. Further protection, especially against the rapid tracking of an atrial tachycardia, can be effected by an automatic change in pacing mode.

Automatic Mode Change

In the DDDR mode of the META-DDDR pacemaker, atrial activities are monitored continuously even within the PVARP. Successive atrial events (eight consecutive beats) within the PVARP will be considered by the pacemaker algorithm as retrograde conduction, and the pacemaker attempts to terminate the retrograde conduction by AV sequential pacing. If multiple P waves occur within the PVARP, atrial tachyarrhythmia is assumed and the pacemaker paces in the VVIR mode. When P waves no longer occur within the PVARP, sinus rhythm is assumed and the pacemaker reverts back to the DDDR mode. Whenever a P wave occurs during the PVARP, a mode switch is effected. Conversely, to avoid excessive mode changes, a number of cycles without a P wave in the PVARP are required to switch back to the DDDR mode. If there have been only one or two P waves in the PVARP, then the same number of "empty" PVARPs are required before the switch back to DDDR, otherwise three are required. In the DDD mode, a similar mechanism is in operation, except that only a 2-ms portion of the PVARP is used for "detection" so that mode switch usually does not occur. This 2-ms window is active at 100 ms into the PVARP. Early reports[49-51] have confirmed the ability of the algorithm to detect atrial fibrillation and appropriate mode switching (Fig. 8). However, judicious programming of the PVARP is crucial to avoid excessive mode switching in the presence of atrial ectopics and nonexercise-related sinus rate changes.[50]

The combination of sensor-determined PVARP (which allows a long PVARP to be used at rest without compromising the upper rate) and automatic mode switching allows protection against retrograde conduction and sensing of atrial tachyarrythmias, although there are a number of potential problems. Mode switching, especially due to frequent atrial ectopics, may result in pacemaker syndrome in those predisposed. The use of a sensor to determine the TARP is theoretically attractive, but this will increase the requirement on the speed and proportionality of response of the sensor. Figure 9 illustrates what would happen to a DDDR pacemaker with sensor-determined shortening of TARP. The

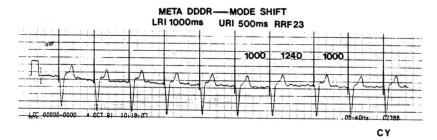

META DDDR——MODE SHIFT
LRI 1000ms   URI 500ms RRF 23

CY

Figure 8. Reversion from DDDR pacing to VVIR pacing in a patient with META-DDDR during spontaneous atrial fibrillation. An intermittent cycle length extension of 240 ms was observed to give an indication of mode switching. Reproduced with permission from Futura Publishing Co.[50]

rate of shortening of the sinus cycle length (PP interval) after exercise is dependent on the condition of the patient and the type of exercise involved. In general, a rate-response half-time of 10–20 seconds occurs in those individuals without chronotropic incompetence.[38] The consequences of a sensor with a delay of 20 seconds in response to exercise is shown in this example. In the worst case scenario, if the PP interval shortens rapidly by 300 ms within the first 20 seconds of a sprint exercise, a long TARP (RP_1) programmed at rest would not be shortened fast enough by the sensor to track the normal sinus activity. This will result in transient AV dissociation, although 1:1 AV tracking will ultimately be established with the proceed of exercise. Thus, a shorter TARP (RP_2) has to be programmed at rest to accommodate for this sudden sinus rate "jump," and the use of a slow sensor may limit the usefulness of sensor-mediated TARP shortening in the rejection of pacemaker-mediated tachycardia. In the META-DDDR pacemaker, we have found that this problem can be minimized by asking the patient to undergo a burst exercise, and to program the baseline PVARP such that 1:1 P wave tracking occurs even with sudden shortening of PVARP[50] (Fig. 10). Although this is, in general, satisfactory for most patients, it is important to recognize that VA conduction is dynamic and changes during exercise may not be directly inferred from resting data[56] so that PVARP shortening by the sensor during exercise must also take into the account of potential prolongation of VA conduction time in some patients. Thus, further refinement on this algorithm and the sensor (and perhaps using a sensor combination) is necessary to maximize the efficacy of this approach.

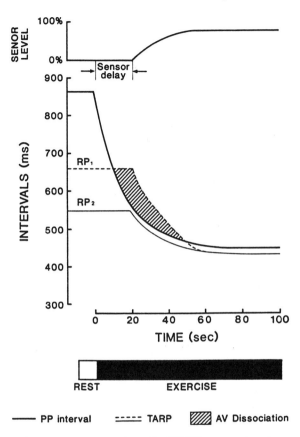

Figure 9. Schematic representation of a DDDR pacemaker that uses a sensor to shorten the total atrial refractory period (TARP) during exercise. A delay of 20 sec is assumed to occur before the sensor can detect the onset of exercise and begin the shortening of the TARP. On the other hand, the sinus response is immediate (denoted by the immediate shortening of the PP interval) at exercise onset from an arbitrary resting PP interval of 860 ms. If a long TARP (RP_1 = 660 ms) is programmed at rest, the PP interval will fall below 660 ms and hence results in AV dissociation before the sensor has time to adjust the TARP. At the end of 20 sec, the sensor starts to shorten the TARP, and the RP_1 will shorten until it is shorter than the PP interval at about 50 sec and allows 1:1 AV tracking. The hatched area thus represents the time for which AV dissociation will occur. By using a shorter TARP at rest (RP_2 = 550 ms), AV dissociation will not occur as the sensor now has sufficient time to shorten the TARP. Reproduced with permission from Futura Publishing Co.[52]

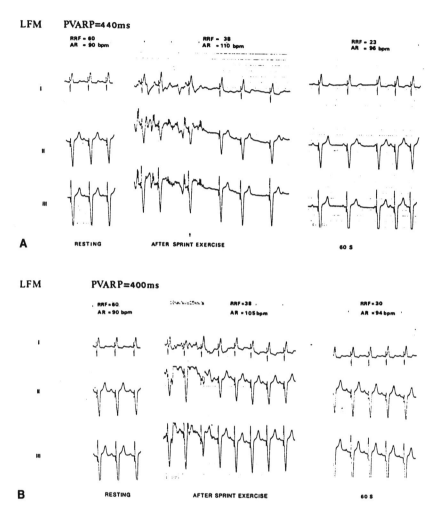

Figure 10. Determination of the baseline PVARP using a 15-second sprint exercise in one patient. (A) At a PVARP of 440 ms, AV dissociation occurred during and immediately after sprint exercise, as the shortening of the PVARP lags behind the rapid increase in sinus rate. (B) A repeat of the sprint exercise using a shorter PVARP (400 ms). This allows full tracking of the P wave during and after exercise. Reproduced with permission from Futura Publishing Co.[50]

Management of Special Problems

A number of special situations may be encountered during the follow-up of patients with DDDR pacemakers. At present, the sensors incorporated in DDDR pacemakers utilize conventional electrodes (with the exception of stroke volume sensor). Thus, the implantation technique is identical to DDD pacing. Complications related to DDDR pacing may be due to the sensor, the DDD mode, or specifically due to their interactions. These are separately discussed below.

General Anesthesia and Electrocautery

During general anesthesia and Caesarian section, appropriate rate responses have been reported with activity[57] and minute ventilation sensing pacemakers.[58] However, a case of artificial hyperventilation-induced rapid pacing occurred in another patient with a minute ventilation sensing pacemaker during general anesthesia.[59] Electrocautery used during cardiothoracic surgery in a patient with an impedance-based minute ventilation sensing pacemaker could be falsely picked up by the impedance sensor, and inappropriate pacing at the upper rate could occur.[60] These reports suggest that patients with DDDR pacemakers should probably be left in the DDD mode during general anesthesia. As radiofrequency ablation of cardiac arrhythmias utilized energy with a frequency similar to electrocautery, it is also advisable to program impedance-sensing pacemakers to the non-rate-adaptive motion during this procedure.

Technical Failure

A number of technical problems have been observed in some early devices. A software problem in calculating rate profile was observed with the RX2000 programmer for the accelerometer-based DDDR pacemaker (Relay). This resulted in representation of the rate above the programmed upper rate. This error occurred in the rate profile but did not actually take place in the patient. An insulation failure in the atrial negative terminal of the pulse generator of a minute ventilation sensing DDDR pacemaker (META-DDDR) observed in one batch of these pacemakers can result in output failure, and sensor-mediated tachycardia could also occur at the maximum programmed rate. We have also encountered a pro-

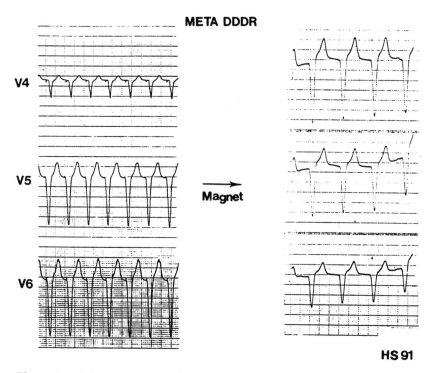

META DDDR

Magnet

HS 91

Figure 11. Upper rate ventricular pacing (150 bpm) in a patient with META-DDDR pacemaker resulting from a programmer software failure. It was not possible to alter the rate by the programmer, but the system was responsive to magnet application which resulted in a better-tolerated magnet rate of 99 bpm.

grammer software problem with the same pacemaker. Using the 5603 programmer with a 4.5 software version to assess the rate-responsive factor during exercise, a sudden break in the telemetry link resulted in the pacemaker pacing at the maximum rate limit with complete loss of telemetry function (Fig. 11). The system was responsive only to magnet application, which converts the DDDR pacemaker to asynchronous ventricular pacing. The pulse generator had to be replaced. These defects are now corrected in the current META-DDDR pacemakers.

Atrial Arrhythmia Induction

In a DDD pacemaker, the atrial escape interval is fixed at the LRI. An atrial ectopic or an early P wave falling within the PVARP will not be followed by a closely coupled atrial paced event that occurs only when the lower rate interval (LRI) times out[61] (Fig. 12A). On the other hand, the "LRI" is continuously changed by the sensor in the DDDR mode. Thus, an atrial ectopic beat may be followed closely by a paced atrial event governed by the sensor[61] and lead to the induction of atrial fibrillation (Fig. 12B). The occurrence of an atrial arrhythmia may be lessened with rate-adaptive shortening of the AVI so that the TARP period is shortened. On the other hand, in some pacemakers with a separate SURI that is programmed shorter than the URI, sensor-driven pacing can actually occur within the PVARP without atrial sensing, and the potential for atrial arrhythmia induction is an important consideration (Fig. 5D). Indeed, the reported incidence of atrial arrhythmias in DDDR pacing during FDA trial ranged from 8% to 10%,[62] although these studies were not designed to investigate this problem and the types and per-

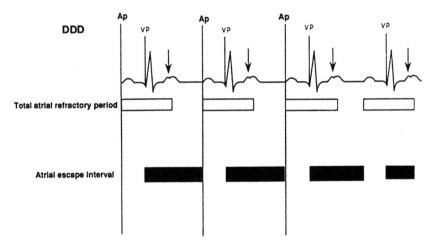

Figure 12. Potential atrial arrhythmia induction in a DDDR pacing system. Reproduced with permission from the authors and Futura Publishing Co.[60] (A) Depicted DDD pacemaker response to a sinus tachycardia. Every second P wave falls within the total atrial refractory period and is therefore not sensed (arrows). The first two nonsensed P waves are followed by an atrial stimulus at the end of the atrial escape interval. The third P wave is not sensed and this is followed by a sensed spontaneous atrial depolarization occurring just before the atrial escape interval timer expires. In both circumstances, there is little chance for atrial competition, and the atrial pacing outputs occur long after the vulnerable period of the preceding nonsensed P waves. Continued.

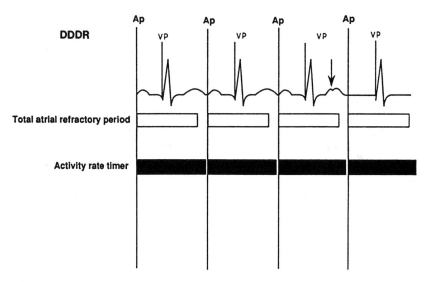

Figure 12. (B) The response of a DDDR pacemaker to a spontaneous atrial depolarization within the TARP is shown here, with a single premature atrial depolarization for simplicity. The spontaneous P wave (arrow) is followed very closely by an atrial output stimulus. This is because the activity-driven atrial output occurs far earlier than the expiration of the atrial escape interval. This may occur particularly at faster sensor-modulated rates and can potentially result in an atrial stimulus falling into the vulnerable period of atrial repolarization. There is a similar potential for atrial competition when sinus tachycardia results in spontaneous P waves falling into the TARP.

sistence of these arrhythmias are not known. The incidence of atrial arrhythmias was investigated with Holter recordings in 10 patients with DDDR pacemakers. With the patient acting as his or her own control, there was no significant increase of atrial arrhythmias in the DDDR mode compared with the DDD mode.[63]

Conclusion

The basic use of the sensor is to boost the pacing rate of DDD pacing in patients with chronotropic incompetence, and thus careful programming of the sensor is fundamental in the follow-up of DDDR pacemakers. There is now increasing use of the sensor for purposes other than rate augmentation, such as automatic adjustment of the conventional DDD parameters to allow for more physiological hemodynamic response during exercise. The use of the sensor in a DDDR pacemaker for the control of atrial arrhythmias and endless-loop tachycardia is a nonelectrical approach to the problems of pacemaker-mediated tachycardias.

References

1. Sutton R. DDDR pacing (editorial). PACE 1990;13:385–387.
2. Wilkoff BL, Shimokochi DD, Schaal SF. Pacing rate increase due to application of steady external pressure on an activity sensing pacemaker (abstr). PACE 1987;10:423.
3. Lau CP, Ritchie D, Butrous GS, Ward DE, Camm AJ. Rate modulation by arm movements of the respiratory dependent rate responsive pacemaker. PACE 1988;11:744–752.
4. Lau CP, Ward DE, Camm AJ. Single chamber cardiac pacing with two forms of respiration controlled rate responsive pacemakers. Chest 1989;95:352–359.
5. De Cock CC, Panis JHC, Van Eenigl MJ, Roos JP. Efficacy and safety of rate responsive pacing in patients with coronary artery disease and angina pectoris. PACE 1989;12:1405–1411.
6. Lau CP, Rushby J, Leigh-Jones M, Tam CYF, Poloniecki J, Ingram A, Sutton R, et al. Symptomatology and quality of life in patients with rate responsive pacemakers: a double-blind crossover study. Clin Cardiol 1989;12:505–512.
7. Oto MA, Muderrisoglu H, Ozir MB, Korkmaz ME, Karamehmetoglu A, Oram A, Oram E, et al. Quality of life with rate ersponsive pacemakers: a randomized cross-over study. PACE 1991;14:800–806.
8. Bubien RS, Kay GN. A randomized comparison of quality of life and exercise capacity with DDD and VVIR pacing modes (abstr). PACE 1990;13:524.
9. Lau CP, Wong CK, Cheng CH, Leung WH. Importance of heart rate modulation on cardiac hemodynamics during post-exercise recovery. PACE 1990;13:1277–1285.
10. Jutzy RV, Florio J, Isaeff DM, Marsa RJ, Bansal RC, Jutzy KR, Levine PA. Comparative evaluation of rate modulated dual chamber and VVIR pacing. PACE 1990;13:1838–1846.
11. Sulke N, Chambers J, Dritsas A, Sowton E. A randomized double-blind crossover comparison of four rate-responsive pacing modes. J Am Coll Cardiol 1991;17:696–706.
12. Markewitz A, Hemmer W. What's the price to be paid for rate response: AV sequential versus ventricular pacing? PACE 1991;14:1782–1786.
13. Alt E. A protocol for treadmill and bicycle stress testing designed for pacemaker patients. Stimucoeur 1987;15:33–35.

14. Wilkoff BL, Covey J, Blackburn G. A mathematical model of the cardiac chronotropic response to exercise. J Electrophysiol 1989;3:176–180.
15. Lau CP, Leung WH, Wong CK, Cheng CH, Tai YT. Adaptive rate pacing at submaximal exercise: the importance of the programmed upper rate. J Electrophysiol 1989;3:283–288.
16. Hayes DL, Holmes DR Jr, Vlietstra RE, Olson MJ. Changing experience with dual chamber (DDD) pacemakers. J Am Coll Cardiol 1984;4:556–559.
17. Carleton RA, Passovoy M, Graettinger JS. The importance of the contribution and timing of left atrial systole. Clin Sci 1966;30:151–159.
18. Lascault G, Bigonzi F, Frank R, Abergel E, Klimczak K, Fontaine G, Grosoglat Y. Non-invasive study of dual chamber pacing by pulsed Doppler. Prediction of the hemodynamic response by echocardiographic measurement. Eur Heart J 1989;10:250–255.
19. Mehta D, Gilmour S, Ward DE, Camm AJ. Optimal atrioventricular delay at rest and during exercise in patients with dual chamber pacemakers: a noninvasive assessment by continuous wave Doppler. Br Heart J 1989;61:161–166.
20. Haskell RJ, French WJ. Optimum AV interval in dual chamber pacemakers. PACE 1986;9:670–675.
21. Daubert C, Ritter P, Mabo P, Ollitrault J, Descaves C, Gouffault J. Physiological relationship between AV interval and heart rate in healthy subjects: applications to dual chamber pacing. PACE 1986;9:1032–1039.
22. Ritter Ph, Vai F, Bonnet JL, Pioger G, Ochetta E, Rognoni G, Aina F, et al. Rate adaptive atrioventricular delay improves cardiopulmonary performance in patients implanted with a dual chamber pacemaker for complete heart block. Eur JCPE 1991;1:31–38.
23. Sulke N, Chambers J, Sowton E. The effects of different AV delay programming in DDDR paced patients during out of hospital activity (abstr). PACE 1991;14:650.
24. Rosenqvist M, Isaaz K, Botvinick EH, Dae MW, Cockrell J, Abbott JA, Schiller NB, et al. Relative importance of activation sequence compared to atrioventricular synchrony in left ventricular function. Am J Cardiol 1991; 67:148–156.
25. Harper GR, Pina IL, Kutallk SP. Intrinsic conduction maximizes cardiopulmonary performances in patients with dual chamber pacemakers. PACE 1991;14:1787–1791.
26. Chirife R, Ortega DF, Salazar AI. Non-physiological left heart AV intervals as a result of DDD and AAI "physiological" pacing. PACE 1991;14:1752–1756.
27. Lau CP, Mehta D, Toff W, Stott RJ, Ward DE, Camm AJ. Limitations of rate response of activity sensing rate responsive pacing to different forms of activity. PACE 1988;11:141–150.
28. Zegelman M, Winter UJ, Alt E, Treese N, Kreuzer J, Henry L, Mugica J, et al. Effect of different body-exercise modes on the rate response of the temperature-control pacemaker Nova MR. Thor Cardiovasc Surg 1990;38: 181–185.

29. Lau CP, Butrous GS, Ward DE, Camm AJ. Comparative assessment of exercise performance of six different rate adaptive right ventricular cardiac pacemakers. Am J Cardiol 1989;63:833–839.

30. Hayes DL, Von Feldt L, Higano ST. Standardized informal exercise testing for programming rate adaptive pacemakers. PACE 1991;14:1772–1776.

31. Lau CP, Tse WS, Camm AJ. Clinical experience with Sensolog 703: a new activity sensing rate responsive pacemaker. PACE 1988;11:1444–1455.

32. Mahaux V, Waleffe A, Kulbertus HE. Clinical experience with a new activity sensing rate modulated pacemaker using autoprogrammability. PACE 1989; 12:1362–1368.

33. Hayes DL, Higano ST. Utility of rate histograms in programming and follow-up of a DDDR pacemaker. Mayo Clin Proc 1989;64:495–502.

34. Lau CP. Activity sensing rate responsive pacing (letter). PACE 1990;13:819–820.

35. Lau CP, Tai YT, Fong PC, Li JPS, Leung SK, Chung FLW, Song S. Clinical experience with an accelerometer based activity sensing dual chamber rate adaptive pacemaker. PACE 1992;15:334–343.

36. Lau CP, Antoniou A, Ward DE, Camm AJ. Initial clinical experience with a minute ventilation sensing rate modulated pacemaker: improvements in exercise capacity and symptomatology. PACE 1988;11:1815–1822.

37. Sulke N, Pipilis A, Bucknall C, Sowton D. Quantitative analysis of contribution of rate response in three different ventricular rate responsive pacemakers during out of hospital activity. PACE 1990;13:37–44.

38. Loeppky JA, Greene ER, Hoekenger DE, Caprihan A, Luft UC. Beat-by-beat stroke volume assessment by pulsed Doppler in upright and supine exercise. J Appl Physiol 1981;50:1173–1182.

39. Miyamoto Y. Transient changes in ventilation and cardiac output at the start and end of exercise. Jpn J Physiol 1981;31:149–164.

40. Clarke M, Allan A. Rate-responsive atrial pacing resulting in pacemaker syndrome (abstr). PACE 1987;10:1209.

41. Lau CP, Wong CK, Cheng CH, Leung WH. Importance of heart rate modulation on cardiac hemodynamics during post-exercise recovery. PACE 1990;13:1277–1285.

42. Swinehart JM, Recker RR. Tachycardia and nightmares. Nebr Med J 1973; 58:314–315.

43. Nordlander R, Hedman A, Pehrsson JK. Rate responsive pacing and exercise capacity (editorial). PACE 1989;12:749–751.

44. Kristensson B, Karlson O, Ryden L. Holter-monitored heart rhythm during atrioventricular synchronous and fixed-rate ventricular pacing. PACE 1986; 9:511–518.

45. Lee MT, Baker R. Circadian rate variation in rate-adaptive pacing systems. PACE 1990;13:1797–1801.

46. Higano ST, Hayes DL, Eisinger G. Sensor-driven rate smoothing in a DDDR pacemaker. PACE 1989;12:922–929.

47. Higano ST, Hayes DL. P wave tracking above the maximum tracking rate in a DDDR pacemaker. PACE 1989;12:1044–1048.

48. Hanich DL, Midei MG, McElroy BP, Brinker JA. Circumvention of maximum tracking limitations with a rate modulated dual chamber pacemaker. PACE 1989;12:392–397.
49. Lau CP, Tai YT, Fong PC, Li JBS, Chung FLW. Clinical experience with a minute ventilation sensing rate adaptive pacemaker: upper rate behavior and the adaptation of PVARP (abstr). PACE 1990;13:1201.
50. Lau CP, Tai YT, Fong PC, Li JPS, Chung FLW. Atrial arrhythmias management with sensor controlled atrial refractory period and automatic mode switching in patients with minute ventilation sensing dual chamber rate adaptive pacemakers. PACE 1992, in press.
51. Vanerio G, Patel S, Ching E, Trohman RG, Wilkoff BL, Castle L, Maloney JD, et al. Early clinical experience with a minute ventilation sensor DDDR pacemaker. PACE 1991;14:1815–1820.
52. Lau CP. Sensors and pacemaker mediated tachycardias (editorial). PACE 1991;14:495–498.
53. Barold SS, Falkoff MD, Ong LS. Pacemaker endless loop tachycardias: termination by simple techniques other than magnet application. Am J Med 1988;85:817–822.
54. Lau CP, Li JPS, Wong CK, Cheng CH, Chung FLW. Sensor initiated termination of pacemaker mediated tachycardia in a DDDR pacemaker. Am Heart J 1991;121:595–597.
55. Lee MT, Adkins A, Woodson D, Vandegriff J. A new feature for control of inappropriate high tracking rate in DDDR pacemakers. PACE 1990;13: 1852–1855.
56. Cazeau S, Daubert C, Mabo P, Ritter P, Lelong B, Pouillot L, Paillard F. Dynamic electrophysiology of ventriculoatrial conduction: implications for DDD and DDDR pacing. PACE 1990;13:1646–1655.
57. Anderson C, Oxhoj H, Arnsbo P, Lybecker H. Pregnancy and caeserean section in a patient with a rate-responsive pacemaker. PACE 1989;12:386–391.
58. Lau CP, Lee CP, Wong CK, Leung WH, Cheng CH. Rate responsive pacing with a minute ventilation sensing pacemaker during pregnancy and delivery. PACE 1990;13:158–163.
59. Madsen GM, Anderson C. Pacemaker-induced tachycardia during general anaesthesia: a case report. Br J Anaesth 1989;63:300–361.
60. van Hemel NM, Hamerlijnck RPHM, Pronk KJ, Van der Veen EDP. Upper limit ventricular stimulation in respiratory rate responsive pacing due to electrocautery. PACE 1989;12:1720–1723.
61. Feuer JM, Shandling AH, Euestad MH. Sensor-modulated dual chamber cardiac pacing: too much of a good thing too fast (editorial)? PACE 1990; 13:816–818.
62. Transcript of the Circulatory System Devices Panel of the Food and Drug Administration. June 30, 1989, pp 90–123, pp 160–172.
63. Spencer WH III, Markowitz T, Alagona P. Rate augmentation and atrial arrhythmias in DDDR pacing. PACE 1991;12:1847–1851.

Chapter 19

Automatic Mode Switching During Antibradycardia Pacing in Patients Without Supraventricular Tachyarrhythmias

S. SERGE BAROLD

Introduction

Conventional or specially designed pacemakers can convert automatically to another pacing mode in a variety of circumstances. Automatic switching of the pacing mode of single and dual chamber devices may be classified as shown in Table 1.

1. Apparent. A VDD pulse generator effectively paces in the VVI mode in the presence of sinus bradycardia slower than the programmed lower rate, while a DDI pacemaker appears to function in the VVI mode in the presence of an atrial tachyarrhythmia when the atrial channel consistently senses P or f waves beyond the postventricular atrial refractory period (PVARP). During DDDR pacing, a particular dual chamber mode may effectively function in another mode according to circumstances (discussed later).

2. Temporary. When the mechanism causing the automatic change of pacing mode no longer exists, the pulse generator reverts immediately to its original pacing mode. In this way, a VVI pacemaker may revert

New Perspectives in Cardiac Pacing, Vol. 3, edited by S. Serge Barold and Jacques Mugica, Mount Kisco, NY, Futura Publishing Co., © 1993.

TABLE 1
Automatic Switching of Pacing Mode

Apparent:	* VDD to VVI with sinus bradycardia * DDI to VVI with long periods of sensing atrial activity
Temporary:	* VVI to VOO or DDD to DOO with electromagnetic interference * DDD to VVI or DDDR to VVIR with supraventricular tachyarrhythmias (fallback or automatic mode switching)
Permanent until Reprogrammed:	* DDD reset to VVI or VOO with electromagnetic interference or elective replacement point
Permanent and Unresponsive to Reprogramming:	* Component malfunction * End-of-life

to the VOO mode and a DDD pacemaker to the VOO or DOO mode as a temporary response to sensed electromagnetic interference (EMI) or other extraneous signals (interference mode)[1] (Fig. 1). Additionally, a pacemaker in the DDD mode may respond to an atrial rate faster than the programmed upper rate by automatic conversion to a fallback mode (such as VVI) with a gradual or sudden reduction of the pacing rate to a predetermined level[2]; reversion to the DDD mode subsequently occurs when the atrial rate drops below the programmed upper rate. These fallback responses are described in detail in the next chapter on optimal antibradycardia pacing in patients with paroxysmal supraventricular tachyarrhythmias. Tachycardia-terminating pacemakers also belong to this group, but a discussion of their function is beyond the scope of this chapter.

3. Permanent until reprogrammed (pacemaker reset). The DDD mode can be converted to the VVI or VOO mode, and the VVIR mode to the VVI mode as a permanent (unless reprogrammed) response to the sensed EMI or as an indicator of the elective replacement time (ERT)[3,4] (Fig. 2).

4. Permanent and unresponsive to reprogramming. Conversion to the reset mode with inability to reprogram the pulse generator to its original

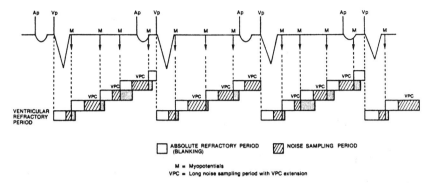

Figure 1. Conversion of the Medtronic Symbios dual chamber pacemaker from the DDD to the DOO mode upon repetitive myopotential (M) oversensing by the ventricular channel. When M signals are sensed by the ventricular channel in the noise sampling period (beyond the absolute refractory period), a new and complete ventricular refractory period (VRP) is initiated. The VRP is automatically extended when the pulse generator detects two ventricular events without an intervening P wave (VPC extension). The overlapping VRPs cause the pulse generator to pace asynchronously at the lower rate. The stippled parts indicate where the VRP would have terminated had sensing not occurred in the noise sampling period. (Reproduced with permission from Barold SS et al: Timing cycles of DDD pacemakers. In: Barold SS, Mugica J (eds.). New Perspectives in Cardiac Pacing, Futura Publishing Co., Mt. Kisco, NY, 1988, p 69.)

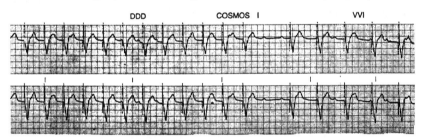

Figure 2. ERI activation during spontaneous pacing in the DDD mode of Intermedics Cosmos I (283-01) DDD pulse generator. The pulse generator was originally found to be reset in the VVI mode. The pulse generator then was reprogrammed to the DDD mode, and it functioned temporarily in the DDD mode. However, the relatively fast pacing rate (VDD cycles) required a higher battery current drain that caused decrease of the available battery voltage to a value below the trip point, thereby causing abrupt conversion to the reset VVI mode. (Reproduced with permission from Barold SS et al: Elective replacement indicators of simple and complex pacemakers. In: Barold SS, Mugica J (eds.). New Perspectives in Cardiac Pacing. 2, Futura Publishing Co., Mt. Kisco, NY, 1991, p 493.)

mode may occur with advanced battery depletion (end-of-life) or component malfunction (including damage from defibrillation, therapeutic radiation, and electrocautery).[1,3,4]

Pacemaker Reset

At the ERT, many contemporary special function pacemakers reset to a simpler mode. A DDD pulse generator can reset to the VVI or VOO mode (according to the manufacturer) and rate-modulated single chamber devices (VVIR or AAIR) to the non-activity mode (VVI or AAI), while automatic tachycardia-terminating pulse generators can reset to the non-antitachycardia mode.[3,4] In the case of battery depletion of a DDD pulse generator, the reset function is designed to prevent the circuit (available battery) voltage from falling for as long as possible below the dangerous end-of-life (EOL) point. The reset VVI or VOO mode at a fixed stimulation frequency automatically reduces battery current drain, increases available battery voltage, and results in conservation of battery capacity. After being reset at the ERT point, a DDD pulse generator can generally continue to function in the VVI mode for up to 6 months. As a rule, the ERT precedes the EOL by wide margins of safety, seldom less than 3 months under normal conditions. The reset mode is latched (permanent unless reprogrammed) to eliminate the possibility of oscillating or see-sawing between the DDD and the VVI or VOO mode when the voltage falls below or rises above the critical level used for activation of the ERT indicator.

Reset from Electromagnetic Interference

Coded instructions relayed via the programmer to the pulse generator are stored in volatile memory susceptible to the influence of EMI. Sophisticated pacemakers require good communication between the internal microprocessor and memory location. When this line of communication is interrupted by strong EMI, the microprocessor becomes "confused" and cannot function properly. This situation is roughly analogous to a personal computer receiving inappropriate instructions whereupon it locks up and does not respond to commands. One way to correct such a problem with a personal computer involves turning the power off and then on again. Obviously, in a biological environment under similar circumstances, a pacemaker cannot be allowed to turn itself off and then on again. Rather, the pulse generator converts automatically to a mode (reset) not dependent upon memory for its function so as to avoid erratic behavior during EMI.

Strong interference even if momentary such as electrocautery or defibrillation (including catheter ablation with defibrillator or radiofrequency energy) may cause reset of DDD and VVIR pacemakers to the VVI or VOO mode, a condition sometimes called "power-on-reset" (POR).[1,5–9] POR describes the function of a pulse generator with only its preprogrammed instructions (pacing mode and parameters) stored in the nonvolatile or nonerasable memory known as ROM (read only memory). POR represents the power-on or "turn-on" parameters designed in the ROM circuit that will be in effect when a voltage source is attached to the circuit and a current is induced. Conceptually, in the event of a "power-down" state, the memory registers (random access memory or RAM) lose their function below a certain critical voltage. Should power be restored, i.e., power-on reset (POR), the pulse generator returns to those factory preset conditions stored only in the ROM memory, i.e., the reset state whose function is not dependent upon RAM memory. In the reset state, some pulse generators employ the same pacing mode and rate setting for both the ERT indicator and POR states. In devices with different ERT indicator and POR parameters, sources of interference such as electrocautery may either activate the ERT indicator or a full POR state consequent to loss of programmed RAM memory.

Levels of Reset

Some pulse generators possess two levels of reset: the ERT indicator and the backup mode. Because of the extreme dependence of sophisticated pacemaker circuits on both the stored programming instructions and internal timing, some pulse generators utilize an independent but rudimentary pacemaker circuit to oversee the basic timing and pacing functions. Such a backup rudimentary circuit depends neither on the volatile memory (RAM) nor on the crystal-controlled clock that provides very accurate timing pulses necessary to run the logic circuitry. Such a backup circuit is less susceptible to failure mechanisms likely to disturb the function of the main pacing and timing operations. For example, the timing function controlled by the "crystal clock" (the time control in all contemporary multiprogrammable devices) is quite susceptible to disruption if the voltage level falls below the ERT trip point. In the case of the Intermedics (Freeport, TX) DDD pacemakers, the backup circuit is a simple RC oscillator with its own preprogrammed or factory-set outputs indelibly etched in nonvolatile memory, much like an old non-programmable VVI pacemaker.[3] The independent circuit was designed to protect against failure in the main timing circuit. The sensing amplifier is shared by both the backup and the main pacing circuits. Because the backup mode of the Intermedics DDD pulse generators does not utilize the memory from the main pacing circuit, there is no magnet response. Occasionally in Intermedics Cosmos DDD pulse generators (such as models 283-01 and 283-02), battery depletion may cause reset to the backup mode that is activated at a lower battery voltage than the ERT indicator. When the pulse generator is close to the ERT point but still functioning in the DDD mode, programming or telemetry transmission may occasionally reset the pulse generator to the backup mode rather than to the ERT point.

Polarity of Reset Mode

In the case of DDD pulse generators with programmable electrode configuration (bipolar vs. unipolar), the reset mode is often unipolar.[4] This response assures a complete circuit by pacing between the tip electrode and the pacemaker can or casing regardless of lead configuration. If unipolar/bipolar programmable devices were to reset to the bipolar mode, a no output condition would result if a unipolar lead were in place.

In patients with an implanted cardioverter/defibrillator (ICD) and a DDD pulse generator with programmable polarity (unipolar vs. bipolar), but functioning in the *bipolar* mode, the delivery of a defibrillating shock may reset the pulse generator to the *unipolar* reset or backup VVI or VOO mode.[10,11] Conversion to the unipolar mode may subsequently interfere with the function of the ICD. An ICD possesses an automatic gain control to guarantee sensing of small electrograms during ventricular fibrillation as compared to the larger signals available in sinus rhythm. An ICD increases its sensitivity automatically as the amplitude of the sensed electrogram decreases. Upon sensing large unipolar pacemaker stimuli as in the VOO mode, the ICD by virtue of its automatic gain control forces its sensitivity to a relatively insensitive setting so that smaller signals associated with ventricular tachycardia or fibrillation may not be detected. In the VVI mode (although the spontaneous normal rhythm inhibits the pulse generator), the development of ventricular fibrillation can produce electrographic signals too small to be sensed by the implanted pacemaker, thereby leading to intermittent or regular release of large unipolar ventricular stimuli capable of interfering with the detection of ventricular fibrillation or tachycardia by an ICD.[12-14] Thus in the presence of both an ICD and a pulse generator with programmable polarity, a patient who develops ventricular fibrillation could be successfully defibrillated by the ICD, but if the shock resets the pulse generator to the unipolar mode, the large unipolar stimuli may then prevent detection of subsequent episodes of ventricular fibrillation with catastrophic consequences.[11,15] This disturbance is probably very rare and further observations are required to determine whether it is clinically important. Ideally, pacing capability should be incorporated into a single device cardioverter/defibrillator. When this is not feasible or available, a committed bipolar pacing system (without programmable polarity) or a unipolar sense and committed bipolar pace system should be used to patients with an ICD assuring that pacemaker reset will always be in the bipolar mode.

Magnet Response

In some pulse generators, there will be no response to magnet application in the reset mode.[4] With continuous sensing and inhibition in the VVI mode, the lack of magnet response should not be interpreted as component failure or a lead problem associated with a no output situation.

Investigation of Pacemaker Reset

Pacemaker reset may occur before implantation due to cold exposure.[16] Battery depletion is the primary but not the only cause of reset. Other causes of reset should be evaluated by simple maneuvers using the pacemaker programmer.[3]

Telemetry of available battery voltage and impedance makes the diagnosis of battery depletion easy by indicating high battery impedance. Although in the DDD mode the available battery voltage may have dipped below 2.4 V (trip point), reset to the VVI mode increases the available battery voltage to above 2.4 V, e.g., 2.56 V. In the future, a pulse generator may respond differently as the ERT is approached. A DDDR pacemaker could switch itself automatically to the VVIR or simpler DDD mode with or without automatic reduction of the upper rate to conserve battery capacity. When reset is due to EMI, the available battery voltage should be normal (approximately 2.8 V) and battery impedance either in the normal range or slightly raised according to the age of the battery.

A large current drain associated with moderate elevation of battery impedance may cause a substantial drop in available battery voltage of sufficient value to activate the ERT indicator. In this way, the ERT indicator could be activated by increasing battery current drain during follow-up programming of higher rates and/or outputs even when the battery impedance measures a few Kohms, far less than the 20–40 Kohms usually associated with activation of the ERT of single chamber pacemakers.[3] If not understood, this situation could lead to inappropriate pulse generator replacement.

In pulse generators without telemetry of available battery voltage and impedance, the differentiation between POR and ERT may be difficult or impossible when the POR and ERT states exhibit identical parameters.[3,5] In such a case, the response of the ERT indicator to a high current drain forms the basis of the so-called "battery stress test" in the DDD mode by increasing the pacing rate and/or output of both channels. In the POR or reset state due to sensing EMI, reprogramming will always be successful. Only the battery voltage in a very "recent" ERT state can recover enough to allow reprogramming of the pulse generator to the DDD mode. Battery depletion is confirmed if the pacemaker reverts back to the reset mode within 15–30 minutes. If a pacemaker with battery depletion has been in the VVI ERT mode for a lengthy period, reprogramming will be impossible. If the pulse generator cannot be programmed out of the reset mode to the DDD or other mode (without excessive rates and/or outputs), substantial battery depletion or component failure is present and the pulse generator should be replaced.

DDX Mode

Many DDD pulse generators offer automatic extension of the PVARP (for one cycle only) after a sensed ventricular event (outside the AV delay) that the pacemaker interprets as a ventricular extrasystole, i.e., two ventricular events without any intervening sensed P wave. PVARP extension is based on the concept that most episodes of endless-loop tachycardia (pacemaker-mediated tachycardia) are initiated by ventricular extrasystoles with retrograde ventriculoatrial (VA) conduction. The so-called DDX mode (really the temporary automatic conversion to the DVI mode) in effect functions like a PVARP extension after a ventricular extrasystole.[17] In the DDX mode, the atrial channel does not necessarily remain refractory for only one complete cycle (Fig. 3). The pacemaker will continue to function in the DVI mode until delivery of an atrial stimulus (either spontaneously or after application of the magnet) restores DDD pacing (Fig. 4). Consequently, with activation of the DDX mode, the DVI mode may continue indefinitely as long as the interval between two consecutive sensed ventricular events is shorter than the pacemaker atrial escape (pacemaker VA) interval.[18] The DDX mode with automatic conversion to the DVI mode may be useful in rare patients with very long retrograde ventriculoatrial conduction times. Under certain circumstances, the DDX mode like excessive extension of the

DDX MODE, LOWER RATE = 45 ppm, AV = 165 ms, UPPER RATE = 145 ppm

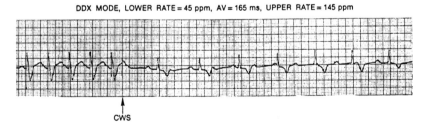

CWS

Figure 3. DDX mode of operation of the 283 AFP Pacesetter DDD pulse generator (Pacesetter-Siemens, Sylmar, CA). Initiation of DVI pacing by chest wall stimulus (CWS) sensed by the ventricular channel of the DDD pacemaker. The pacemaker interprets the CWS as a ventricular extrasystole and initiates the DVI mode which will continue indefinitely until the emission of an atrial stimulus whereupon the DDD mode returns automatically (see Fig. 4).

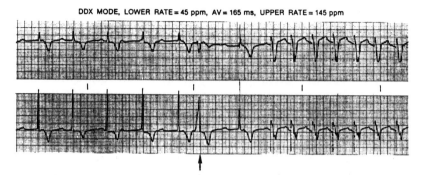

DDX MODE, LOWER RATE = 45 ppm, AV = 165 ms, UPPER RATE = 145 ppm

Figure 4. DDX mode of operation of the 283 AFP Pacesetter DDD pulse generator. The programmed parameters are shown above the ECG. Two ECG leads were recorded simultaneously. The DDX mode of operation initiated the DVI mode after sensing of a ventricular extrasystole. The DVI mode can terminate only with the emission of an atrial stimulus. The atrial stimulus is not released as long as the RR interval of the AV junctional escape rhythm (approximately 1,000 ms) remains shorter than the atrial escape interval (1,333 − 165 = 1,168 ms.). A ventricular extrasystole (arrow) induces a longer pause that allows the release of an atrial stimulus at the termination of the atrial escape interval. The atrial stimulus produces a pseudopseudofusion beat and terminates the DVI mode, with the return of P-wave tracking in the DDX (or DDD) mode. (Reproduced with permission from Barold SS et al: Electrocardiography of DDD pacemakers. A. Basic concepts, upper rate response, retrograde ventriculoatrial conduction and differential diagnosis of pacemaker tachycardias. In: Saksena S, Goldschlager N (eds.). Electrical Therapy for Cardiac Arrhythmias. Pacing, Antitachycardia Devices, Catheter Ablation, W.B. Saunders, Philadelphia, PA, 1990, p 255).

PVARP may itself paradoxically induce susceptibility to endless loop tachycardia.[19]

DDDR Pacemakers

Functional Mode versus Programmed Mode (Table 2)

A particular programmed pacing mode in a DDDR pacemaker may effectively function in another mode according to circumstances.[20–22] The upper rate response of a DDDR pulse generator depends on the

TABLE 2
DDDR Pacemakers
Automatic Switching of Pacing Mode
Functional Mode vs. Programmed Mode

1. DDIR to VVIR (as DDD to VVI under specific circumstances)
2. DDIR to DVIR when SDI ≤ TARP
3. DDDR to DVIR when SDI ≤ TARP (only in pacemakers capable of programming TARP > common atrial-driven URI and sensor-driven URI)
4. DDDR to DDIR when atrial-driven URI = sensor driven URI. When P-P < SDI = atrial-driven URI = sensor-driven URI (provided TARP < URI), no pauses occur at the end of a Wenckebach cycle and DDDR mode effectively becomes DDIR.
5. DDDR to DDIR when sensor-driven URI < atrial-driven URI.
   a. P-P < SDI < atrial-driven URI (provided TARP < atrial-driven URI). The atrial-driven URI does not time out and the Vp-Vp interval is controlled by SDI.
   b. P-P < SDI = atrial-driven URI (provided TARP < atrial-driven URI). The atrial-driven URI times out and response looks like 4 (above) with no pause at the end of the Wenckebach cycle.
6. Apparent switching to DDD mode during sensor-controlled DDDR pacing. When sensor-driven URI < atrial-driven URI (provided TARP < atrial-driven URI), the relationship P-P interval = SDI < atrial-driven URI produces apparent P wave tracking.

SDI = sensor-driven interval; URI = upper rate interval; TARP = total atrial refractory period; PVARP = postventricular atrial refractory period; P-P = interval between two consecutive P waves; Vp-Vp = interval between two consecutive ventricular paced beats.

interplay of four variables: P-P interval, total atrial refractory period (TARP), atrial-driven upper rate interval (URI), and sensor-driven URI.

The relationship between the sensor-driven URI and the atrial-driven URI may take one of three forms: (1) sensor-driven URI > atrial-driven URI, i.e., the sensor-driven upper rate is slower than the atrial-driven upper rate. There appears to be no real clinical use for a sensor-driven upper rate slower than an atrial-driven upper rate except perhaps to attenuate the effect of sudden deceleration of the sinus rate after effort.[20] As a rule, sensor-driven URI > atrial-driven URI should not be programmed,[20] and this combination will not be discussed further. (2) Sensor-driven URI = atrial-driven URI (common upper rates), and (3) sensor-driven URI < atrial-driven URI, i.e., sensor-driven upper rate faster than the atrial-driven upper rate.

The following abbreviations and definitions will be used in the discussion of DDDR pacemakers.

Abbreviations: Ap = atrial paced event, As = atrial sensed event, Vp = ventricular paced event, Vs = ventricular sensed event, P-P interval refers to the interval between two consecutive P waves in sinus rhythm, SDI = sensor driven interval, LRI = lower rate interval, AEI = atrial escape interval.

Definitions: The *atrial*-driven upper rate interval (URI) refers to the shortest Vs-Vp or Vp-Vp where the second Vp is triggered by a sensed *atrial* event. The second Vp can only be released at the completion of the atrial-driven *ventricular* URI initiated by a preceding Vs or Vp. Obviously a DDD device possesses only one URI, i.e., the atrial-driven URI. The *sensor*-driven URI refers to the shortest Vs-Vp or Vp-Vp where the second Vp is controlled by *sensor* activity. The second Vp can only be released at the completion of the sensor-driven *ventricular* URI initiated by a preceding Vs or Vp.

A DDDR pacemaker can switch its functional pacing mode in the following situations.

DDIR Mode to VVIR Mode

In the DDIR mode when the P-P interval is shorter than the SDI, P waves march through the pacing cycle until one falls in the PVARP and is unsensed. The pulse generator then emits an atrial stimulus at the end of the sensor-driven AEI, a situation functionally equivalent to the VVIR mode with AV dissociation and occasional atrial extrasystoles, the latter being due to occasional atrial stimulation[20] (Fig. 5).

DDIR Mode to DVIR Mode

In the DDIR mode with AV = 150 ms, PVARP = 350 ms, and LRI = 1,000 ms, the atrial sensing window is equal to LRI − TARP = 500 ms. As the sensor-driven LRI (or SDI) shortens with exercise, the atrial sensing window also shortens. Eventually, when the SDI reaches 500 ms (corresponding to a rate of 120 per minute), the programmed parameters obliterate the atrial sensing window and the pacemaker then functions in the DVIR mode.

DDIR

SENSOR · DRIVEN INTERVAL = 500 ms
AV = 150 ms
PVARP = 200 ms

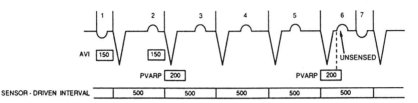

Figure 5. Diagrammatic representation of the DDIR mode. The sinus rate is faster than the sensor-driven rate, i.e., the P-P interval < SDI (500 ms). In the DDI or DDIR mode, the ventricular paced rate (or the Vp-Vp interval) always remains constant and equal to the programmed lower rate interval or sensor-driven (lower rate) interval. The first atrial stimulus captures the atrium. The pulse generator senses the subsequent P waves (2 to 5). The P waves march through the pacing cycle with progressive prolongation of the AV interval. The sixth P wave falls in the 200 ms PVARP and is therefore unsensed. The pacemaker delivers its next atrial stimulus (which captures the atrium and generates the seventh P wave) at the end of the sensor-driven AEI (500 − 150 = 350 ms). Because the ventricular pacing rate (or Vp-Vp interval) remains constant, the DDIR mode is functionally equivalent to the VVIR mode (with AV dissociation) with the occasional occurrence of atrial extrasystoles (premature beats) when the pulse generator delivers Ap relatively close to the preceding (unsensed) P wave which is in the PVARP.

DDDR Mode to DVIR Mode

Obviously in the conventional DDD mode, the relationship TARP > atrial-driven URI cannot exist because the atrial-driven URI can only be longer than or equal to the TARP. On this basis, in a DDDR device with a common upper rate, one could easily conclude that the two upper rates (atrial-driven and sensor-driven) are inextricably linked and cannot be dissociated. As in the conventional DDD mode, some DDDR pulse generators with a common upper rate interval (e.g., Intermedics Relay[23]) permit programming of the TARP to a value equal to or shorter than but not longer than the atrial-driven URI (the latter being equal to the sensor-driven URI) (Fig. 6). Yet, in any DDD or DDDR pulse generator, it should be electronically possible to program the TARP to a value equal

DDDR UPPER RATE INTERVALS

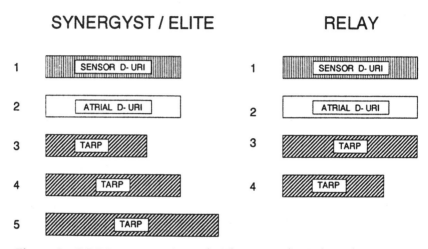

Figure 6.   DDDR upper rate intervals. The Intermedics Relay pulse generator has a common URI. The TARP can be programmed to a value shorter than or equal to the atrial-driven URI (common URI). In the Relay unit, the TARP cannot be programmed to a value longer than the atrial-driven or common URI. The Medtronic Synergyst II and Elite pulse generators also have a common URI. However, these devices (including the new Elite II) allow the TARP to be programmed to a value *longer* than the common URI. When TARP > common URI, the atrial-driven URI becomes equal to the TARP and therefore becomes functionally longer than the sensor-driven URI. The new Medtronic Elite II device (but not the Elite I) allows programming of the sensor-driven URI independently of the atrial-driven URI.

to, shorter than, or longer than the common URI. Indeed, in the Medtronic DDDR devices (Synergyst II and Elite[24,25]), the TARP can be programmed to a value *longer* than the common URI (Fig. 6). Obviously if the TARP ≥ common URI, a Wenckebach upper rate response (with extension of the AV interval) cannot occur. When TARP > common URI, the actual atrial-driven URI becomes equal to the duration of the TARP. This manipulation allows programming of a sensor-driven upper rate faster than the atrial-driven upper rate. The latter corresponds to the interval provided by the TARP and represents the rate at which fixed-ratio pacemaker AV block will supervene. Thus the atrial-driven URI can be *functionally* separated from the sensor-driven URI by programming a TARP longer than the common URI, i.e., atrial-driven URI = TARP > sensor-driven URI. In this way, fixed-ratio pacemaker AV block (e.g., 2:1) will occur at atrial rates slower than the programmed sensor-driven upper rate. This approach may be useful in limiting the atrial-driven upper rate in patients with paroxysmal supraventricular tachyarrhythmias. In a DDDR pacemaker with common URI < TARP, when SDI ≤ TARP, the atrial channel paces asynchronously and the DDDR mode functions like the DVIR mode. For example, in such a DDDR pacemaker, if AV = 200 ms, PVARP = 400 ms, TARP = 600 ms, the pacemaker functions in the DVIR mode when the SDI ≤ 600 ms because the atrial sensing window becomes obliterated (Fig. 7).

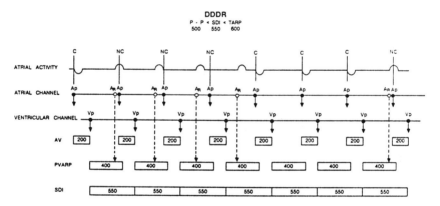

Figure 7. Diagrammatic representation of pacing in the DDDR mode with a common URI = 450 ms, AV = 200 ms, PVARP = 400 ms, TARP = 600 ms, SDI = 550 ms. Provided the pulse generator allows programming TARP > common URI, these parameters indicate that atrial-driven URI (600 ms = TARP) > sensor-driven URI (450 ms = programmed common URI). There is an atrial sensing window beyond the PVARP, but it closes with SDI ≤ TARP. In this example, because SDI < TARP, the pulse generator cannot sense spontaneous atrial activity (AR). Atrial pacing is asynchronous and Ap competes with AR producing a response functionally equivalent to the DVIR mode. Therefore, both Ap-Ap and Vp-Vp intervals remain constant. C = capture, NC = no capture (Ap in atrial myocardial refractory period).

DDDR Mode to DDIR Mode During the Wenckebach Upper Rate Response

As in the DDD mode, a Wenckebach upper rate response can only occur when TARP < atrial-driven URI. Any Wenckebach upper rate response without a pause at the termination of the cycle (when the P wave falls within the PVARP) is functionally equivalent to the DDIR mode. In turn, the DDIR mode functions as a pseudo-VVIR device with occasional "atrial extrasystoles" due to atrial capture from the release of Ap whenever a P wave falls in the PVARP and is unsensed.[20]

A. Atrial-Driven Upper Rate Interval = Sensor-Driven Upper Rate Interval

In a pulse generator with equal atrial-driven URI and sensor-driven URI, shortening of the SDI (i.e., sensor-driven LRI) on exercise brings it closer to the atrial-driven or common URI.[26] The pacing mode begins to resemble the DDIR mode (Fig. 8). When the difference between the common URI and the SDI becomes small, the Wenckebach pause becomes inconspicuous so that the pacing mode looks like the DDIR mode (constant rate of ventricular pacing) with an occasional hardly discernible slight prolongation of the Vp-Vp interval at the end of the Wenckebach sequence. When the SDI = atrial-driven URI = sensor-driven URI, no pauses occur at the end of the Wenckebach cycle and the pacing mode becomes effectively DDIR. In this situation, the Vp-Vp interval becomes equal to the atrial-driven URI (Fig. 5).

B. Sensor-Driven Upper Rate Interval Shorter than Atrial-Driven Upper Rate Interval

The capability of programming different atrial-driven and sensor-driven upper rate intervals has added new complexity to the interpretation of DDDR pacemaker function[21,22,27-33] (Fig. 9).

1. P-P Interval Shorter than Sensor-Driven Interval

When the atrial rate exceeds the sensor-driven rate, (P-P interval < SDI), the SDI can also become shorter than the atrial-driven URI (i.e., P-P interval < SDI < atrial-driven URI), a

DDDR WENCKEBACH UPPER RATE RESPONSE

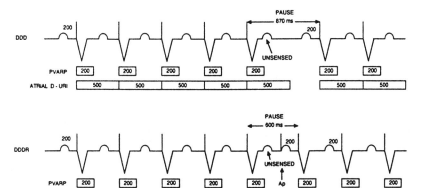

Figure 8. Diagrammatic representation of DDD and DDDR pacing with pacemaker Wenckebach AV block. Lower rate interval = 1,000 ms, atrial-driven URI = 500 ms, PVARP = 200 ms, AV interval = 200 ms (As-Vp = Ap-Vp in both the DDD and DDDR modes). A Wenckebach upper rate response occurs because the atrial-driven URI > TARP. Top: DDD pacing with typical Wenckebach upper rate response. The pulse generator does not sense the sixth P wave in the PVARP, but senses the succeeding P wave so that the pause at the end of the Wenckebach cycle measures approximately 870 ms. Bottom: In the DDDR mode with the same basic parameters as in the DDD mode above, SDI = 600 ms > atrial-driven URI. The pulse generator does not sense the sixth P wave in the PVARP. The pause at the end of the Wenckebach sequence is shorter than in the DDD mode above because the SDI = 600 ms and sensor-driven AEI = 400 ms. Thus, Ap occurs earlier (and closer to the preceding P wave in the PVARP) because its release is sensor-controlled. The pause at the end of the Wenckebach sequence therefore shortens to the 600 ms SDI.

relationship that cannot occur when the sensor-driven URI and the atrial-driven URI are common and cannot be dissociated.

(a) *Sensor-Driven Interval Shorter than Atrial-Driven Upper Rate Interval*

In the absence of atrial activity, when the SDI < atrial-driven URI, a pulse generator delivers an atrial stimulus (Ap) at the termination of the sensor-driven AEI and an accompanying ventricular stimulus (Vp) at the completion of the Ap-Vp interval.

DDDR UPPER RATE INTERVALS

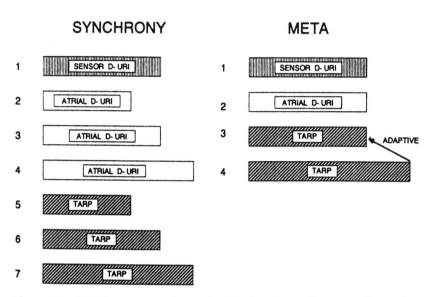

Figure 9. DDDR upper rate intervals. The Synchrony (Pacesetter-Siemens) DDDR pulse generator allows programming of the atrial-driven URI independently of the sensor-driven URI. The TARP cannot be programmed to a value *longer* than the atrial-driven URI. In the Telectronics Meta DDDR pulse generator, the atrial-driven URI (when the TARP assumes its shortest value) and sensor-driven URI are equal (an exception is discussed in the next chapter). The TARP is adaptive and shortens with increasing sensor activity. When SDI becomes equal to the common URI, the TARP also becomes equal to the common URI. Because TARP ≥ atrial URI, no Wenckebach pacemaker AV block can occur. Furthermore, fixed-ratio pacemaker AV block cannot occur because when P-P < the prevailing TARP, the pulse generator is automatically converted to the VVIR mode (see Chapter 20).

Vp occurs at the end of the SDI initiated by the preceding ventricular event, but before completion of the atrial-driven URI, also initiated by the same preceding ventricular event (Fig. 10). If a sensed P wave (As) occurs before the expected emission of Ap (controlled by the SDI), the pulse generator inhibits the subsequent release of sensor controlled Ap (Fig. 10). Although the pulse generator omits Ap, it delivers Vp on time according to

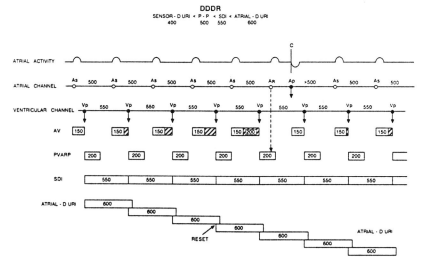

Figure 10.   Diagrammatic representation of pacing by a DDDR pulse generator with a sensor-driven URI (400 ms) < atrial-driven URI (600 ms). Sensor-driven URI (400 ms) < P-P interval (500 ms) < SDI (550 ms) < atrial-driven URI (600 ms). As-Vp = Ap-Vp = 150 ms, PVARP = 200 ms, TARP = 350 ms, TARP < P-P < atrial-driven URI. The maximal increment of the AV interval during the Wenckebach upper rate response is 600 − 350 = 250 ms. The first P wave initiates an AV interval of 150 ms. The second P wave initiates an AV interval extended beyond 150 ms to conform to the atrial-driven URI. The atrial-driven URI does not time out because the SDI is shorter than the atrial-driven URI. Thus, the delivery of Vp is sensor-controlled and the Vp-Vp interval is controlled by the sensor or the SDI. The AV interval cannot fully extend to the completion of the atrial-driven URI because an earlier Vp (sensor-controlled) terminates the AV interval. This response may be called a ventricular paced repetitive aborted Wenckebach upper rate response. The sixth P wave falls in the PVARP and is therefore unsensed (AR). The next Ap released at the end of the sensor-driven AEI (550 − 150 = 400 ms) occurs 400 ms from the previous Vp, close to the sixth P wave, but capable of atrial capture. There is no pause at the end of the Wenckebach sequence because the Vp-Vp interval is controlled by sensor activity or the SDI and not the atrial-driven URI which is therefore continually reset by the earlier Vp. On the right, the process then repeats itself.

the SDI at that given time. Consequently, the As–Vp interval extends beyond its programmed value, a response analogous to the classic pacemaker Wenckebach upper rate behavior (possible only if atrial-driven URI > TARP).

In this response, when the P-P interval < SDI < atrial-driven URI, P waves march through the pacing cycles and initiate As–Vp intervals of progressively longer duration until a P wave falls in the PVARP and is unsensed, a behavior resembling the classic DDD pacemaker Wenckebach AV block upper rate response. However, there is no pause in the cycle that contains the P wave in the PVARP because release of the subsequent Ap and Vp is sensor-controlled according to the SDI and the sensor-driven AEI (Fig. 10). The Vp-Vp interval, therefore, remains constant and equal to the prevailing SDI (either longer than the sensor-driven URI or equal to it) but shorter than the atrial-driven URI. The constant sensor-driven Vp-Vp interval with the occasional emission of Ap (when P is unsensed in the PVARP) resembles DDIR pacing (Fig. 5). In other words, when P-P < sensor-driven URI < atrial-driven URI, the atrial-driven URI does not time out because the SDI or the sensor-driven URI usurps control of the paced ventricular rate. The modified pacemaker Wenckebach upper rate response may be called a ventricular paced repetitive aborted Wenckebach upper rate response because the atrial-driven URI never times out. In this response, SDI obviously times out and when SDI becomes equal to the sensor-driven URI, the latter also times out.

(b) *Sensor-Driven Interval Equal to the Atrial-Driven Upper Rate Interval*

When P-P < atrial-driven URI = SDI, a Wenckebach upper rate response will also occur with no pause at the end of the sequence in the cycle containing the unsensed P wave within the PVARP, as in Figure 10. The Vp-Vp interval remains equal to the SDI and to the atrial-driven URI. Therefore, two intervals (SDI and atrial-driven URI) time out, but the sensor-driven URI does not. The effect is therefore identical to the situation where the atrial-driven URI = sensor-driven URI when TARP < P-P < atrial-driven URI = sensor-driven URI = SDI, as discussed in section A (atrial-driven URI = sensor-driven URI). The scenario in A also creates a typical Wenckebach upper rate response without a pause at the end of the sequence. In the response described in section A, all three intervals (atrial-driven URI, sensor-driven URI, and SDI) time out at the end of every Vp-Vp cycle (Figs. 5 and 8).

2. *Apparent Switching to DDD Mode During Sensor-Controlled DDDR Pacing: P-P Interval Equal to the Sensor-Driven Interval*

In the DDDR mode, if atrial sensing produces sustained inhibition of Ap, pacemaker behavior resembles P-wave tracking seen in the simpler DDD mode, a situation called "apparent tracking" by Higano and Hayes.[21] When TARP < P-P = SDI < atrial-driven URI, sustained apparent P-wave tracking occurs at a rate faster than the atrial-driven upper rate and the extended As-Vp interval remains constant (Fig. 11). When SDI < atrial-driven URI, the P waves start an AV interval, but unlike the Wenckebach response in the DDD mode, the pulse generator never completes the AV interval (though it is extended to some extent) because the pulse generator emits Vp at the completion of the SDI causing continual reset of the atrial-driven URI by the sensor-controlled Vp (Figs. 10 and 11). The Vp-Vp interval is sensor-driven and the atrial-driven URI does not time out. This response with AV interval prolongation mimicking the DDD mode resembles another situation during DDDR pacing where the TARP < P-P interval = atrial-driven URI = sensor-driven URI (Fig. 12). In Figure 12, both atrial-driven URI and sensor-driven URI time out simultaneously so that the atrial-driven URI actually times out and the DDD mode is real (Fig. 12) rather than apparent as in Figure 11.

Automatic Mode Switching During Exercise

On exercise, the DDDR mode could be switched automatically to the VVIR mode provided it is previously shown that loss of AV synchrony is well tolerated.[34,35] This pacemaker response may be useful in selected patients, particularly in those where the atrial contribution to cardiac output becomes negligible during exercise. VVIR pacing during exercise avoids atrial competition, decreases battery current drain, and increases battery life.

DDDR
ATRIAL D - URI LONGER THAN SENSOR D - URI

ATRIAL D - URI = 600 ms
SENSOR D - URI = 400 ms
TARP = 350 ms
SDI = 450 ms

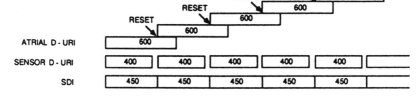

ATRIAL D - URI > SENSOR D - URI > TARP

Figure 11. Diagrammatic representation of pacing with a DDDR pulse generator showing apparent P-wave tracking and apparent switching to the DDD mode. Atrial-driven URI > sensor-driven URI. As-Vp = Ap-Vp = 150 ms. The sinus rate is equal to the sensor-driven rate (P-P interval = SDI = 450 ms). The pulse generator senses the last three spontaneous P waves (As). A sensed P wave initiates an AV interval of 150 ms, but at the completion of the 150 ms AV interval, the atrial-driven URI (600 ms) has not yet timed out. Consequently, the pacemaker extends the AV interval to conform to the atrial-driven URI (600 ms). The latter does not time out because the pulse generator emits Vp at the termination of the 450 ms SDI initiated by the preceding ventricular event. The As-Vp interval is stretched to 250 ms. (In the absence of sensor activity or SDI, the As-Vp interval would have stretched to 400 ms to conform to the atrial-driven URI.) Delivery of the last three ventricular stimuli is sensor-controlled. The atrial-driven URI is repeatedly reset by the early delivery of sensor-controlled Vp, producing apparent P-wave tracking at a rate faster than the programmed atrial-driven upper rate. Although this form of apparent P-wave tracking resembles that shown in Figure 12, the mechanism is different. In Figure 11, delivery of Vp is sensor-controlled and the DDD mode is apparent, while in Figure 12, delivery of Vp is controlled by the atrial-driven URI and the DDD mode is real. In Figure 12, the sinus rate is equal to the common URI while in Figure 11, P-P = SDI.

DDDR

ATRIAL D - URI = SENSOR D - URI

URI = 400 ms
TARP = 350 ms
SDI = 450 ms

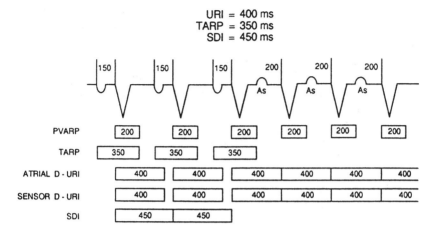

URI > TARP

Figure 12. Diagrammatic representation of pacing by a DDDR pulse generator with a common URI (atrial-driven URI = sensor-driven URI). As-Vp = Ap-Vp = 150 ms. The sinus rate on the right is equal to the programmed upper rate, i.e., P-P interval = atrial-driven URI = sensor-driven URI = 400 ms. On the right, the As-Vp interval remains constant, but extended (by 50 ms) to conform to the atrial-driven URI. The SDI (450 ms) is longer than the common URI (400 ms). Therefore, the pulse generator releases Vp at the completion of the atrial-driven URI. Delivery of the Vp is not sensor-controlled. Although this response resembles that in Figure 11, the timing cycles and control of Vp are different. The last three cycles represent a true DDD mode in contrast to Figure 11.

Automatic Switching From Single Chamber Atrial to Dual Chamber Pacing

AAI or AAIR pacing ensures that rapid ventricular pacing rates cannot occur with supraventricular tachyarrhythmias. AAI or AAIR can be accomplished safely in a substantial proportion of patients with the sick sinus syndrome, even in the presence of atrial tachyarrhythmias. However, some workers have indicated that the Wenckebach point (the atrial rate at which AV block occurs) may change from day to day, and indeed a given value does not always predict the subsequent development of AV block.[36] Furthermore, the AV interval may not shorten or may actually lengthen on exercise in some patients with AAIR pacemakers, particularly with concomitant antiarrhythmic therapy, a situation (P wave close to preceding QRS complex) that can lead to unfavorable hemodynamics similar to the pacemaker syndrome with VVI pacing.[37,38] For this reason, in patients with sick sinus syndrome and relatively normal AV conduction, a DDD or DDDR pulse generator could be safely programmed to the AAI/AAIR mode with the capability of switching automatically to the dual chamber mode whenever a given number of PR or AV intervals exceed a certain programmable value. With improvement of AV conduction and reversion of the PR interval to a shorter value, the pacemaker could be switched back automatically to the AAI/AAIR mode, thereby conserving battery capacity and optimizing left ventricular function by providing normal ventricular depolarization from a conducted atrial paced event.[39,40] Preliminary experience with the Chorus II DDD pulse generator (ELA Medical, Montrouge, France) that provides the DDD/AMC mode (automatic mode conversion) capable of switching from the DDD to the AAI mode and back to DDD mode (according to circumstances) has so far been satisfactory.[41]

Automatic Switching From Bipolar to Unipolar Mode

Although not strictly a change in the pacing mode, automatic switching of polarity from bipolar to unipolar is pertinent to the present discussion. A pulse generator with automatic switching of polarity was recently designed by Intermedics, Inc. (Freeport, TX). In case of a fracture or other lead defect in a bipolar lead, the pulse generator could switch automatically to unipolar pacing with the intact electrode. The Intermedics Cosmos II DDD pulse generator monitors the presence of an intact (normal) bipolar lead impedance in each chamber when programmed to the bipolar mode. Detection of a high bipolar impedance in the ventricular lead results in automatic conversion to the unipolar DOO mode using the tip electrode because most lead problems occur first in the outer coil linked to the proximal electrode.[42] Detection of a high bipolar impedance in the atrial lead only converts the pulse generator automatically to the VVI mode. Loss of capture during bipolar pacing can then be exposed upon application of the magnet because this maneuver causes pacing at the programmed (bipolar) polarity.[42] The switching mechanism also offers protection against inadvertent programming of the bipolar mode with a unipolar lead. Theoretically, if there is undersensing with a bipolar lead, a smart pacemaker could automatically switch to the polarity providing the larger signal. A smart pacemaker could also determine the lowest pacing threshold from a particular electrode and could then switch from one polarity to another to achieve pacing at the lower output.

References

1. Barold SS, Falkoff MD, Ong LS, et al. Interference in cardiac pacemakers: Exogenous sources. In: El-Sherif N, Samet P (eds.), Cardiac Pacing and Electrophysiology, W.B. Saunders, Philadelphia, PA, 1991, p 608.
2. Barold SS, Falkoff MD, Ong LS, et al. Upper rate response. In: Barold SS, Mugica J (eds.). New Perspectives in Cardiac Pacing, Futura Publishing Co., Mt. Kisco, NY, 1988, p 121.
3. Sanders R, Barold SS. Understanding elective replacement indicators and automatic parameter conversion mechanism in DDD pacemakers. In: Barold SS, Mugica J (eds.). New Perspectives in Cardiac Pacing, Futura Publishing Co., Mt. Kisco, NY, 1988, p 203.
4. Barold SS, Schoenfeld MH, Falkoff MD, et al. Elective replacement indicators of simple and complex pacemakers. In: Barold SS, Mugica (eds.). New Perspectives in Cardiac Pacing. 2, Future Publishing Co., Mt. Kisco, NY, 1991, p 493.
5. Barold SS, Schoenfeld MH. Pacemaker elective replacement indicators. PACE 1989;12:990.
6. Nathan AW, Bennett DH, Ward DE, et al. Catheter ablation of atrioventricular conduction. Lancet 1984;1:1280.
7. Lamas GA, Antman EM, Gold JP, et al. Pacemaker backup mode reversion and injury during cardiac surgery. Ann Thorac Surg 1986;41:155.
8. Levine PA, Balady GJ, Lazar HL, et al. Electrocautery and pacemakers: Management of the paced patient subject to electrocautery. Ann Thorac Surg 1986;41:313.
9. Chin MC, Rosenqvist M, Lee MA, et al. The effect of radiofrequency catheter ablation on permanent pacemakers. An experimental study. PACE 1990; 13:23.
10. Calkins H, Brinker J, Veltri EP, et al. Clinical interactions between pacemakers and automatic implantable cardioverter/defibrillators. J Am Coll Cardiol 1990;16:666.
11. Luceri RM, Brownstein SL, Habal SM, et al. Device-device and drug-device

interactions. In: Barold SS, Mugica J (eds.). New Perspectives in Cardiac Pacing. 2, Futura Publishing Co., Mt. Kisco, NY, 1991, p 527.
12. Kim SG, Furman S, Waspe LE, et al. Unipolar artifacts induced failure of an automatic implantable cardioverter/defibrillator to detect ventricular fibrillation. Am J Cardiol 1986;57:880.
13. Bardy GH, Ivey TD, Stewart R, et al. Failure of the automatic implantable defibrillator to detect ventricular fibrillation. Am J Cardiol 1986;58:1107.
14. Cohen AI, Wish MH, Fletcher RD, et al. The use and interaction of permanent pacemakers and the automatic implantable cardioverter/defibrilator. PACE 1988;11:704.
15. Medtronic Tech Note 90-6. The use of (U/B) polarity programmable IPG's in conjunction with AICD, Medtronic, Inc., Minneapolis, MN, 1990.
16. Barold SS, Falkoff MD, Ong LS, et al. Resetting of DDD pulse generators due to cold exposure. PACE 1988;11:736.
17. Barold SS, Falkoff MD, Ong LS, et al. Electrocardiography of contemporary DDD pacemakers. A. Basic concepts, upper rate response, retrograde ventriculoatrial conduction and differential diagnosis of pacemaker tachycardias. In: Saksena S, Goldschlager N (eds.). Electrical Therapy for Cardiac Arrhythmias. Pacing, Antitachycardia Devices, Catheter Ablation, W.B. Saunders, Philadelphia, PA, 1990, p 225.
18. Satler LF, Rackley CE, Pearle DL, et al. Inhibition of a physiologic pacing system due to its antipacemaker mediated tachycardia mode. PACE 1985; 8:806.
19. DenDulk K, Wellens HJ. Failure of the post-ventricular premature beat DVI mode in preventing pacemaker circus movement tachycardia. Am J Cardiol 1984;54:1371.
20. Ritter Ph. La stimulation DDDR définitive: aspects techniques, Stimucoeur 1990;18:29.
21. Higano ST, Hayes DL. P wave tracking above the maximum tracking rate in a DDDR pacemaker. PACE 1989;12:1044.
22. Higano ST, Hayes DL, Eisinger G. Advantage of discrepant upper rate limits in a DDDR pacemaker. Mayo Clin Proc 1989;64:932.
23. Physician Manual, Relay DDDR pulse generator model 293-03 and 294-04, Intermedics, Freeport, TX, 1991.
24. Synergyst II 7070/7071 activity responsive dual chamber pacer with telemtry, Technical Manual, Medtronic, Inc., Minneapolis, MN, 1989.
25. Technical Manual, Elite 7074/75/76/77 activity responsive dual chamber pacemaker with telemetry, Medtronic, Inc., Minneapolis, MN, 1991.
26. Higano ST, Hayes DL, Eisinger G. Sensor-driven rate smoothing in a DDDR pacemaker. PACE 1989;12:922.
27. Levine PA, Hayes DL, Wilkoff BL, et al. Electrocardiography of rate-modulated pacemaker rhythms, Siemens-Pacesetter, Inc., Sylmar, CA, 1990.
28. Hayes DL, Higano ST, Eisinger G. Electrocardiographic manifestations of a dual-chamber, rate-modulated (DDDR) pacemaker. PACE 1989;12:555.
29. Physician Manual, Pacesetter Synchrony 2020T rate-modulated polarity programmable dual-chamber pacemaker, Pacesetter Systems, Inc., Sylmar, CA, USA, 1988.

30. Hanich RF, Midei MG, McElroy BP, et al. Circumvention of maximum tracking limitations with a rate-modulated dual chamber pacemaker. PACE 1989;12:392.
31. Vey G, Werner K. Interaction of sensor-driven pacing and intrinsic atrial activity in dual chamber rate-responsive pacemakers. PACE 1989;12:1577.
32. Hayes DL, Higano ST. DDDR pacing. Follow-up and complications. In: Barold SS, Mugica J (eds.). New Perspectives in Cardiac Pacing. 2, Futura Publishing Co., Mt. Kisco, NY, 1991, p 473.
33. Stroobrandt R, Willems R, Vandenbulcke F, et al. DDDR pacemakers: A framework for the understanding of atrial and ventricular based device timing. Eur J Cardiac Pacing Electrophysiol 1991;2:151.
34. Spencer W, Markowitz T. DDD/VVIR. A new mode of cardiac pacing for exercise. PACE 1990;13:1211.
35. French WJ, Haskell RJ, Wesley GW, et al. Physiological benefits of a pacemaker with dual chamber pacing at low rate and single chamber rate responsive pacing during exercise. PACE 1988;11:1840.
36. Haywood GA, Ward J, Ward DE, et al. Atrioventricular Wenckebach point and progression to atrioventricular block in sinoatrial disease. PACE 1990; 13:2054.
37. DenDulk K, Lindemans FW, Brugada P, et al. Pacemaker syndrome with AAI rate variable pacing: Importance of atrioventricular conduction properties, medication and pacemaker programmability. PACE 1988;11:1226.
38. Mabo P, Pouillot C, Kermarrec A, et al. Lack of physiological adaptation of the atrioventricular interval to heart rate in patients chronically paced in the AAIR mode. PACE 1991;14:2133.
39. Girodo S, Ritter P, Pioger G, et al. Improved dual chamber mode in paroxysmal atrioventricular conduction disorders. PACE 1990;13:2059.
40. Physician manual, Chorus II 6234 implantable dual-chamber pulse generator: DDDMO, ELA Medical, Montrouge, France, 1992.
41. Ritter P. Personal communication, 1992.
42. Risser T, Drumm GW. A safety feature for protecting against loss of output with bipolar lead fracture. Eur J Cardiac Pacing Electrophysiol 1992;2:A64.

Chapter 20

Optimal Antibradycardia Pacing in Patients with Paroxysmal Supraventricular Tachyarrhythmias: Role of Fallback and Automatic Mode Switching Mechanisms

S. Serge Barold, Harry G. Mond

Introduction

In the last few years, many important retrospective but nonrandomized studies focusing mainly on the sick sinus syndrome (SSS) have demonstrated the benefits of atrial pacing. Compared to single chamber atrial or dual chamber pacing, single chamber ventricular pacing in SSS leads to a greater incidence of (1) pacemaker syndrome, (2) chronic atrial fibrillation, embolization, and stroke, (3) increase in heart size and left atrial size, (4) congestive heart failure, and (5) mortality.[1-28] Preliminary but mounting evidence suggests that atrial pacing may also prevent attacks of paroxysmal atrial fibrillation in the bradycardia-tachycardia syndrome other than the type associated with vagally induced atrial fibrillation in which atrial pacing alone is often effective.[1] Until recently, the presence of paroxysmal atrial arrhythmias constituted a contraindication to DDD (DDDR) pacing to avoid atrial tracking of rapid atrial rates during paroxysmal atrial tachyarrhythmias. However, the bradycardia-

New Perspectives in Cardiac Pacing, Vol. 3, edited by S. Serge Barold and Jacques Mugica, Mount Kisco, NY, Futura Publishing Co., © 1993.

tachycardia form of SSS now represents an important indication for DDD (DDDR) pacing.[29]

Patients with alternating bradycardia and tachycardia pose a challenge in terms of choosing an optimal pacing mode that also provides atrial pacing. Three clinical scenarios should be considered. (1) Sick sinus syndrome. In the bradycardia-tachycardia syndrome, second or third degree AV block is unusual while atrial chronotropic incompetence and retrograde VA conduction are common. Although some of these patients may be treated safely with only AAI (AAIR) pacing with or without antiarrhythmic agents,[30–32] implantation of a DDD, especially a DDDR, pulse generator provides greater flexibility should antiarrhythmic agents eventually cause substantial depression of sinus and/or AV nodal function.[33–35] (2) Intractable atrial flutter/fibrillation with iatrogenic complete AV block after His bundle ablation. Such patients often retain normal atrial chronotropic function and retrograde ventriculoatrial (VA) conduction is rare. (3) Spontaneous AV block and drug refractory paroxysmal supraventricular tachyarrhythmias.

Pacing with Conventional Pulse Generators

Pacing in patients with alternating bradycardia and tachycardia can be accomplished with conventional DDD or DDDR pulse generators programmed to a variety of modes or responses that often compromise optimal pacemaker function or physiology to avoid tracking of rapid atrial rates. Several approaches can be used (Table 1).

TABLE 1

Alternating Bradycardia and Tachycardia Antibradycardia Pacing with Conventional Pacemakers

---
* VVI/VVIR
* AAI/AAIR
* DDI/DDIR
* DDD with slow upper rate
* DDD with retriggerable atrial refractory period
* DDDR mode with slow atrial-driven upper rate and faster sensor-dependent upper rate

Retriggerable Atrial Refractory Period

A DDD pulse generator with a retriggerable atrial refractory period will switch itself automatically to the DVI mode upon sensing a fast atrial rate (Fig. 1). In such a case, an atrial signal sensed in the noise sampling period (or terminal portion) of the postventricular atrial refractory period (PVARP) does not start a new AV interval, but reinitiates an entirely new *total* atrial refractory period (AV interval + PVARP).[36] Atrial tachycardia faster than the programmed upper rate (i.e., P-P < total atrial refractory period) leads to asynchronous atrial pacing, i.e., the DVI mode (at the lower rate) because the atrial refractory periods overlap until such time that the P-P interval becomes longer than the total atrial refractory period.[36,37] The process of overlapping atrial refractory periods therefore represents temporary mode switching to the DVI mode and resembles the function of a dual demand pacemaker for the termination of reentrant tachycardia by competitive asynchronous pacing. A pulse generator with a retriggerable atrial refractory period may exhibit

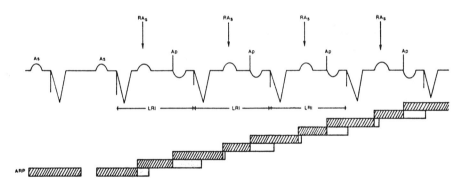

Figure 1. Diagrammatic representation of the retriggerable atrial refractory period (ARP) of the Siemens 674 DDD pulse generator. As = atrial sense event outside ARP; RAs = atrial sense event within ARP; Ap = atrial paced event. The first 125 ms of the PVARP represents the absolute refractory period during which signals cannot be sensed. The second part of the PVARP (and AV interval) consist of the noise sampling period. P waves falling within the noise sampling period may be sensed, and although they do not initiate a new AV interval, they retrigger a full ARP. Continual retriggering of the ARP causes the DDD pulse generator to operate in the atrial asynchronous mode at the lower rate, i.e., DVI mode when P-P interval < ARP. (Reproduced with permission.[46])

a Wenckebach (AV block) upper rate response only if the upper rate interval exceeds the total atrial refractory period (TARP), but a fixed ratio AV block upper rate response (i.e., 2:1) cannot occur. In certain circumstances, an atrial extrasystole falling relatively late in the PVARP will reinitiate a new total atrial refractory period without disrupting the atrial escape interval, so that subsequent delivery of the atrial stimulus close to the atrial extrasystole may precipitate an atrial tachyarrhythmia. Parenthetically, certain pulse generators utilize retriggerable ventricular refractory periods to deal with sensed interference, e.g., myopotentials, by the ventricular channel. In this way, a VVI pulse generator functions in the VOO mode while a DDD pulse generator functions in the DOO mode (because continual reinitiation of the ventricular refractory period by oversensing causes simultaneous reinitiation of the PVARP).[38]

DDI and DDIR Modes

In dual chamber pulse generators with ventricular-based lower rate timing (lower rate interval controlled by ventricular events—constant atrial escape interval), the DDI mode is equivalent to the DDD mode with the upper rate (interval) equal to the lower rate (interval).[39,40] Thus, in dual chamber pulse generators (with ventricular-based timing) without a specifically programmable DDI mode, the latter can be obtained simply by programming identical upper and lower rates in the DDD mode.[39,40] In the DDI mode (ventricular-based), the pacemaker avoids competitive atrial pacing by sensing atrial activity (which therefore inhibits release of the atrial stimulus at the completion of the atrial escape interval). Unlike the ventricular response of traditional DDD and VDD modes, the paced ventricular rate in the DDI mode cannot exceed the programmed lower rate (the functional equivalent of no atrial tracking). For this reason, the DDI mode has gained popularity for the treatment of patients with alternating bradycardia and tachycardia and has achieved modest success, especially in patients with chronotropic incompetence.[41]

In the DDI mode, AV synchrony is maintained in only two situations: (1) when the programmed lower rate exceeds the spontaneous atrial rate so that both channels pace sequentially, and (2) in patients with SSS and *relatively normal AV conduction* if the spontaneous atrial rate exceeds the programmed lower rate (P-P interval < lower rate interval). The conducted QRS inhibits the pulse generator and there will be no advantage over DDD pacing, particularly in the presence of atrial tachyar-rhythmias that conduct to the ventricle. In contrast, AV synchrony does not occur in the DDI mode in patients with AV block when the sinus rate exceeds the programmed lower rate. In the latter case, the P waves sensed by the atrial channel gradually march through the pacing cycles, moving closer and closer to the preceding paced ventricular beat. The

DDIR

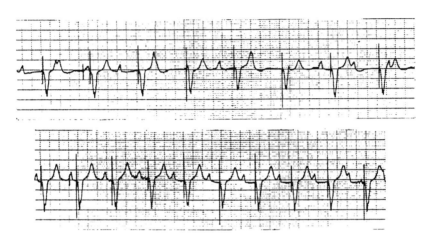

Figure 2.   Electrocardiograms of a patient who developed the pacemaker syn-drome with the DDIR mode. A dual chamber pulse generator was implanted after His bundle ablation for intractable paroxysmal atrial fibrillation. Top: The DDIR mode at rest functions at the programmed lower rate of 60/min, slower than the prevailing sinus rate. Note that sinus P waves march through the cardiac cycle producing AV dissociation. The P wave following the first ventricular paced beat falls in the 300 ms postventricular atrial refractory period (PVARP) and is unsensed, thereby allowing the release of an atrial stimulus at the end of the atrial escape interval initiated by the first ventricular paced complex. Bottom: On exercise, when the sinus rate is slightly faster than the sensor-driven rate, sinus P waves march through the cardiac cycle, producing AV dissociation. The pulse generator does not sense the P wave following the first ventricular paced beat because it falls in the PVARP. This allows emission of an atrial stimulus at the termination of the sensor-driven atrial escape interval initiated by the first ventricular paced beat. (Reproduced with permission from Barold SS et al., Car-diac Pacing Update: Guidelines in Choosing Pacemakers and Optimal Pacing Modes. In: Progress in Cardiology, Zipes DP, Rowlands DJ (eds.), Lea and Febiger, Philadelphia, PA, 1992, p 171.)

pacemaker functions like the VVI mode (with AV dissociation) except when a P wave falling in the PVARP is unsensed, whereupon the pulse generator delivers an atrial stimulus at the termination of the atrial escape interval (Fig. 2). Thus with a normal sinus mechanism and AV block, the DDI mode presents no real hemodynamic advantage over VVI pacing. A comparable situation can occur in the DDIR mode on exercise in patients with complete AV block when the sinus rate exceeds the sensor-driven interval and the pacemaker functions essentially like the VVIR mode[41] (Fig. 2, lower strip). The loss of AV synchrony at low levels of exercise in the DDIR mode may be hemodynamically important in some patients, especially those with left ventricular dysfunction. AV dissociation physiology in the DDI or the DDIR mode can sometimes lead to the pacemaker syndrome at rest and/or on exercise.[41] Consequently, the DDI or DDIR mode cannot be recommended as first-line therapy in patients with AV block and paroxysmal supraventricular tachyarrhythmias unless there is atrial chronotropic incompetence. Patients with AV block and a normal sinus mechanism fare better with retained AV synchrony using DDD or appropriately programmed DDDR devices designed with a protective algorithm for the recognition of supraventricular tachyarrhythmias and prevention of rapid ventricular paced rates. DDIR pacing can be useful in patients with atrial chronotropic incompetence, high degree or complete AV block, and paroxysmal supraventricular tachyarrhythmias. The DDI and DDIR modes can also be useful as *temporary* pacing modes in DDD or DDDR pacemakers equipped with automatic mode switching in response to supraventricular tachyarrhythmias (discussed later).

DDD or DDDR Mode with Slow Atrial-Driven Upper Rate

A slow upper rate of an atrial tracking pacemaker can be used when the DDI mode is unavailable. If the upper rate is close to the lower rate and the sinus rhythm is faster than the upper rate, pacing resembles the DDI (DDIR) mode (fixed R–R intervals at the relatively long upper rate interval, i.e., Wenckebach upper rate response) until the P wave falls in the PVARP and a pause typical of the Wenckebach upper rate response occurs.

DDDR Mode with Slow Atrial-Driven and Fast Sensor-Dependent Upper Rate

To avoid tracking relatively fast atrial rates, a DDDR pulse generator with a relatively slow atrial-controlled upper rate and a faster sensor-controlled upper rate can be used to provide a faster ventricular pacing rate on exercise.[42] Separation of the two upper rates cannot be accomplished in DDD pulse generators with common atrial-driven and sensor-driven upper rate intervals when the TARP cannot be programmed to a value *longer* than the common (atrial- or sensor-driven) upper rate interval.

Dissociation of Atrial-Driven and Sensor-Driven Upper Rate Intervals

1. Dissociation of the atrial-driven and sensor-driven upper rates can be easily accomplished in pulse generators allowing separate programming of these two upper rate intervals. For example, in the presence of paroxysmal supraventricular tachyarrhythmias, the atrial-driven upper rate could be programmed to 100/min to limit the ventricular paced response to sensed supraventricular tachycardia and the sensor-driven upper rate could be programmed to 150/min to provide rate increase on exercise (Pacesetter-Siemens Synchrony and Medtronic Elite II DDDR pacemakers).

2. Long TARP in pulse generators with a common upper rate. In pulse generators with a common upper rate, i.e., identical sensor-driven and atrial-driven upper rate intervals, dissociation of the two upper rates can actually be accomplished by a maneuver that at first appears paradoxical. (See previous chapter.) The desired upper rate is programmed first and is then considered the sensor-driven upper rate. A long PVARP is then programmed so that the TARP now becomes *longer* than the programmed (common) upper rate interval. The duration of the TARP now limits the atrial-driven upper rate so that 1:1 AV synchrony occurs until the P-P interval becomes shorter than the TARP, whereupon fixed-ratio 2:1 AV block supervenes. Functional separation of the upper rates cannot be achieved in DDDR pulse generators with common atrial-driven and sensor-driven upper rates if the device does not permit programming TARP > common URI. Obviously a Wenckebach upper rate

response cannot occur when common URI ≤ TARP because it requires URI > TARP. In this way, fixed-ratio AV block (e.g., 2:1) occurs at atrial rates *slower* than the programmed sensor-driven upper rate. With such an arrangement, when SDI < TARP, atrial pacing can occur in the PVARP to conform to the relatively fast sensor-driven rate or shorter sensor-driven interval.

AAI or AAIR Mode

Programming a dual chamber pulse generator to the AAI or AAIR mode if AV conduction is relatively normal provides another way of dealing with bothersome supraventricular tachyarrhythmias.

Diagnosis of Inappropriate Tachycardia by Dual Chamber Pacemakers

Many available DDD and DDDR pacemakers cannot reliably differentiate a physiologic increase in atrial rate with exercise or emotion from an inappropriately high atrial rate due to endless loop tachycardia, myopotential oversensing by the atrial channel, paroxysmal atrial tachycardia, etc.

Contemporary pacemakers use a large variety of elaborate algorithms to terminate endless loop tachycardia, and most are very effective. We believe that with contemporary dual chamber pacemakers, endless loop tachycardia should be prevented altogether or immediately terminated at its onset. A smart pacemaker should automatically lengthen its PVARP in situations predisposing to endless loop tachycardia. A smart pacemaker will eventually be capable of differentiating anterograde from retrograde P waves, and when this occurs it will eliminate the use of a long PVARP to contain relatively slow retrograde VA conduction.

A DDDR pacemaker receives signals from two sources: the atrium provides the P wave and the independent (nonatrial) sensor provides information concerning the need to increase the pacing rate according to changing activity. A smart DDDR pacemaker can differentiate physiologic from nonphysiologic rate variations. This discrimination can be achieved in the passive sensor mode with the pulse generator itself not necessarily functioning in the rate-adaptive mode. Data from these two inputs can be used to determine whether a high atrial rate is appropriate or not, thereby providing a relatively easy way for the pulse generator to make the diagnosis of abnormal sinus bradycardia on exercise, physiologic, and pathologic atrial tachycardias. In the face of atrial tachycardia, if the sensor of a DDDR pacemaker determines that physiologic tachycardia should not be present,[43] the PVARP could be increased for only one or two cycles (or the AV interval decreased for one beat[44] or a single ventricular stimulus could be dropped), whereupon endless loop tachycardia would terminate immediately. The pacemaker would therefore identify the tachycardia as an endless loop tachycardia. Alternatively, the pacemaker could switch its pacing mode automatically to avoid rapid ventricular pacing secondary to endless loop tachycardia. If the tachycardia persists, the pulse generator then identifies it as not being endless loop tachycardia and responds to the tachycardia according to a predetermined algorithm, i.e., automatic mode switching, fallback, etc.

Pacemaker Response to Inappropriate Atrial Rates: Fallback and Automatic Mode Switching

The response of antibradycardia pacemakers to rapid nonphysiologic atrial rates has become important now that dual chamber pacemakers are recommended for patients with alternating bradycardia and tachycardia, as emphasized earlier.

Traditional fallback mechanisms introduced some time ago in certain DDD pacemakers provide a reasonably satisfactory degree of protection against rapid ventricular pacing rates in supraventricular tachycardia. In fallback, when the atrial rate exceeds the programmed upper rate (for a given duration that may be programmable), the pulse generator activates a mechanism that produces a slower ventricular pacing rate with or without maintaining the same pacing mode (Fig. 3). During traditional fallback, a DDD pulse generator functions either in the VVI mode with uncoupling of atrial activity from the ventricular paced complexes (actually the VDI mode because atrial sensing is maintained) or stays in the DDD mode so that the ventricular pacing rate drops *gradually* to a programmed fallback rate anywhere between the upper and lower rates according to design or programmability.[44–47] The pulse generator automatically returns to its previous DDD mode (or DDDR) with 1:1 AV synchrony when the sensed atrial rate drops below the programmed upper rate. VVI pacing during supraventricular tachyarrhythmia such as

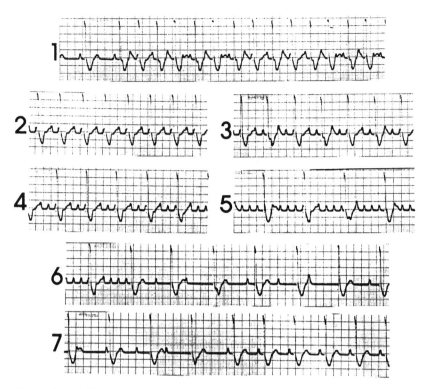

Figure 3. Fallback mechanism of the CPI 925 Delta DDD pulse generator to the VVI mode. Eight cycle onset and 4 ms/cycle. 1 = onset of supraventricular tachycardia (SVT); 2 = 20 sec after onset of SVT; 3 = 40 sec after onset of SVT; 4 = 1 min after onset of SVT; 5 = 2 min after onset of SVT stops; 6 = SVT stops; 7 = pacemaker resynchronization. (Reproduced with permission.[46])

atrial fibrillation does not cause serious hemodynamic impairment because the pacemaker syndrome requires organized atrial systole (antegrade or retrograde) for its development.

Van Wyhe[45] reported the successful use of DDD pacemakers with a fallback mechanism in the VVI mode (CPI Delta 925) in patients with paroxysmal atrial tachycardia (e.g., atrial flutter/fibrillation, etc.) after His bundle ablation. Theoretically, on physical exertion, if sinus tachycardia exceeds the programmed upper rate of the pacemaker, conversion to the VVI fallback mode will lead to loss of AV synchrony and a drop in the ventricular pacing rate at a time when it is most needed. This problem can be minimized or eliminated by appropriate programming of the pulse generator with an upper rate above the patient's sinus node response on exercise, but below the atrial rate observed during supraventricular tachycardia.[45]

Intelligent pulse generators with a fallback mechanism should have extensive programmability of (1) fallback rate (the slowest ventricular paced rate that will be maintained as long as the spontaneous atrial rate exceeds the programmed upper rate), (2) number of events at the upper rate required to initiate the fallback mechanism, (3) deceleration of the fallback response in terms of prolongation of the pacing cycles in ms/cycle until attainment of the programmed fallback rate (Fig. 4). The capability of rapid or immediate conversion to the fallback rate or mode

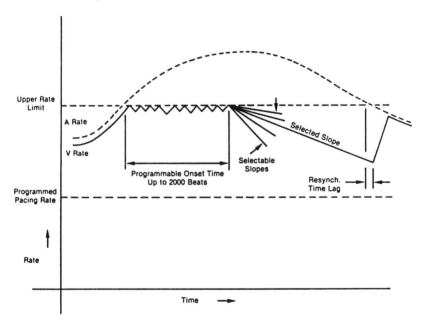

Figure 4.   Diagrammatic representation of a fallback response without AV synchrony. One-to-one P-wave-triggered ventricular pacing occurs up to the upper rate limit. The pacemaker then responds with Wenckebach upper rate limitation. After a programmed onset time, the fallback response is initiated and the ventricular rate gradually decreases (programmable slope) to the fallback rate (programmed lower rate). When the atrial rate falls below the programmed upper rate, the pacemaker restores 1:1 P-wave-triggered ventricular pacing after a resynchronization time lag. A = atrial; V = ventricular. (Reproduced with permission.[46])

should be programmable. (4) Fallback response. Dual chamber pulse generators can respond to supraventricular tachycardia by (a) maintaining the same pacing mode and slowing the paced ventricular rate, and (b) conversion to another pacing mode with consequent control of the ventricular pacing rate by virtue of the new pacing mode, a response now called automatic mode switching (AMS, a trademark of Telectronics). AMS is not a new concept, but it has recently gained popularity as more and more patients with bradycardia and paroxysmal supraventricular tachyarrhythmias become candidates for dual chamber pacemakers. An intelligent DDDR pulse generator should have the capability of AMS to one of the following pacing modes according to design or programmability: DDD (with a slower upper rate) and nonatrial tracking modes such as DDI, DDIR, VVI, or VVIR. Although some DDD pulse generators are designed to maintain a semblance of AV synchrony during the fallback mechanism by using the DDD (by continually reducing the upper rate interval) or DDI mode, the constantly changing AV intervals during this process probably provide little or no hemodynamic benefit.

Proposed Classification of Pacemaker Fallback Responses

The advent of rate-adaptive pacing has introduced new complexity into the fallback mechanisms for three reasons. (1) The pacemaker receives information from two sources: the atrium via the atrial lead, and the nonatrial sensor; (2) the fallback response consists of a change in rate and/or mode; and (3) the fallback response may or may not be driven by sensor activity, i.e., rate-adaptive or non-rate-adaptive. Tables 2 and 3 show a proposed classification of pacemaker fallback mechanisms.

Automatic Mode Switching of the Telectronics Meta DDDR Pacemaker

The Telectronics Meta DDDR pulse generator (Telectronics, Englewood, CO) is a minute ventilation rate-adaptive device that responds to supraventricular tachycardia with automatic and immediate switching to the VVIR mode at the onset of tachycardia when the atrial cycle length becomes shorter than the prevailing total atrial refractory period.[47-56] The Meta DDDR pulse generator initiates AMS upon the detection of early *atrial* activity only in the PVARP (Fig. 5) beyond the 100 ms atrial

TABLE *2*
Classification of Fallback Mechanisms

		Input			
Mode	*Class*	*Atrial*	*Nonatrial Sensor*	*Rate Adaptive Response**	*Availability (See Table 3)*
DDDR	1	+	−	− (B)	−
DDD	1	+	−	− (B)	+
DDDR	1	+	−	+ (A)	+
DDD**	1	+	−	+ (A)	+
DDDR	2	+	+	− (B)	+
DDD	2	+	+	− (B)	−
DDDR	2	+	+	+ (A)	−
DDD	2	+	+	+ (A)	−

+ = Yes

− = No

Class 1: Input from atrial sensor only.

Class 2: Input from atrial and nonatrial sensors.

* Response: This classfication can be expanded by including the type of fallback response. Rate only (R) or mode switching (M) as shown in Table 3. + Rate-adaptive response (A). − No rate-adaptive response (B).

** Sensor-controlled or rate-adaptive response occurs automatically when fallback mechanism is activated, i.e., automatic switching from DDD to VVIR mode.

blanking window. Lack of sensor input in the presence of atrial tachycardia plays no role in the initiation of AMS, i.e., the initiation of AMS depends upon a critical atrial cycle length and *not* sensor activity (Fig. 6). In the AMS mode, in contrast to traditional fallback mechanisms, conversion to the VVIR mode allows control of the ventricular rate by sensor input (Figs. 7 and 8). According to Table 2, the fallback response of the Meta DDDR pacemaker to supraventricular tachyarrhythmias can be classified as an M Class 1A fallback. Once AMS is in effect, the pulse generator does not strictly function in the VVIR mode as atrial events are continuously monitored, i.e., VDI or VDIR mode.

The Meta DDDR pacemaker exhibits automatic AV delay shortening dependent on a metabolic indicated rate (MIR) interval (calculated pacing rate interval determined by the algorithm during both atrial pacing and sensing). The MIR interval is dependent on the programmed rate-

TABLE *3*

Fallback and Automatic Mode Switching

Mode	Sensor	Classification	Examples
DDD	–	M class 1B	CPI Delta, Telectronics Quadra, ELA Chorus I & II
		R class 1B	Intermedics Cosmos I
Generic DDDR	+	M or R class 1B	
DDDR	MV	M class 1A	Telectronics Meta*
DDDR	MV	M class 1A	ELA Chorus RM (in the DDD mode, 2 options are available—M class 1A and M class 1B)**
DDDR	Accelerometer	M class 1A	CPI Vigor
DDDR	Accelerometer	R class II B	Intermedics Relay

MV = minute ventilation.

R = Rate only.

M = Mode only.

* It could be argued that the Meta DDDR pacemaker possesses a class 2 fallback because the total atrial refractory period is sensor controlled. For the sake of simplicity, the Meta DDDR pacemaker is best classified as having a class 1 fallback. This example illustrates the complex parameter interrelationships of contemporary DDDR devices.

** Sensor-controlled or rate-adaptive response occurs automatically with activation of the fallback mechanism, i.e., automatic mode change from DDD to VVIR.

response factor, the upper and lower pacing rates, and the measured transthoracic impedance changes. Shortening of the PVARP on exercise is also dependent on the MIR interval and the programmable indices. PVARP shortening depends on the PVARP at rest (PVARP base) and the atrial tracking interval (ATI = interval for P wave sensing) that follows the PVARP. As the atrial pacing or sensing rate increases, the ATI shortens according to the change in the MIR interval. If the pulse generator calculates that the ATI will disappear before the upper rate is reached, then PVARP shortening occurs in a linear fashion to maintain an ATI window and hence retain normal atrial sensing up to the upper

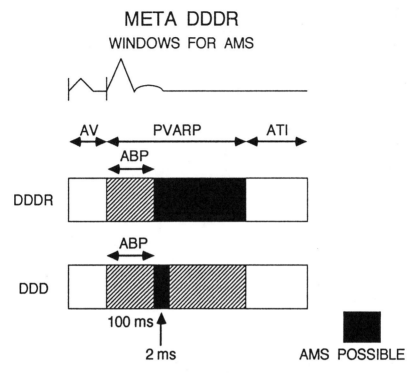

Figure 5. Timing intervals of the Telectronics 1250 Meta DDDR pulse generator showing the windows for automatic mode switching (AMS). In the DDDR mode (and DDIR, VDDR), the first 100 ms of the postventricular atrial refractory period (PVARP) consists of an absolute refractory period (atrial blanking). Atrial sensing within the PVARP beyond the absolute refractory period will evoke AMS. When the pulse generator is programmed to the DDD mode, the AMS window occupies a very narrow 2-ms window immediately after the absolute refractory period in the first part of the PVARP.

rate limit. When programmed to the DDDR or VDDR mode, the Meta DDDR pacemaker monitors atrial electrical activity within a designated PVARP window immediately following a nonprogrammable 100-ms atrial blanking period (Fig. 5). When the pacemaker detects a single atrial event in the PVARP, it omits the succeeding atrial stimulus and also ignores other atrial signals in the ATI beyond the PVARP, resulting in automatic mode switching (AMS) with effective VVIR pacing. With the

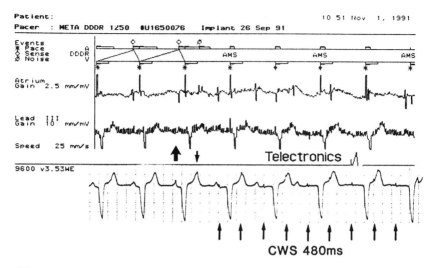

Figure 6. Meta DDDR pacemaker showing automatic mode switching (AMS) with chest wall stimulation (CWS) sensed by the atrial channel. The Telectronics printout demonstrates simultaneously from above: the event recording, the calibrated atrial electrogram, and the surface ECG lead 2. High quality ECG below the printout was recorded simultaneously. The first (thick) arrow pointing up indicates the onset of CWS. The first CWS falls within the P wave and does not disturb the basic rhythm. The arrow pointing down corresponds with the first CWS sensed by the pacemaker within the PVARP (beyond the 100-ms atrial blanking period) with consequent initiation of automatic mode switching (AMS). The 480-ms interval between two CWS signals was shorter than the prevailing total atrial refractory period at that time. The symbol for noise denotes sensing of noise or atrial activity within the PVARP and if appropriately timed it triggers AMS.

present algorithm, once AMS has occurred, an atrial rate monitor documents atrial electrical events detected in the PVARP. The pulse generator automatically reverts back to the DDDR mode if no atrial electrical events occur in the PVARP for up to three cycles. (AMS to the VVI mode can also occur with DDD and VDD pacing during a 2-ms AMS window immediately following the 100-ms absolute atrial refractory period.)

In the Meta DDDR pacemaker, the atrial-driven upper rate interval (URI) is programmable and equal to the sensor-driven URI. In a DDD pulse generator with a Wenckebach upper rate response, the URI must

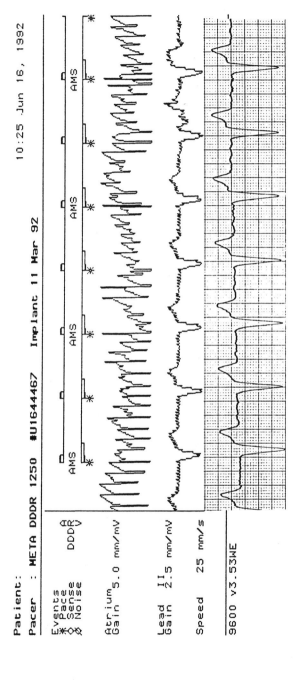

Figure 7. Meta DDDR Pulse generator showing automatic mode switching (AMS) with atrial fibrillation in a patient at rest. The Telectronics printout was recorded with the same format as in Figure 6. A high quality ECG below the printout was recorded simultaneously. Sensing of f waves in the postventricular atrial refractory period perpetuates AMS.

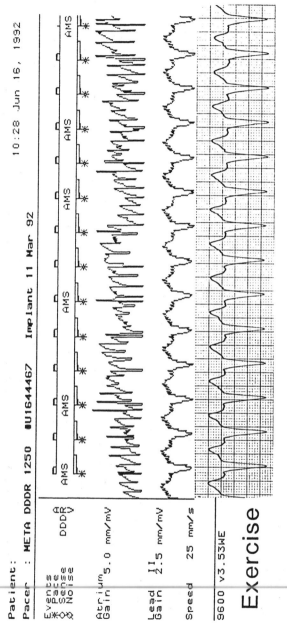

Figure 8. Meta DDDR pulse generator showing automatic mode switching (AMS) in the same patient as in Figure 7, but now on exercise (same format as in Figure 6.) A high quality ECG below the printout was recorded simultaneously. During AMS in the VVIR mode, the pacemaker increases its rate.

be longer than TARP. In the DDDR mode of the Meta DDDR pacemaker, a Wenckebach (AV block) upper rate response cannot occur because the prevailing TARP never becomes shorter than the upper rate interval (common sensor- and atrial-driven URI). (In software unavailable in the United States, it is possible to program an ATI at the programmed upper rate. In this circumstance, the atrial-driven URI becomes longer than the TARP and a Wenckebach-like AV interval extension can occur but the first P wave falling within the PVARP produces AMS.) At rest, the pulse generator will maintain 1:1 AV synchrony up to an atrial rate that yields a P-P interval shorter than the resting TARP (longest TARP duration). On exercise, in contrast to rest, shortening of the TARP (because both AV and PVARP shorten) allows 1:1 AV synchrony according to the MIR interval with faster atrial rates or shorter P-P intervals. Finally, when the pulse generator functions with a sensor-driven interval equal to the sensor-driven URI, the TARP becomes equal to the programmed atrial-driven URI (Fig. 9). While conventional DDDR pulse generators respond to a P-P cycle shorter than the TARP with a fixed-ratio 2:1 AV block, the Meta DDDR pacemaker cannot respond in this fashion because the P wave within the PVARP causes AMS.

The Meta DDDR pacemaker responds to single atrial extrasystoles and ventricular extrasystoles with retrograde ventriculoatrial conduction, a distinct disadvantage because continual AMS may result in significant hemodynamic changes, particularly if retrograde VA conduction follows ventricular pacing (Fig. 10). The pulse generator possesses a protective mechanism to prevent continual AMS with persistent VVIR pacing when retrograde P waves fall consistently within the PVARP. The pulse generator alters its function after eight consecutive modified VVIR cycles (secondary to sensing of eight consecutive P waves within the PVARP, but not necessarily retrograde P waves) so that the duration of the ninth pacemaker cycle automatically lengthens by 240 ms (Fig. 11). Cycle prolongation guarantees return of AV synchrony by favoring P-wave sensing or by the delivery of a delayed but effectual atrial stimulus sufficiently removed from the previous retrograde P wave to avoid stimulation within the atrial myocardial refractory period (generated by the preceding retrograde P wave). Prolongation of the pacing cycle by 240-ms periods after eight cycles can also be seen with atrial fibrillation causing AMS.

AMS can occur with sinus tachycardia when the P-P interval becomes shorter than the prevailing TARP (Figs. 12 and 13). Factors pre-

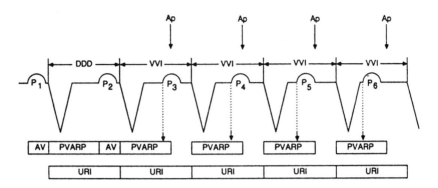

Figure 9. Diagrammatic representation of DDDR pacing with the Telectronics Meta DDDR pulse generator showing the upper rate response when the sensor-driven interval (SDI) is equal to the programmed upper rate interval (URI). The pulse generator has a common upper rate (atrial-driven URI = sensor-driven URI). The atrial rate is faster than the programmed upper rate. With appropriate programming, the total atrial refractory period (TARP) gradually shortens with exercise (increased sensor activity) so that when SDI = URI, TARP = URI. The first (P_1) and second (P_2) P waves are sensed outside the postventricular atrial refractory period (PVARP) and both initiate an AV interval as programmed. The third P wave (P_3) occurs in the PVARP, but is sensed by the atrial channel whereupon the pulse generator inhibits release of the next Ap (atrial stimulus), producing a modified VVIR cycle. The VVIR cycles are sensor-driven and equal to the programmed URI because SDI = URI. The fourth, fifth, and sixth P waves fall in the PVARP and also inhibit release of Ap.

disposing to AMS in patients with normal sinus mechanism include an upper rate programmed too low, an excessively long PVARP base, and/or auto AV (adapt) interval (Fig. 12). Programming a lower rate-response factor also favors AMS during normal sinus rhythm by restricting shortening of the AV interval and PVARP on exercise. AMS can also occur during normal sinus rhythm in the early phase of exercise (such as running on the spot, sprinting, or walking up stairs) when the sinus rate transiently exceeds the ability of the pulse generator to change the MIR and its dependent parameters, particularly if the patients hold their breath. A similar situation could occur with fright or panic. AMS during normal

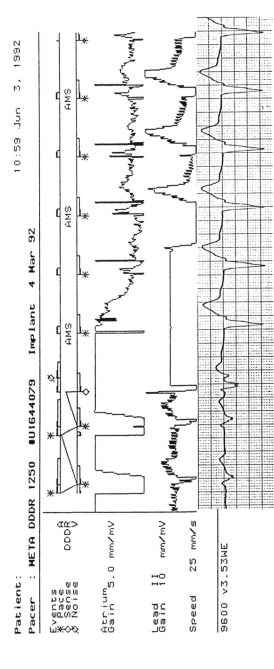

Figure 10. Meta DDDR pulse generator with automatic mode switching (AMS) response due to sensing of retrograde P waves within the postventricular atrial refractory period (PVARP). (The same format as in Figure 6 was used. The high quality ECG below the printout was recorded simultaneously.) The third beat is a ventricular extrasystole associated with retrograde ventriculoatrial (VA) conduction. The retrograde P wave falls within the PVARP (beyond the 100-ms atrial blanking period) and therefore induces AMS. Subsequent ventricular paced beats during AMS perpetuate retrograde VA conduction and therefore AMS itself because the retrograde P waves continue to fall within the PVARP. The pacemaker terminates this sequence after sensing eight consecutive P waves within the PVARP, as shown and explained in Figure 11.

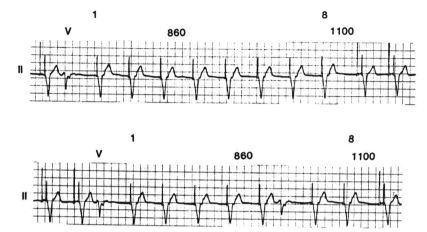

Figure 11. Top: Meta DDDR pacemaker showing automatic mode switching (AMS) initiated by a ventricular extrasystole (V) with retrograde ventriculoatrial (VA) activity sensed in the postventricular atrial refractory period (PVARP). Subsequent ventricular paced beats in the VVIR mode perpetuate retrograde VA conduction and AMS. After sensing eight consecutive retrograde P waves within the PVARP, the pacemaker alters its function as follows: (a) automatic prolongation of the next pacing interval (actually the sensor-driven atrial escape interval) by 240 ms; (b) automatic uncoupling of the AMS function, thereby allowing successful atrial pacing with immediate termination of retrograde VA conduction. Bottom: Same patient as in top figure. The ECG shows that automatic prolongation of the pacing cycle (sensor-driven atrial escape interval) during AMS depends on sensing eight consecutive atrial events within the PVARP rather than the occurrence of eight consecutive ventricular paced cycles.

sinus rhythm can be minimized or prevented by careful programming of the pulse generator, bearing in mind that a low rate-responsive factor and an excessively long base PVARP constitute very important causes of AMS during sinus rhythm (Fig. 13).

Inappropriate AMS can also occur with oversensing of the farfield ventricular electrogram by the atrial channel during the PVARP (Fig. 14). Farfield interference appears to be more common with paced rather than sensed QRS complexes, with unipolar sensing configuration and high atrial sensitivity. This problem can generally be overcome by analysis of the atrial electrogram and appropriate adjustment of atrial sensitivity and sensing polarity. On the other hand, when the atrial channel of the Meta DDDR pacemaker (programmed to unipolar sensing) detects

META DDDR

LOWER RATE INTERVAL = 1000 ms
UPPER RATE INTERVAL = 414 ms (145 / min)
PVARP (BASE) = 400 ms
ATRIAL SENSITIVITY = 0.5 mV

VVIR

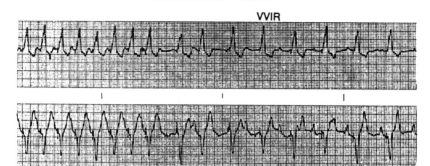

Figure 12. Two-lead ECG showing pacing with the Telectronics Meta DDDR pacemaker during treadmill exercise. On the left, there is 1:1 atrioventricular (AV) synchrony. When the sinus rate generates a P-P interval shorter than the prevailing total atrial refractory period at that given point in time, the pulse generator automatically reverts to the VVIR mode (AMS) at a relatively slow rate controlled by sensor activity. The sudden slowing of the paced ventricular rate and loss of AV synchrony may not be tolerated in some individuals. Appropriate programming (upper rate and/or sensor response) and testing should prevent or minimize such a nonphysiologic response.

myopotentials in the PVARP, AMS may provide protection against rapid ventricular pacing rates triggered by this type of interference in contrast to the relative lack of such protection in the DDD mode (Fig. 15).

Vaneiro et al.[52] recently reported their experience with 28 patients who received Meta DDDR pulse generators. Of the 28 patients, five had chronotropic incompetence and 16 (57%) had paroxysmal atrial fibrillation. Twenty-six of the patients underwent an exercise test and 18 had at least one 24-hour Holter monitor. During stress testing, seven patients reported symptoms; four had severe dyspnea (three of these episodes were associated with AMS), near-syncope occurred in two patients due to a marked drop in blood pressure, while one patient experienced angina pectoris (although not specifically mentioned in the report, hypotension

META DDDR

LOWER RATE INTERVAL = 1000 ms
UPPER RATE INTERVAL = 375 ms (160 / min)
PVARP (BASE) = 280 ms
ATRIAL SENSITIVIY = 0.5 mV

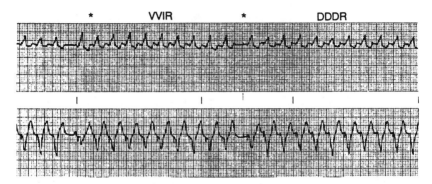

Figure 13. Two-lead ECG showing pacing with the Telectronics Meta DDDR pacemaker during treadmill exercise (same patient as in Figure 12). Appropriate programming allows a smoother transition to the VVIR mode during the upper rate response. After eight cycles with a sinus P wave detected in the postventricular atrial refractory period, the pacemaker lengthens its atrial escape interval by 240 ms, permitting the release of an atrial stimulus. This is followed by DDDR sequential pacing on the right. The asterisks indicate small bipolar stimuli not seen in the upper strip.

and angina were most probably related to AMS). AMS was frequent and detected in 16 of the 26 patients (57%). AMS was detected in 11 patients during an exercise test (42% of the entire group) and was due to sinus tachycardia in seven and paroxysmal atrial tachycardia in four. AMS was also documented in nine patients (50%) during Holter recordings (in only four patients was this due to paroxysmal atrial fibrillation, in three it was due to episodes of retrograde conduction associated with ventricular extrasystoles, and in two it was due to sinus tachycardia). AMS due to farfield sensing was also observed in one patient. Vaneiro et al.[52] emphasized that AMS is very sensitive and works well in the presence of paroxysmal atrial tachyarrhythmia, but it is not very specific because it also occurs in the presence of sinus rhythm (about half of AMS events

META DDDR

LOWER RATE INTERVAL = 1000 ms
UPPER RATE INTERVAL = 414 ms (145 / min)
PVARP (BASE) = 400 ms

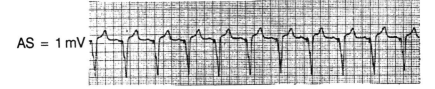

AS = 1 mV

META DDDR

LOWER RATE INTERVAL = 1000 ms
UPPER RATE INTERVAL = 414 ms (145 / min)
PVARP (BASE) = 400 ms
ATRIAL SENSITIVITY = 0.5 mV

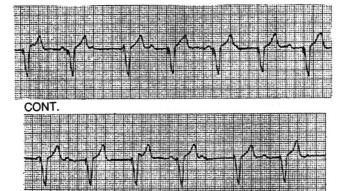

CONT.

Figure 14. Top: Meta DDDR pacemaker showing normal atrial tracking when the atrial sensitivity (AS) is 1 mV. Bottom: Meta DDDR pacemaker showing farfield sensing. Same patient as in top figure. The atrial sensitivity was increased to 0.5 mV. The atrial channel senses the tail-end of the paced QRS complex as a farfield signal. The latter falls within the PVARP beyond the atrial blanking period and therefore induces automatic mode switching (AMS). The pacemaker then paces in the VVIR mode at the base rate of 60/min. Note that the atrial escape interval is increased by 240 ms after eight pacing cycles, during which the farfield QRS signal is sensed within the PVARP.

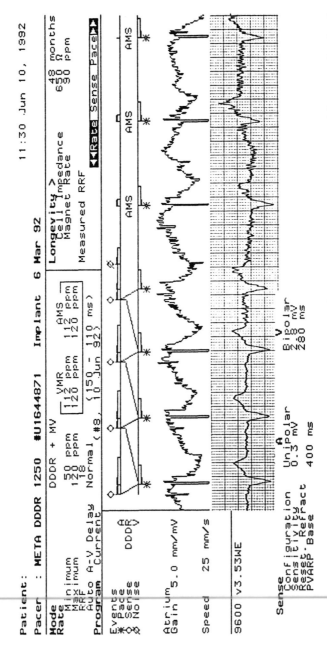

Figure 15. Meta DDDR pacemaker with automatic mode switching (AMS) response to myopotential oversensing by the atrial channel (programmed for unipolar sensing). (The format is the same as in Figure 6. The high quality ECG below the printout was recorded simultaneously.) AMS induced by the detection of myopotential interference by the atrial channel within the postventricular atrial refractory period prevents triggering of rapid ventricular rates.

TABLE 4
Automatic Mode Switching Teletronics Meta DDDR
Problems
* AMS after isolated atrial or ventricular extrasystoles with retrograde VA conduction
* Sequence of VVIR pacing with retrograde VA conduction is too long
* AMS due to farfield sensing of the ventricular paced QRS complex
* AMS during sinus tachycardia
* Dyspnea on exercise with VVIR mode
* VVIR pacemaker syndrome on exercise

---

occurred during sinus rhythm). Despite these shortcomings, severe symptoms associated with AMS were rare and more common in patients with impaired left ventricular function. Vaneiro et al.[52] concluded that "further modifications of the algorithm may be necessary to enhance the performance of this pacemaker" (Table 4).

Future generations of the Meta DDDR and other pulse generators providing AMS will possess more refined and efficient AMS mechanisms and more extensive programmability of the number of cycles before AMS goes into effect to avoid VVIR pacing after single atrial or ventricular extrasystoles. The necessity to detect eight consecutive P waves before extension of the pacing cycle may be too long and will undoubtedly be reviewed in new algorithm development. Programmability or lengthening the atrial blanking period should minimize farfield sensing.

As with the Meta DDDR pulse generator, the new Chorus RM DDDR device (ELA Medical, Montrouge, France) provides an M type 1A fallback response. According to its design, the Chorus RM DDDR pacemaker should behave similarly to the Meta DDDR unit in response to paroxysmal supraventricular tachyarrhythmias. Reports on the clinical performance of the Chorus RM DDDR device are eagerly awaited.

Combined Sensor and Atrial Inputs for the Diagnosis and Control of Paroxysmal Supraventricular Tachyarrhythmias with Dual Chamber Rate-Adaptive Pacemakers

An intelligent DDDR pacemaker should respond to inappropriate atrial rates by comparing atrial and sensor activity so that AMS and rate changes are directly controlled by atrial and sensor inputs. This concept is being incorporated into new generations of DDDR pacemakers. The Intermedics Relay DDDR pacemaker (Intermedics, Freeport, TX) detects nonphysiologic supraventricular tachycardia in this manner (relatively fast atrial rate, but no sensor activity) and responds with a sudden change in the pacing rate without a change in the pacing mode. This response is called the conditional ventricular tracking limit (CVTL).[60-64] Thus, CVTL is not an AMS algorithm, but a limitation of the paced ventricular rate in situations considered nonphysiologic by the sensor. The CVTL is 35 ppm above the lower rate but never less than 80 ppm (Figs. 16, 17). If, in the absence of patient activity, the sensed atrial rate

CVTL WITHOUT PATIENT ACTIVITY

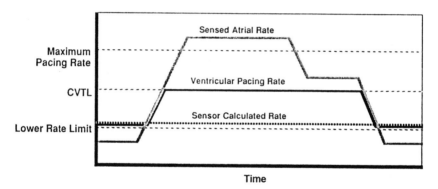

**Without patient activity,
system will pace no faster than CVTL**

Figure 16.   Diagrammatic representation of the conditional ventricular tracking limit (CVTL) of the Intermedics Relay DDDR pacemaker. When programmed "on," the CVTL limits the maximum tracking rate to 35 beats above the programmed lower rate whenever the sensor believes the patient is at rest. Thus, without sensor activity, the ventricular pacing rate will never exceed the CVTL, no matter how high the sensed atrial rate. Supraventricular tachyarrhythmia occurring when the patient is at rest will therefore induce only a limited ventricular paced response at the CVTL. The top horizontal dotted line is the programmed maximum rate and the bottom horizontal dotted line represents the programmed lower rate. The middle horizontal dotted line is the CVTL rate. (Courtey of Intermedics.)

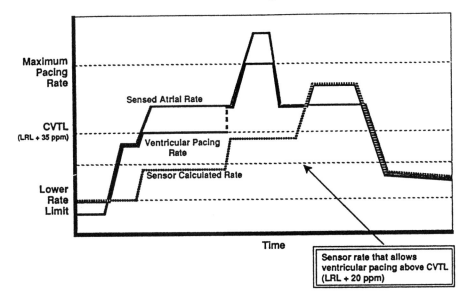

Maximum Pacing Rate

CVTL
(LRL + 35 ppm)

Lower Rate Limit

Sensed Atrial Rate

Ventricular Pacing Rate

Sensor Calculated Rate

Time

Sensor rate that allows ventricular pacing above CVTL (LRL + 20 ppm)

Figure 17. Diagrammatic representation of the conditional ventricular tracking limit (CVTL) function of the Intermedics Relay DDDR pacemaker. The horizontal dotted lines depict the same information as in Figure 16 except for a new horizontal dotted line between the CVTL and the lower rate limit. This particular horizontal dotted line represents the sensor-driven rate threshold (lower rate + 20 ppm) where the pacemaker will automatically uncouple the CVTL function and restore 1:1 AV synchrony up to the programmed upper rate. In other words, when the sensor-indicated rate exceeds the sum of the lower rate plus 20 ppm, the pacemaker switches off the CVTL function and the ventricular pacing rate can increase beyond the CVTL. When the sensor-indicated rate is less than the sum of the lower rate plus 20 ppm, the pacemaker interprets this information as lack of activity with resultant activation of the CVTL function and limitation of the paced ventricular rate. On the right, when the sensed atrial rate falls below the sensor-driven rate, rate-adaptive AV sequential pacing occurs. (Courtesy of Intermedics.)

is faster than the CVTL, the ventricular response becomes limited to the CVTL. The sensor-driven rate controls the upper rate response according to circumstances. (1) If the sensor-driven rate exceeds the programmed lower rate by 20 ppm or more (Fig. 17), ventricular pacing is released from the CVTL and 1:1 AV synchrony occurs up to the programmed upper rate (Fig. 17). (2) When the sensor-driven rate exceeds the pro-

MPI (RELAY)

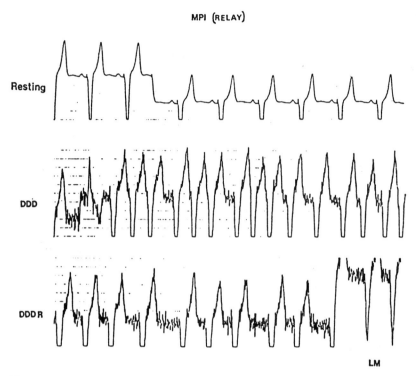

Figure 18. Selected ECG recordings of a patient with a Relay DDDR pacemaker during myopotential interference (MPI) in the DDD and DDDR modes. The top panel shows normal DDD pacing at an atrial sensitivity of 0.8 mV. In the DDD mode, MPI was tracked and resulted in intermittent pacing near the maximum rate (150 beats/min) During DDDR pacing, the pacemaker tracks the MPI at the conditional ventricular tracking limit at a rate of 85 beats/min. (Reproduced with permission from Lau et al.[51])

grammed lower rate by a value less than 20 ppm, the CVTL functions as if there is no patient activity (Fig. 17–19). (3) If the patient's rate is close to the CVTL at rest, at the onset of exercise (with little sensor activity), AV dissociation may occur with hemodynamic disadvantage. (4) At the end of exercise, with the abrupt loss of sensor activity and a persistent increase in sinus rate, the pulse generator can activate CVTL with loss of AV synchrony. (5) If an atrial tachyarrhythmia occurs at the onset of exercise, the pulse generator will disable the CVTL (if sensor-

AF RESPONSE

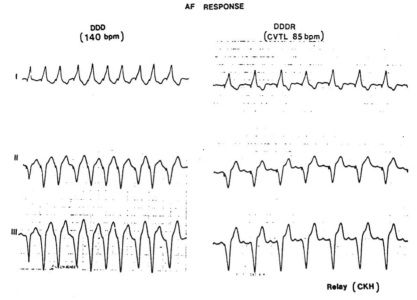

Figure 19. Ventricular responses in a patient with a Relay DDDR pacemaker during spontaneous atrial flutter (AF). The upper rate was 150 bpm and the atrial sensitivity was at 0.8 mV. Irregular ventricular tracking at 140 bpm occurred in the DDD mode. The rate was regularized and reduced to 85 bpm when DDDR mode was programmed such that the conditional ventricular tracking response (CVTL) was activated. (Reproduced with permission from Lau et al.[51])

driven rate > lower rate by 20 ppm) and the tachycardia will persist until the patient returns to rest and the sensor-indicated rate exceeds the programmed lower rate by less than 20 ppm. Similarly, the nervous anticipation of exercise can increase the sinus rate beyond the CVTL and cause AV dissociation before or at the onset of exercise (Fig. 20). The limitations of the present Intermedics CVTL system in the Relay DDDR system are obvious, especially in terms of its relative lack of flexibility and the CVTL rate not being equal to the lower rate. Nevertheless, the Relay DDDR represents the first pacemaker with an advanced fallback mechanism controlled by input from both atrial and nonatrial sensor sources. The next generation of the Relay DDDR system will undoubtedly contain more extensive programmability of (1) CVTL rates and (2)

WENCKEBACH IN SR   (CVTL 85 bpm)

SR 92 bpm

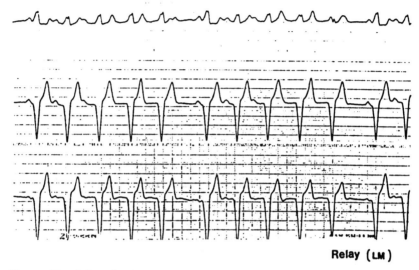

Relay (LM)

Figure 20.   Selected ECG recordings of a patient with a Relay DDDR pacemaker showing the development of Wenckebach-like response in the DDDR mode at rest because of sinus tachycardia. Sinus rate (SR) was 92 bpm in this instance, which exceeded the CVTL of 85 bpm. 1:1 tracking was resumed by increasing the CVTL to 95 bpm. (Reproduced with permission from Lau et al.[51])

threshold sensor-driven rates triggering the CVTL function, e.g. (lower rate + n) bpm where n is programmable.

Conclusion

The responses of dual chamber systems to paroxysmal supraventricular tachyarrhythmias need to be improved. Present devices represent transitional designs that will soon be replaced by more intelligent devices with algorithms based on data from the atrium and one or more sensors. Such intelligent pacemakers will soon become more refined and commonplace and will possess extensive programmability of the fallback mechanisms to provide a large variety of responses to limit the paced ventricular rate during paroxysmal supraventricular tachyarrhythmia. New indications for automatic AMS will undoubtedly emerge. Advanced technology will allow AMS and fallback functions to be customized according to the changing needs of the individual patient.

References

1. Barold SS, Mugica J. Stimuler ou détecter l'oreillette sauf contreindication. Règle d'or de la stimulation cardiaque des années 90. Stimucoeur 1992;20: 129.
2. Hesselson AB, Parsonnet V, Bernstein AD, et al. Deleterious effects of long-term single-chamber ventricular pacing in patients with sick sinus syndrome: The hidden benefits of dual chamber pacing. J Am Coll Cardiol 1992;19: 1542.
3. Sasaki Y, Furihata A, Suyama K, et al. Comparison between ventricular inhibited pacing and physiologic pacing in sick sinus syndrome. Am J Cardiol 1991;67:772.
4. Kosakai Y, Ohe T, Kamakura S, et al. Long term follow-up of incidence of embolism in sick sinus syndrome after pacing. PACE 1991;14:680.
5. Sutton R, Kenny RA. The natural history of sick sinus syndrome. PACE 1986;9:1110.
6. Markewitz A, Schad N, Hemmer W, et al. What is the most appropriate stimulation mode in patients with sinus node dysfunction? PACE 1986;9: 1115.
7. Zanini R, Facchinetti AI, Gallo G, et al. Morbidity and mortality of patients with sinus node disease. Comparative effects of atrial and ventricular pacing. PACE 1990;13:2079.
8. Santini M, Alexidou G, Ansalone G, et al. Relation of prognosis in sick sinus syndrome to age, conduction defect and modes of permanent cardiac pacing. Am J Cardiol 1990;65:735.
9. Biaconi L, Boccadamo R, DiFlorio A, et al. Atrial versus ventricular stimulation in sick sinus syndrome. Effect on morbidity and mortality. PACE 1989;12:1236.
10. Grimm W, Langenfeld H, Maisch T, et al. Symptoms, cardiovascular risk profile and spontaneous ECG in paced patients. A 5-year follow-up study. RBM 1990;12:93.
11. Vanerckelens F, Sigmund M, Lambertz H, et al. Atrial fibrillation in different pacing modes. J Am Coll Cardiol 1991;17:272A.
12. Rosenqvist M, Brandt J, Schüller H. Long-term pacing in sinus node disease: Effects of stimulation mode on cardiovascular morbidity and mortality. Am Heart J 1988;116:16.
13. Rosenqvist M. Atrial pacing for sick sinus syndrome. Clin Cardiol 1990;13: 43.

14. Stangl K, Seitz K, Wirtzfeld A, et al. Differences between atrial single chamber pacing (AAI) and ventricular single chamber pacing (VVI) with respect to prognosis and antiarrhythmic effect in patients with sick sinus syndrome. PACE 1990;13:2080.
15. Sethi KK, Bajaj V, Mohna JC, et al. Comparison of atrial and VVI pacing modes in symptomatic sinus node dysfunction without associated tachyarrhythmias. Indian Heart J 1990;42:143.
16. Jutila C, Klein R, Shivley B. Deleterious long-term effects of single chamber as compared to dual chamber pacing. Circulation 1990;32:(Suppl. III):III-182.
17. Alpert MA, Curtis JJ, Sanfelippo JF, et al. Comparative survival after permanent ventricular and dual chamber pacing for patients with chronic high degree atrioventricular block with and without preexisting congestive heart failure. J Am Coll Cardiol 1986;7:925.
18. Albert MA, Curtis JJ, Sanfelippo JF, et al. Comparative survival following permanent ventricular and dual chamber pacing for patients with chronic symptomatic sinus node dysfunction with and without heart failure. Am Heart J 1987;113:958.
19. Linde-Edelstam C, Gullberg B, Nordlander R, et al. Longevity in patients with high degree atrioventricular block paced in the atrial asynchronous or the fixed rate ventricular inhibited mode. PACE 1992;15:304.
20. Nürberg M, Frohner K, Podczeck A, et al. Is VVI pacing more dangerous than AV sequential pacing in patients with sick sinus node syndrome? PACE 1991;14:674.
21. Witte J, v.Knorre GH, Volkmann HJ, et al. Survival rate in patients with sick sinus syndrome in AAI/DDD vs. VVI pacing. PACE 1991;14:680.
22. Feuer JM, Shandling AH, Messenger JC, et al. Influence of cardiac pacing mode on the long-term development of atrial fibrillation. Am J Cardiol 1989;54:1376.
23. Sgarbossa EB, Pinski SL, Castle LW, et al. Determinants of chronic atrial fibrillation and stroke in paced patients with sick sinus syndrome. PACE 1992;15:511.
24. Grimm W, Langenfeld H, Maisch B, et al. Symptoms, cardiovascular risk profile, and spontaneous ECG in paced patients: a five-year follow-up study. PACE 1990;13:2086.
25. Snoeck J, Decoster H, Verherstraeten M, et al. Evolution of P wave characteristics after pacemaker implantation. PACE 1990;13:2091.
26. Theodorakis G, Kremastinos D, Karavolias G, et al. The early and longterm complications in DDD versus VVI pacing. Eur J Pacing Electrophysiol 1992;2:(Suppl. 1A):A75.
27. Snoeck J, Decoster H, Marchand K, et al. Which factors influence the occurrence of atrial fibrillation after VVI pacemaker implantation? Eur J Pacing Electrophysiol 1992;2:(Suppl. 1A):A69.
28. Ishikawa T, Kimura K, Miyazaki N, et al. Prevention effects of pacemakers on atrial fibrillation in patients with tachycardia-bradycardia syndrome. Eur J Pacing Electrophysiol 1992;22:(Suppl. 1A):A27.

29. Clarke M, Sutton R, Ward D, et al. Recommendations for pacemaker prescription for symptomatic bradycardia. Report of a working party of the British Pacing and Electrophysiology Group. Br Heart J 1991;66:185.
30. Rydén L. Atrial inhibited pacing. An underused mode of cardiac stimulation. PACE 1988;11:1375.
31. Rosenqvist M, Obel IWF. Atrial pacing and the risk for high-grade AV block. Time for a change in attitude? PACE 1989;12:97.
32. Brandt J, Anderson H, Fåhreus T, et al. Natural history of sinus node disease treated with atrial pacing in 213 patients. Implications for selection or stimulation mode. J Am Coll Cardiol 1992;20:633.
33. Griffin JC. The optimal pacing mode for the individual patient: The role of DDDR. In: New Perspectives in Cardiac Pacing. 2, Barold SS, Mugica J (eds), Futura Publishing Co., Mt. Kisco, NY, 1991, p 325.
34. Sutton R. Pacing in atrial arrhythmias. PACE 1990;13:1823.
35. Bodinot B. Stimulation cardiaque à fréquence asservie. Ann Cardiol Angeiol 1990;39:597.
36. Diplos 06 Technical Manual. Biotronik, Lake George, OR, 1990.
37. Ahmed R, Worzewski W, Ingram A, et al. A new pacemaker algorithm preventing atrial tracking during atrial flutter/fibrillation in DDD pacing. Eur Heart J 1991;12:(Abstr, Suppl.):414.
38. Barold SS, Falkoff MD, Ong LS, et al. Timing cycles of DDD pacemakers. In: Barold SS, Mugica J (eds.) New Perspectives in Cardiac Pacing, Futura Publishing Co., Mt. Kisco, NY, 1988, p 69.
39. Barold SS. The DDI mode of cardiac pacing. PACE 1987;10:480.
40. Barold SS, Falkoff MD, Ong LS, et al. All dual chamber pacemakers function in the DDD mode. Am Heart J 1988;119:1353.
41. Vanerio G, Maloney JD, Pinski SL, et al. DDIR versus VVIR pacing in patients with paroxysmal atrial tachyarrhythmias. PACE 1991;14:1630.
42. Higano ST, Hayes DL, Eisinger G. Advantage of discrepant upper rate limits in a DDDR pacemaker. Mayo Clin Proc 1989;64:932.
43. Mugica J, Barold SS, Ripart A. The smart pacemaker. In: New Perspectives in Cardiac Pacing. 2, Barold SS, Mugica J (eds.). Futura Publishing Co., Mt. Kisco, NY, 1991, p 545.
44. Lascault G, Frank G, Girodo S, et al. Tachycardias atriales et stimulation double chambre. Utilité potentielle de l'algorithme de repli. Stimucoeur 1990;18:8.
45. VanWyhe G, Sra J, Rovang K, et al. Maintenance of atrioventricular sequence after His bundle ablation for paroxysmal supraventricular rhythm disorders. A unique use of the fallback mode in dual chamber pacemakers. PACE 1991;14:410.
46. Barold SS, Falkoff MD, Ong LS, et al. Upper rate response of DDD pacemakers. In: Barold SS, Mugica J (eds.). New Perspectives in Cardiac Pacing, Futura Publishing Co., Mt. Kisco, NY, 1988, p 121.
47. Hidden F, Saoudi N, Köning R, et al. Fallback algorithm in DDD pacing mode. Clinical benefit and possible interactions. Eur J Cardiac Pacing Electrophysiol 1992;2:A-26.

48. Meta DDDR Model 1250 multiprogrammable minute ventilation volume rate responsive pulse generator with telemetry. Physician's Manual, Telectronics Englewood, CO, 1990.
49. Ilvento J, Fee JA, Shewmaker AA. Automatic mode switching from DDDR to VVIR. A management algorithm for atrial arrhythmias in patients with dual chamber pacemakers. PACE 1990;13:1199.
50. Gibson S, Paul V, Ward D, et al. Differentiation of atrial arrhythmias from sinus rhythm by DDDR pacemakers. Eur Heart J 1990;11:313.
51. Lau CP, Tai YT, Fong PC, et al. The use of implantable sensors for the control of pacemaker mediated tachycardias: A comparative evaluation between minute ventilation sensing and acceleration sensing dual chamber rate adaptive pacemakers. PACE 1992;15:34.
52. Vaneiro G, Patel S, Ching E, et al. Early clinical experience with a minute ventilation sensor DDDR pacemaker. PACE 1991;14:1815.
53. Lau CP, Tai YT, Fong PC, et al. Atrial arrhythmia management with sensor controlled atrial refractory period and automatic mode switching in patients with minute ventilation sensing dual chamber rate adaptive pacemakers. PACE 1992;15:1504.
54. Clementy J, Rouves D, Dulhoste MN, et al. DDD pacing after AV ablation for paroxysmal atrial fibrillation: First results. Eur J Cardiac Pacing Electrophysiol 1992;2:A65.
55. Sweesy M, Batey R, Forney R, et al. Automatic mode change in a DDDR pacemaker for supraventricular tachyarrhythmias. PACE 1991;14:737.
56. Davis M, Pitney M, May C. Automatic mode switching and program selection in a rate adaptive dual chamber pacemaker. PACE 1991;14:664.
57. Brinker J, Simmons T, Kay N, et al. Initial experience with a minute ventilation based dual chamber rate adaptive pacemaker. PACE 1991;14:663.
58. Ujhazy A, Telectronics, Englewood, Colorado. Personal communication, 1992.
59. Manuel du practicien. Chorus RM 7034. Generateur d'impulsion cardiaque asservi double-chambre-implantable DDDR. ELA Medical, Montrouge, France, 1992.
60. Physician Manual. Relay DDDR pulse generator model 293–03 and 294–04, Intermedics, Freeport TX, 1991.
61. Lee MT, Adkins A, Woodson D, et al. A new feature for control of inappropriate high rate tracking in DDDR pacemakers. PACE 1990;13(Part II):1852.
62. Lau CP, Tai YT, Fong PC, et al. Clinical experience with an activity sensing DDDR pacemaker using an accelerometer sensor. PACE 1992;15:334.
63. Mahaux V, Verboven Y, Waleffe A, et al. Initial experience with a new sensor driven algorithm limiting ventricular pacing rate during supraventricular tachycardia. PACE 1992;15:577.
64. Brunner U, Mahaux V, Benitez J. Worldwide clinical experience with a new accelerometer based rate adaptive pacing system. Eur J Cardiac Pacing Electrophysiol 1992;2:A20.

Chapter 21

Optimal Pacing Mode in Specific Situations: Coronary Artery Disease, Cardiomyopathy, and Cardiac Transplantation

JEFFREY A. BRINKER

Introduction

Discussions of indications for and specific modes of permanent cardiac pacing traditionally focus on the underlying rhythm disturbance. While the primary goal of pacing therapy remains that of providing a minimum heart rate in patients having constant or recurrent transient bradyarrhythmia, the increasing sophistication of pacing systems provides other opportunities to improve the clinical state. In this regard, much attention has been directed at optimizing hemodynamics in patients requiring pacing therapy. The ability to maintain appropriate AV sequencing and provide rate adaptability (either by P synchronous pacing or the utilization of biosensor technology) has fostered the concept of "physiologic" pacing to mimic the normal condition. When programmed appropriately, such devices have been shown to be beneficial in terms of exercise capacity and the feeling of general well-being when compared to standard ventricular fixed rate pacing (VVI) in the bradyarrhythmic patient.[1-4]

New Perspectives in Cardiac Pacing, Vol. 3, edited by S. Serge Barold and Jacques Mugica, Mount Kisco, NY, Futura Publishing Co., © 1993.

TABLE *1*
Pacing in Specific Clinical Scenarios: Considerations

A. Indication(s)	B. Preferred Mode(s) of Pacing
1. Bradycardia	1. Single chamber
2. Tachycardia	2. Dual chamber
3. Unique applications	A. tracking
A. improve hemodynamics	B. nontracking
B. monitor cardiac function	C. Preferred Programming
C. detect disease processes	D. Special Implant Considerations

The ability to stimulate the heart at various rates, coordinate atrial and ventricular events, and convey information about the heart (e.g., electrograms, event registry, sensor indices) has broadened the utility of today's pacing systems. These devices may be used to prevent or terminate tachyarrhythmias, improve hemodynamics by adjusting the AV interval or providing an alternative ventricular contraction pattern in patients without underlying bradyarrhythmia, and to facilitate diagnosis or therapy (Table 1). This chapter examines the expanded role of permanent pacemaking in several unique clinical entities with emphasis on hemodynamic optimization.

Hemodynamic Overview

The normal physiologic interrelationships between the heart, the vascular system, and metabolic need are extremely complex. In the simplest terms, the cardiovascular system functions to supply oxygen and nutrients to individual cells and remove their waste products. The amount of blood pumped by the heart per unit time (cardiac output) should be rapidly adaptable to the body's metabolic requirements, which may vary widely in accordance to a variety of physiologic and pathophysiologic challenges. An optimal hemodynamic state would result when the cardiac output is perfectly matched to the instantaneous metabolic requirement in the most efficient manner possible. For the purposes of this discussion, optimal hemodynamics will be assumed to be that most closely approaching the "normal" state. Attention will be directed toward those factors that may be influenced by pacemaker therapy.

The cardiac output (CO) is directly related to the amount of blood ejected by each ventricular contraction (stroke volume, SV) and the frequency of such contraction (heart rate, HR). Thus,

$$CO \text{ (in cc/min)} = SV \text{ (in cc)} \times HR \text{ (beats/min)}$$

Stroke volume is dependent on three variables: the resistance to ventricular ejection, afterload; ventricular filling prior to ejection, preload; and the inotropic state of the heart muscle, contractility. Elevation of heart rate (up to 300%) is the predominant mechanism of increasing cardiac output during exercise. Although stroke volume may also be increased by a combination of increased contractility, increased preload (by increased venous return), and decreased afterload (by a fall in peripheral resistance), the effect of these changes relative to that brought about by increased heart rate is modest.

The role of the atrial contribution to ventricular filling (preload) has been somewhat controversial.[5-7] It would appear that a properly timed atrial contraction facilitates ventricular filling by acting as a booster pump and assists closure of the AV valves, thereby preventing regurgitation.[8,9] The contribution of atrial systole to ventricular filling depends on the diastolic properties of the latter chamber (Fig. 1) as well as on the strength of the atrial contraction. Less compliant ventricles require higher filling pressures to maintain stroke volume. Loss of the atrial contribution would be more detrimental in patients having stiffer ventricles (e.g., aortic stenosis, hypertrophic cardiomyopathy, hypertension, etc.) (Fig. 2) than in those with large dilated failing hearts (e.g., congestive cardiomyopathy). At rest, the atrial contribution to cardiac output may vary from 10% to 40%, depending on the above factors. With exercise, however, venous return is augmented and the benefits of atrial systole are dwarfed by those of increased heart rate.[10] There is mounting evidence, however, that an appropriate AV relationship may be important during exercise as well. Blanc et al.[11] demonstrated that maintenance of AV sequencing prevented a rise in atrial natriuretic factor seen during exercise in patients with rate-matched ventricular pacing, suggesting increased atrial distension (pressure) with the latter. Jutzy et al.[12] found improved exercise performance in chronotropically incompetent patients with DDDR compared to VVIR pacing. The role of the atrium in optimizing exercise hemodynamics in paced patients is underestimated unless the AV interval is appropriately shortened,[13] possibly accounting for the discrepancy of previous studies. Based on these data, it would seem pru-

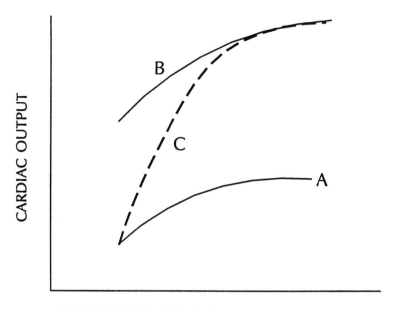

LEFT VENTRICULAR END-DIASTOLIC PRESSURE

Figure 1. Idealized representation of ventricular function curves relating cardiac output to left ventricular filling. Curve A demonstrates the depressed contractility and relatively flat contour of congestive cardiomyopathy. Curve B is representative of the normal heart, while curve C demonstrates the close relationship between cardiac output and filling pressure of a stiff ventricle (e.g., hypertrophic cardiomyopathy).

dent to utilize dual chamber systems that can provide automatic AV interval adjustment with rate and also with respect to whether the atrial event is paced or sensed.[14]

A particularly deleterious situation may exist when atrial and ventricular contractions coincide, resulting in underfilling of the ventricles and the generation of high atrial pressures. While this may occur at times in patients without pacemakers (Fig. 3), it most often results from ventricular pacing accompanied by retrograde activation of the atria. The symptom complex associated with this phenomenon includes hypotension and congestion and is the most frequent etiology of "pacemaker syndrome."[15,16] While associated primarily with VVI(R) pacing, a similar situation may occur with DDD or AAIR modes unless care is taken

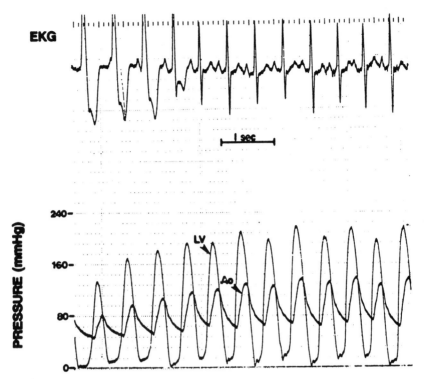

Figure 2. Simultaneous left ventricular (LV) and aortic (AO) pressure tracings in a patient with aortic stenosis demonstrating a marked decrease in pressure with ventricular pacing. Note that pressure increases even during pacing as atrial activity begins to assume a more normal relationship to that of the ventricle (from Plack RH, Porterfield JK, Brinker JA. Complete heart block developing during aortic valvuloplasty. Chest 1989;96:1201- 1203).

to program the devices in accordance to the peculiarities of the individual patient's conduction both at rest and during exercise.[17]

A number of factors influence the choice of a pacing mode for the individual patient (Table 2). The most important decision occurs at the time of implant because the device selected initially will define the range of future programming options. While one might advocate exclusive use of the most sophisticated "universal" device capable of being programmed to any mode as the occasion arises, this is neither practical nor fiscally responsive.[18] While this chapter focuses on the role of pacing in

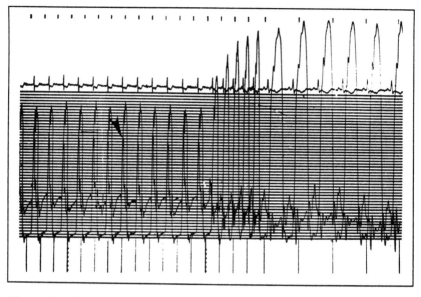

Figure 3. Pacemaker syndrome without a pacemaker. Hemodynamic effects of simultaneous atrial and ventricular contraction in a patient with junctional rhythm converting simultaneously to a sinus mechanism. Ventricular pressure (scale 0–100 mm Hg) increases from 90 to 150 while right atrial pressure (scale 0–25 mm Hg) decreases with disappearance of cannon A waves (arrow). Time lines are at 1-second intervals (from Brinker JA. Pursuing the perfect pacemaker. Mayo Clin Proc 1989;64:587–591).

several unique clinical scenarios, there are some hemodynamic axioms that apply to most patients receiving a pacing system (Table 3). From the point of view of hemodynamics alone, patients requiring pacemaker therapy for a bradyarrhythmia should have a device that allows for rate modulation and maintenance of appropriate AV sequencing. This assumes that the atria are electrically and mechanically functional. If the sinus mechanism is intact, a DDD pacemaker will suffice. When native rate adaptation is inadequate, a sensor driven device should be considered. There is increasing evidence that normal activation of the ventricles is superior to that of right ventricular apical pacing.[19] Thus, in patients without AV conduction disturbance, atrial pacing seems appropriate. Single chamber ventricular pacing should be avoided except when pro-

TABLE *2*

Factors Influencing the Choice of Pacing Mode

Site(s) of conduction disturbance
    –at present and anticipated
Chronotropic competence
    –at present and anticipated
Hemodynamic status
Anticipated percent time paced
    –rare, occasionally, frequently, continuously
Concurrent disease and therapy
Cost/benefit ratio
Ease of implant and follow-up/benefit ratio
Anticipated changes in clinical status
Physician/patient bias
Unique anatomic, physical, or psychological factors

tracted supraventricular arrhythmia exists. In such cases (e.g., atrial fibrillation), the capability for rate modulation may be beneficial.

The implantation of any pacing system, regardless of how sophisticated or simple, may result in detrimental effects unless properly programmed. This is obvious for output and sensitivity settings but is important as well for sensor-driven parameters, upper and lower pacing rate limits, and AV intervals. There is no substitute for adequate clinical assessment (at rest and with effort) post implantation and at regular intervals thereafter.

TABLE *3*

Influence of Pacing Mode on Hemodynamics Axioms

A. Maintain appropriate AV mechanical sequence
    1. atrial sense/pace differential
    2. physiologic shortening with increasing rate
B. Restore hemodynamic rate variability
    1. appropriate upper and lower rate limits
    2. close relationship to metabolic demand
    3. Avoidance of inappropriate augmentation and/or decrease in rate
C. Preserve normal ventricular depolarization pattern

Pacing in Specific Clinical Scenarios

Coronary Artery Disease

Patients with coronary artery disease may be asymptomatic, have chronic or acute ischemia, or have a complication of ischemic disease (Table 4). Pacemaker therapy may be required because of pharmacologically induced bradycardia, ischemic heart block or sinoatrial disease, post-bypass arrhythmia, or bradycardia unrelated to the coronary disease. Some patients with transient conduction system disturbances accompanying acute infarction will have prophylactic pacemaker implantation. Pacing may also be indicated to prevent or terminate tachyarrhythmia and, in patients with automatic internal cardioverter/defibrillators, provide for backup post shock pacing should asystole occur.

The pathophysiology of myocardial ischemia relates to an imbalance between the myocardium's demand for nutrients and the blood supply available through obstructed coronary vessels. Medical therapy for angina pectoris is primarily directed at limiting the demand for blood flow by decreasing heart rate, contractility, afterload, and preload with the goal of increasing the efficiency of the heart's work. Should pacemaker therapy be needed, a system capable of maintaining normal AV con-

---

TABLE 4
The Spectrum of Coronary Artery Disease

Nonflow restrictive
Ischemic coronary disease
    acute (unstable angina)
    chronic (stable angina)
    silent ischemia (may accompany stable or unstable angina)
Acute myocardial infarction
Sequelae of coronary artery disease
    ischemic cardiomyopathy
    ventricular septal defect
    mitral regurgitation
    ventricular aneurysm
Postrevascularization
    bypass surgery
    catheter intervention

traction sequencing would result in the greatest cardiac output for a given level of cardiac work.[20] Dual chamber devices should be considered even when AV conduction is normal because of the possible depressant effects at this site of future pharmacologic therapy. Clearly not all patients with coronary disease are the same with regard to ischemic thresholds. In patients with severe angina and in post-acute infarction patients, both the lower and upper pacing rates should be programmed to mimic effective beta blockade (e.g., 50 and 100/min, respectively). In other patients, these rate limits will vary in accordance with the patient's functional capacity and ischemic threshold assessed clinically. Since ischemia can exist without angina, this assessment should be based on exercise testing or ambulatory ECG monitoring. Care should be taken to avoid the possibility of pacer induced tachycardia (i.e., reentrant PMT, tracking of supraventricular tachyarrhythmia, or inappropriate sensor-driven tachycardia). When possible, the AV interval should be prolonged to allow normal ventricular activation, since ventricular pacing interferes with relaxation and filling of the left ventricle[21] and increases the potential for ischemia compared to atrial pacing at the same rate.[22] While too long an interval may compromise the hemodynamic benefits of atrial systole, the relative merits of hemodynamics compared with ischemic potential must be judged on an individual basis. Clinical assessment of the patient is necessary to adjust pacing parameters and drug therapy to provide an adequate anti-ischemic regimen while maintaining reasonable exercise tolerance.

The role of sensor-mediated pacing is not clear in patients with coronary disease. De Cock et al.[23] found that VVIR improved exercise performance without increasing anginal episodes or nitrate consumption when compared to VVI pacing. It is likely that similar results would be obtained with a DDDR device in patients with chronotropic incompetence. While a VVIR system may be easier to implant, it is inferior in terms of hemodynamics to a rate-adaptive dual chamber pacemaker and should be considered primarily in those patients with refractory atrial fibrillation and inadequate chronotropic response. For those few patients in whom it is difficult or impossible to implant an atrial lead, a single lead VDD system may be a more viable option than VVIR. In patients with paroxysmal supraventricular tachyarrhythmias, programming the dual chamber rate-adaptive pacemaker to a nonatrial tracing mode (DDIR) may prove useful.[24] Whenever a rate-modulated device is used, the maximum sensor-driven rate should be in keeping with the patient's

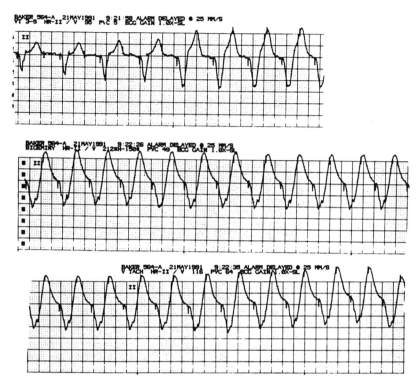

Figure 4. Inappropriate acceleration of an activity-based rate-adaptive pace-maker, resulting in symptoms of chest pain in a patient with coronary artery disease. The acceleration was caused by the patient lying in bed with his chest pressed against a pillow.

clinical status and care should be taken to avoid the possibility of inappropriate acceleration of heart rate (Fig. 4).

Patients with acute myocardial infarction may require permanent pacemaker implantation prior to hospital discharge. Early in acute myocardial infarction complicated by bradycardia, DDD pacing has been shown to be superior to that of VVI.[25] It is likely that these benefits extend at least into the early postinfarct period. It is probably wise to implant a dual chamber system in patients who regain sinus rhythm but have met criteria for prophylactic permanent pacing. Care should be taken when positioning leads in the postinfarct patient because these individuals may be susceptible to sustained tachyarrhythmias. Patients with recent inferior wall infarcts may be at higher risk of perforation by a ventricular lead. Obtaining adequate capture and sensing thresholds in these individuals may also be a problem if there has been considerable right ventricular infarction. In selecting an AV interval, one should be aware that ventricular pacing may mask electrocardiographic changes accompanying ischemia and infarction making the diagnosis of these events more difficult.

Patients with coronary disease may present with ischemic cardiomyopathy. In these cases, the heart may be dilated and exhibit poor systolic function. Symptoms relate to congestive heart failure rather than angina. Often there is little role for revascularization, although transplant surgery may be an option in selected cases. Considerations for pacing are similar to those for congestive cardiomyopathy except that acceleration of the heart rate to improve hemodynamics may be counterproductive if ischemia is provoked.

Coronary artery bypass surgery may be complicated by bradycardia requiring permanent pacemaker implantation with an incidence of 0.8%. Both sinoatrial disease and heart block may be causative. Risk factors include: older age, preexistent left bundle branch block, and a leftward frontal QRS axis.[26] The benefits of temporary dual chamber pacing have been demonstrated in patients post cardiac surgery and would probably extend to those requiring permanent pacing.[27] The persistent need for temporary pacing beyond 4 or 5 days should prompt consideration of a permanent implant. On occasion, an indication for pacing is apparent prior to anticipated surgery. In such instances, temporary pacing should be instituted initially and a permanent system implanted epicardially at the time of heart surgery or subsequently utilizing an endocardial approach.

Cardiomyopathy

The term "cardiomyopathy" implies dysfunction due to disease of the heart muscle itself. The various forms of cardiomyopathy have been classified into three major groups: congestive (dilated), hypertrophic, and restrictive. The groups are differentiated by systolic and diastolic functional abnormalities as well as by morphologic characteristics. A wide variety of disease processes may afflict the heart and result in cardiomyopathy. In some instances, the conduction system is directly effected as well (e.g., sarcoid, amyloid, myotonic dystrophy). The myopathic patient may present with tachy- or bradyarrhythmias or both and pacemakers have an established role in treating these dysrhythmias. They may also be used in novel ways to improve hemodynamics in patients without overt rhythm disturbance.

Dilated (Congestive) Cardiomyopathy

Dilated cardiomyopathy is characterized by a large heart with dilated ventricular cavities exhibiting poor systolic performance. The condition may occur rather acutely following a myocarditis, or more subtly consequent to ethanolism, infiltrative disease, metabolic disorder, infectious process, etc. In most cases, the etiology is undefined and the term "idiopathic" cardiomyopathy is used. Patients may present with symptoms of congestion, hypoperfusion, arrhythmia, or thromboembolism. A variety of drugs may be employed to treat symptoms and improve overall cardiac function and there is some evidence that vasodilators may prolong life.[28] Overall, however, dilated cardiomyopathy has a poor prognosis and continues to be the most frequent indication for heart transplant. The annual incidence of this disorder is 5–8/100,000 and, in the US, it is higher in the black community than in the white community.[29] Signs and symptoms of both right and left heart failure may occur, and compensatory mechanisms to maintain cardiac output result in a tachycardia and venous congestion due to fluid retention. When pacing is required to treat bradyarrhythmia, an argument may be made that the high filling pressures and flat ventricular function curve of the myopathic patient obviate the benefit of dual chamber pacing compared with the simplicity of a VVIR system.[30] Indeed, Rossi et al.[31] found similar advantages for VVIR and atrial-triggered ventricular pacing compared to VVI in patients with heart failure. Others, however, find significant benefit to maintenance of appropriate AV sequencing in this group.[32,33] Even if the mechanical contribution of the atrium was small in these patients, the intact sinus node remains the best indicator of heart rate and should be considered the biosensor of choice.

A further advantage to dual chamber pacing in patients with congestive heart failure is suggested by Alpert et al.[34] These authors found an increased 5-year survival in such patients paced for sinus node dysfunction in a dual chamber mode compared to those paced VVI. While the reason for this is not clear, there is a growing concensus that ventricular pacing for sinus node dysfunction results in a higher incidence of atrial fibrillation and thromboembolism than does atrial or dual chamber pacing. This in turn may influence morbidity and mortality rates.[35–37]

Recently, there has been renewed interest in utilizing pacemakers to improve hemodynamics in patients with dilated cardiomyopathy unassociated with dysrhythmia. As noted above, there is a direct relationship between heart rate and cardiac output, assuming stroke volume remains constant. One would expect, therefore, an increase in cardiac output to be brought about by elevation of heart rate. This is the case in normal and abnormal hearts under experimental conditions.[38] Furthermore, it has been known that the strength of normal heart muscle contraction is increased with the rate of stimulation, although this may not be apparent in myopathic hearts.[39] Iskandrian and Mintz[40] suggested that a "preload mismatch" exists in dilated cardiomyopathy whereby increased left ventricular end-diastolic volume causes overstretching of potentially functional sarcomeres, resulting in a disadvantageous orientation of actin and myosin. They proposed that atrial pacing at a rate of 100–110 bpm may be beneficial in reducing ventricular volume, which in turn might allow "stretched" sarcomeres to return to optimum length, thus increasing their force of contraction.

While atrial pacing may be beneficial for patients with congestive cardiomyopathy and relative bradycardia, the long-term clinical applicability of atrial pacing at high rates is unknown. Certainly, in those patients with coronary disease, ischemia may preclude this approach. Even in the absence of overt coronary obstruction, myopathic hearts have increased mass, and a persistently elevated heart rate may have a detrimental effect, especially in the subendocardial region.

Hochleitner et al.[41] hypothesized that ventricular depolarization is prolonged in the myopathic heart such that the relationship between atrial and ventricular contraction is not optimal even when the P-R interval is normal. These authors shortened the AV interval to 100 ms using a DDD pacemaker in patients with dilated cardiomyopathy and found this to increase left ventricular ejection fraction and blood pressure while decreasing heart size and improving the clinical state. Most of these patients had upper normal P-R intervals prior to pacing, and it is presumed that ventricular contraction was significantly delayed by the extended pathway for depolarization. Thus, shortening the AV interval optimized the relationship between atrial and ventricular contractions, resulting in significant hemodynamic improvement that appears to be sustained. Others have commented on the discrepancy between right-sided electrical and left-sided mechanical events,[42] and it has been recently confirmed that hemodynamics are improved by dual chamber pacing in patients with prolonged P-R intervals.[43]

Pacing therapy may be considered for patients with dilated cardiomyopathy having bradyarrhythmia (absolute or relative), for tachyarrhythmia control, or for improvement of hemodynamics in the absence of dysrhythmia. For the latter indication, a prolonged P-R interval or evidence of delayed ventricular activation should be present. Justification for pacing in these patients would be strengthened by the demonstration of improved hemodynamics with temporary pacing. Dual chamber pacing is indicated except for those with refractory atrial tachyrhythmia. The implantation of a DDDR device provides the greatest flexibility and would allow programming to rate-adaptive nontracking modes should atrial tachyarrhythmias evolve. Automatic adaption of AV delay to rate is important. The dilated right-sided chambers may provide a challenge to lead placement, and active fixation devices are preferred. One may have to accept higher capture thresholds and lower electrogram amplitude than would be ideal because of the underlying pathology.

Hypertrophic Cardiomyopathy

Hypertrophic cardiomyopathy may exist with or without demonstrable obstruction of left ventricular outflow. The disorder is typified by an increased ventricular muscle mass and abnormalities in both systolic and diastolic function. There is a growing consensus that the pathogenesis involves abnormal myocardial-catecholamine interaction. Beta-blocking agents decrease both the ventricular outflow gradient (when present) and diastolic stiffness. Considerable debate exists as to whether the subaortic pressure gradient measured in the basal state or with provocation represents true outflow obstruction.[44,45] It would appear, however, that symptomatic improvement often accompanies measures taken to reduce outflow obstruction (e.g., partial septal resection, beta blockade, mitral valve replacement, etc.).[46]

Heart block in patients with hypertrophic cardiomyopathy may occur spontaneously or result from attempts at operative intervention.

The importance of a properly timed atrial systole is exemplified in these cases by cycle-to-cycle variations in hemodynamics. This is mediated by two interrelated mechanisms: atrial contribution plays an important role in filling the noncompliant ventricle (see Fig. 1), and subvalvular obstruction appears to decrease when left ventricular end-diastolic volume is augmented.[47] The differential effects on hemodynamics brought about by ventricular and atrial pacing have been studied in patients after surgery to relieve outflow obstruction. Ventricular pacing decreases blood pressure and cardiac output while increasing pulmonary artery wedge pressure compared to atrial pacing at a similar rate. Too high an atrial pacing rate, however, causes hemodynamic impairment, presumably due to subendocardial ischemia of the hypertrophied heart.[48] Ischemia may occur at heart rates of 130 per minute or more and is said to be mediated by different mechanisms, depending on whether or not outflow obstruction is present.[49]

A number of recent studies have documented that right ventricular pacing may be an effective way to reduce the left ventricular outflow gradient in patients with symptoms refractory to pharmacologic therapy (Fig. 5).[50–52] This presumably results from the alteration in contraction sequence brought about by the aberrant pathway of ventricular depolarization. Optimal hemodynamics are obtained by dual chamber systems programmed with an AV interval shortened just enough to ensure ventricular pacing but adequate enough to allow an atrial contribution to ventricular filling. Functional improvement parallels the hemodynamics and could appear to be sustained.[53] In some patients, it may be necessary to pharmacologically prolong the P-R interval so that an appropriate P-V interval can be achieved.

The role of this unique application of dual chamber pacing as a therapeutic option in the nonbradyarrhythmic patient with hypertrophic cardiomyopathy remains undefined. At present, it should be employed only in situations in which ventricular outflow obstruction is associated with symptoms refractory to standard pharmacologic therapy. Demonstration of a reduction in gradient by temporary pacing is mandatory before a permanent system can be justified.

If pacing is to be instituted for any reason in hypertrophic cardiomyopathy, attention to hemodynamics is important. Dual chamber pacing with widely programmable AV intervals and rate-adaptive AV interval algorithms should be used in all patients except those with refractory atrial tachyarrhythmias. Care must be taken to avoid inap-

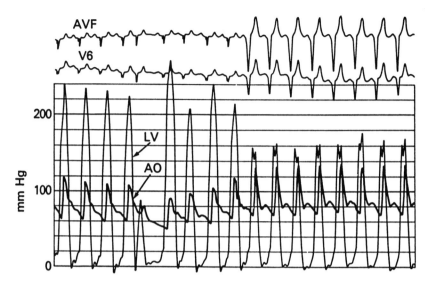

Figure 5. Decrease in pressure gradient and increase in aortic pressure in a patient with IHSS brought about by shortening the AV interval (courtesy of Dr. Fananapazir).

propriately high heart rates so as to prevent the occurrence of ischemia. Sensor-driven pacemakers may be considered when chronotropic incompetence is documented. These devices may also be helpful if appropriate algorithms exist to shorten the AV interval with increasing pacing rates and prevent the tracking of paroxysmal supraventricular tachyarrhythmias.

Cardiac Transplantation

Cardiac transplantation has evolved from an experimental oddity to an accepted form of therapy for patients with end-stage heart disease. Some 1900 such procedures are performed yearly in the US, with the scarcity of donor organs being the major limiting factor. With improved immunosuppression, survival rates of 85% and 60% are seen at 1 and 5 years, respectively. Most heart transplants involve removal of all but the posterior aspects of the recipient's atria to which the donor organ is

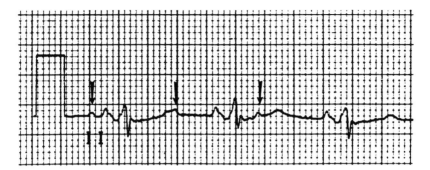

Figure 6. Lead 2 of an electrocardiogram showing both donor and recipient (arrow) atrial activity.

sutured (orthotopic transplant). These remnants of the recipient's heart are electrically isolated from the donor atria and two sets of P waves may be detected on the electrocardiogram (Fig. 6). The surgeon attempts to preserve the now-denervated donor sinus node which, free of parasympathetic tone, drives the donor heart at a relatively high rate. In some patients, however, a profound atrial bradycardia occurs that may require pharmacologic and temporary pacemaker therapy. Such bradycardia may be caused by surgical injury to the sinus node, impaired sinoatrial blood supply, preexisting sinus node disease in the donor, pharmacotherapy, and/or a prolonged period of donor organ ischemia prior to implantation.

The transplanted heart frequently exhibits dysrhythmia.[54] Electrophysiologic studies have revealed a relatively high incidence of sinus node dysfunction evidenced by abnormalities of automaticity and conduction. Because subsidiary pacemakers may be unreliable, sinus node dysfunction may lead to profound clinical sequelae.[55] The incidence of significant atrial bradycardia post transplant appears to be about 15–20%; however, in most cases, this is temporary. The need for permanent pacing depends to a degree on physician preference. Payne et al.[56] implanted permanent pacemakers in 15% of their transplant patients and found that long-term pacing was required in six of these seven individuals. Miyamoto et al., however, found that although 18% of their 401 patients had bradycardia early after transplant, only 4% had permanent devices implanted, and 12 of these 17 (70%) subsequently developed an acceptable intrinsic heart rate.[57]

While the most frequent cause of significant bradycardia after heart transplantation is sinus node dysfunction, some authors have reported a high incidence of AV block. Heart block has been attributed to problems with perioperative myocardial protection and acute rejection.[58] In one series,[59] complete AV block occurred in 21/140 (15%) of patients; however, this was transient in all but three. Permanent pacing (11/140) was instituted in patients with persistent block and in those with subsequently documented infra-Hisian block. This incidence is almost identical to the 7% of patients paced for heart block by Dodinot et al.[58]

Most patients receiving permanent pacing systems after heart transplantation do not require long-term chronotropic support.[60] However, while the need for pacing may be temporary, it is difficult to determine who will ultimately recover and how long this process may take. Postoperative studies of sinus node function are poor predictors of the prevalence of dysfunction at 3 months. It has been suggested that those patients remaining in an escape rhythm throughout the postoperative hospitalization receive a pacemaker.[61] Pharmacologic therapy with oral theophylline has a been proposed as an alternative to pacing in patients with atrial bradyarrhythmias.[62] Potential shortcomings of this approach compared to pacing include the need to take yet another drug on a relatively frequent basis, the systemic effects of the drug, and lack of the rate modulation and telemetric capabilities of pacing. The ultimate role of theophylline for chronotropic support in heart transplant patients requires further study in larger populations.

Choice of a Pacing System

There are many unique aspects to pacing in the transplant patient (Table 5) and these must be considered in choosing the most appropriate pacing system to implant. In the early postoperative period, the heart is relatively noncompliant and, despite the distorted atrial architecture, the atrial contribution to cardiac output is thought to be important. We have found that compared to ventricular pacing, atrial pacing is associated with a significantly greater cardiac output and higher systemic arterial blood pressure (Fig. 7). Diastolic abnormalities will persist in a varying number of patients, especially in those with hypertension.[63] While a single chamber atrial pacemaker may suffice for the treatment of atrial bradycardia, we have felt more comfortable implanting a dual chamber system. The

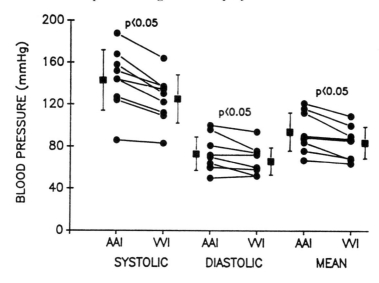

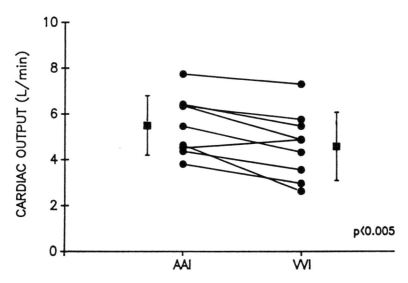

Figure 7. Decreases in blood pressure (top panel) and cardiac output (panel) in heart transplant patients when paced VVI compared to AAI at the same rate (from Midei MG, Baughman KL, Achuff SC, Walford GD, Baumgartner W, Brinker JA. Is atrial activation beneficial in heart transplant recipients? J Am Coll Cardiol 1990;16:1201–1204).

TABLE 5

Pacing the Transplanted Heart: Special Considerations

Immunosuppression increases susceptibility to infection
Complex atrial architecture with electrically isolated recipient and donor
   atria
Denervated heart results in impaired rate response to exercise
Rejection may effect sensing and pacing thresholds
Need for repeated right ventricular biopsies increases potential for lead
   dislodgment

latter would prove beneficial should distal conduction disorders arise in the future and also provides a mechanism for telemetering the ventricular electrogram, which may prove helpful in predicting rejection (see below).

Most transplant patients exhibit at least some impairment of chronotropic response despite normal or slightly elevated levels of catecholamines during exercise. It is assumed that this is the result of denervation of the SA node.[64] A rate-modulated dual chamber system (DDDR) would thus seem advantageous. When AV conduction is intact, some authors have suggested that the neurologically intact recipient atria may serve as the most appropriate biosensor to drive the donor atria. This may be accomplished by using a dual chamber device whose atrial channel is connected to a lead placed in the recipient atrium while the lead from the ventricular channel is implanted in the donor atrium.[65]

A second option is to utilize a bipolar single chamber device programmed to the triggered mode. Unipolar leads from the recipient and donor atria are then connected to the device via a Y adapter.[66] The efficacy of using the recipient atria as a rate modulator must be questioned, however, in view of the relatively high incidence of recipient sinoatrial dysfunction.[55]

Implant Considerations

The decision to implant a pacemaker is often delayed until 3 or more weeks post transplant in order to give the donor atrium adequate time to recover. In all cases, we have utilized a transvenous approach, most often via the left cephalic vein. We have tried to avoid the right side because the right internal jugular vein is used as an access for biopsy.

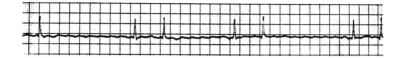

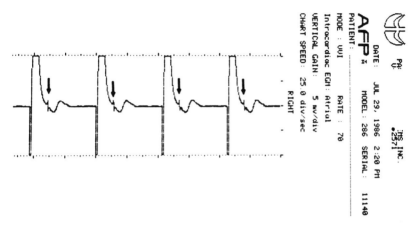

Figure 8. Surface electrocardiogram showing apparent atrial fibrillation (top panel). Atrial electrogram from donor atrium, however, shows retrograde atrial activity with VVI pacing (bottom panel). In this case, the recipient atria were fibrillating while the donor atria demonstrated sinus arrest and a junctional escape rhythm. This resulted in retrograde activation of the donor atria which then causes the coupled "echo" beat.

The electrical independence of the donor and recipient atria must be kept in mind when pacemaker implantation is contemplated. Figure 8a shows a surface electrocardiogram that is consistent with atrial fibrillation. This, however, represents fibrillation of the recipient atria while the donor heart exhibits a junctional escape with retrograde atrial activation and subsequent antegrade conduction, resulting in an "echo" beat. Figure 8b demonstrates retrograde donor atrial activation following each paced ventricular complex.

It is relatively easy to implant both atrial and ventricular leads in the transplanted heart. While Markewitz et al.[67] suggested using a passive-fixation lead in the atrium, we exclusively use active-fixation devices in both chambers of the heart. These allow us to search for the best site in terms of electrical parameters and also provide some protection against dislodgement consequent to repeated right ventricular biopsies. Markewitz suggests that bipolar lead configurations should be used after a patient developed myopotential inhibition during cyclosporine-induced tremors.

Both capture and sensing thresholds may be dramatically altered by episodes of rejection. Usually, however, these measurements are remarkably stable. The consistently low capture thresholds may be the result of concomitant steroid medication that these patients often receive.

Pacing in Heterotopic Transplantation

Heterotopic heart transplantation involves implanting the donor heart in parallel with that of the recipient so that it acts as a ventricular assist device for the latter. This procedure is infrequently employed at present; however, it may still be considered as a bridge to orthotopic transplant when there is mismatch between the size of the donor and recipient organs or when pulmonary hypertension is present and heart-lung transplant is not performed. With heterotopic transplantation, both hearts beat independently and use of a dual chamber pacing system has been suggested to coordinate their activities in an attempt to optimize hemodynamics.[68,69]

Telemetry as a Marker of Rejection

Rejection of the transplanted heart remains a primary concern despite the progress in pharmacotherapy to prevent this. There is considerable benefit in being able to detect the process at a preclinical stage so intensive therapy can be initiated and rejection aborted, thus limiting permanent myocardial damage. While a number of less invasive diagnostic tests have been proposed, none have the specificity and sensitivity of endocardial biopsy. At present, repeated right ventricular biopsy is required as part of routine posttransplant care and as a means of assessing efficacy therapy should rejection occur.

The presence of a pacing wire in the heart affords one the unique ability to gain information via telemetry. Pirolo et al.[70] implanted intramyocardial electrodes in the left and right ventricles in a canine model of heterotopic transplant and found good correlation between measurements of the unipolar peak-to-peak ventricular electrogram amplitude and histologic changes of rejection. The slew rate of the electrogram has also been studied and may complement amplitude.[71] Grace et al.[72] found that a fall in evoked T-wave amplitude correlated well with rejection. It is possible that one or more indices derived from telemetered electrograms may provide a sensitive and specific means of detecting and following the course of rejection. It should also be possible for a specially designed pacemaker to store trends of these measurements to show changes over time.

Summary

The rapid evolution in pacemaker technology has provided the physician with abilities not only to address disorders of rhythm but also to "fine tune" the electrical state of the heart to obtain optimal hemodynamics. It is now apparent the pacemaker may be useful in patients without dysrhythmia in order to achieve improved hemodynamics. It is the physician's responsibility to chose a pacing system wisely with regard to both the rhythm disturbance and the hemodynamics. It is also the physician's responsibility to program the device correctly and to view pacing therapy within the context of available pharmacotherapy.

References

1. Rediker DE, Eagle KA, Homma S, Gillam LD, Harthorne JW. Clinical and hemodynamic comparison of VVI versus DDD pacing in patients with DDD pacemakers. Am J Cardiol 1988;61:323–329.
2. Boon NA, Frew AJ, Johnston JA, Cobbe SM. A comparison of symptoms and intra-arterial ambulatory blood pressure during long term dual chamber atrioventricular synchronous (DDD) and ventricular demand (VVI) pacing. Br Heart J 1987;58:34–39.
3. Karpawich PP, Perry BL, Farooki ZQ, Clapp SK, Jackson WL, Cicalese CA, Green EW. Pacing in children and young adults with nonsurgical atrioventricular block: comparison of single-rate ventricular and dual-chamber modes. Am Heart J 1987;113:316–321.
4. Kruse I, Arnman K, Conradson T-B, Ryden L. A comparison of the acute and long-term hemodynamic effects of ventricular inhibited and atrial synchronized ventricular inhibited pacing. Circulation 1982;65:846–855.
5. Kosowsky BD, Scherlag BJ, Damato AN. Re-evaluation of the atrial con-

tribution to ventricular function: study using His bundle pacing. Am J Cardiol 1968;21:518–524.
6. Burchell HB. A clinical appraisal of atrial transport function. Lancet 1964;1: 775–779.
7. Cohen SI, Frank HA. Preservation of active atrial transport: an important clinical consideration in cardiac pacing. Chest 1982;81:51–54.
8. Ruskin J, McHale PA, Harley A, Greenfield JC. Pressure-flow studies in man: effect of atrial systole on left ventricular function. J Clin Invest 1970;49: 472–478.
9. Skinner NS, Mitchell JH, Wallace AG, Sarnoff SJ. Hemodynamic effects of altering the timing of atrial systole. Am J Physiol 1963;205:499–503.
10. Rossi P, Rognoni G, Occhetta E, Aina F, Prando MD, Plicchi G, Minella M. Respiration-dependent ventricular pacing compared with fixed ventricular and atrial-ventricular synchronous pacing: aerobic and hemodynamic variables. J Am Coll Cardiol 1985;6:646–652.
11. Blanc JJ, Mansourati J, Ritter P, Nitzche R, Pages Y, Genet L, Morin JF. Atrial natriuretic factor release during exercise in patients successively paced in DDD and rate matched ventricular pacing. PACE 1992;15:397–402.
12. Jutzy RV, Florio J, Isaeff DM, Marsa RJ, Bansal RC, Jutzy DR, Levine PA, Feenstra L. Comparative evaluation of rate modulated dual chamber and VVIR pacing. PACE 1990;13:1838–1846.
13. Vogt P, Goy JJ, Fromer M, Kappenberger L. Hemodynamic benefit of atrio-ventricular delay shortening in DDDR pacing (abstr). PACE 1991;14:621.
14. Janosik DL, Pearson AC, Buckingham TA, Labovitz AJ, Redd RM. The hemodynamic benefit of differential atrioventricular delay intervals for sensed and paced atrial events during physiologic pacing. J Am Coll Cardiol 1989;14:499–507.
15. Nishimura RA, Gersh BJ, Vlietstra RE, Osborn MJ, Ilstrup DM, Holmes DR. Hemodynamic and symptomatic consequences of ventricular pacing. PACE 1982;5:903–910.
16. Erlebacher JA, Danner RL, Stelzer PE. Hypotension with ventricular pacing: an atrial vasodepressor reflex in human beings. J Am Coll Cardiol 1984;4: 550–555.
17. Chirife R, Ortega DF, Salazar AI. Non-physiological left heart AV intervals as aresult of DDD and AAI "physiological" pacing. PACE 1991;14:1752–1756.
18. Brinker JA. Pursuing the perfect pacemaker. Mayo Clin Proc 1989;64:587–591.
19. Leclercq C, Mabo P, Le Helloco A, Nicol L, Kermarrec A, Daubert C. The importance of preserving normal intrinsic conduction in permanent cardiac pacing (abstr). PACE 1992;15:511.
20. Zhou JT, Yu GY. Hemodynamic findings during sinus rhythm, atrial and AV sequential pacing compared to ventricular pacing in a dog model. PACE 1987;10:118–123.
21. Zile MR, Blaustein AS, Shimizu G, Gaasch WH. Right ventricular pacing reduces the rate of left ventricular relaxation and filling. J Am Coll Cardiol 1987;10:702–709.

22. Baller D, Wolpers HG, Zipfel J, Bretschneider HJ, Hellige G. Comparison of the effects of right atrial, right ventricular apex and atrioventricular sequential pacing on myocardial oxygen consumption and cardiac efficiency: a laboratory investigation. PACE 1988;11:394–403.

23. De Cock CC, Panis JHC, Van Eenige MJ, Roos JP. Efficacy and safety of rate responsive pacing in patients with coronary artery disease and angina pectoris. PACE 1989;12:1405–1411.

24. Vanerio G, Maloney JD, Pinski SL, Simmons TW, Castle LW, Trohman RG, Wilkoff BL. DDIR versus VVIR pacing in patients with paroxysmal atrial tachyarrhythmias. PACE 1991;14:1630–1638.

25. Murphy P, Morton P, Murtagh JG, Scott M, O'Keeffe DB. Hemodynamic effects of different temporary pacing modes for the management of bradycardias complicating acute myocardial infarction. PACE 1992;15:391–396.

26. Emlein G, Rofino K, Mittleman RS, Vander Salm T, Huang SKS. Severe bradyarrhythmias requiring permanent pacemaker insertion after coronary artery bypass graft surgery: incidence, clinical and electrocardiographic characteristics (abstr). PACE 1992;15:508.

27. Hartzler GO, Maloney JD, Curtis JJ, Barnhorst DA. Hemodynamic benefits of atrioventricular sequential pacing after cardiac surgery. Am J Cardiol 1977;40:232–236.

28. Cohn JN: Current therapy of the failing heart. Circulation 1988;78:1099–1107.

29. Manolio TA, Baughman KL, Rodeheffer R, Pearson TA, Bristow JD, Michels VV, Abelmann WH, Harlan WR. Prevalence and etiology of idiopathic dilated cardiomyopathy (summary of a National Heart, Lung, and Blood Institute workshop). Am J Cardiol 1992;69:1458–1466.

30. Greenberg B, Chatterjee K, Parmley WW, Werner JA, Holly AN. The influence of left ventricular filling pressure on atrial contribution to cardiac output. Am Heart J 1979;98:742–751.

31. Rossi P, Domenica PM, Eraldo 0, Giorgio R, Franco A. Rate-responsive pacing in patients with left ventricular failure. Adv Cardiol 1986;34:115–123.

32. DiCarlo L, Morady F, Krol RB, Baerman JM, de Buitleir M, Schork MA, Sereika SM, Schurig L. The hemodynamic effects of ventricular pacing with and without atrioventricular synchrony in patients with normal and diminished left ventricular function. Am Heart J 1987;114:746–752.

33. Shefer A, Rozeenman Y, Ben David Y, Flugelman MY, Gotsman MS, Lewis BS. Left ventricular function during physiological cardiac pacing: relation to rate, pacing mode, and underlying myocardial disease. PACE 1987;10:315–325.

34. Alpert MA, Curtis JJ, Sanfelippo JF, Flaker GC, Walls JT, Mukerji V, Villarreal D, et al. Comparative survival following permanent ventricular and dual chamber pacing for patients with chronic symptomatic sinus node dysfunction with and without congestive heart failure. Am Heart J 1987;113:958–965.

35. Rosenqvist M, Brandt J, Schuller H. Long-term pacing in sinus node disease:

effects of stimulation mode on cardiovascular morbidity and mortality. Am Heart J 1988;116:16–22.

36. Feuer JM, Shandling AH, Messenger JC. Influence of cardiac pacing mode on the long-term development of atrial fibrillation. Am J Cardiol 1989;64: 1376–1379.

37. Camm AAJ, Katritsis D. Ventricular pacing for sick sinus syndrome: a risky business. PACE 1990;13:695–699.

38. Nitsch J, Seiderer M, Bull U, Luderitz B. Evaluation of left ventricular performance by radionuclide ventriculography in patients with atrioventricular versus ventricular demand pacemakers. Am Heart J 1984;107:906–911.

39. Feldman MD, Alderman JD, Aroesty JM, Royal HD, Ferguson JJ, Owen RM, Grossman W, et al. Depression of systolic and diastolic myocardial reserve during atrial pacing tachycardia in patients with dilated cardiomyopathy. J Clin Invest 1988;82:1661–1669.

40. Iskandrian AS, Mintz GS. Pacemaker therapy in congestive heart failure: a new concept based on excessive utilization of the Frank-Starling mechanism. Am Heart J 1986;112:867–870.

41. Hochleitner M, Hortnagl H, Ng CK, Hortnagl H, Gschnitzer F, Zechmann W. Usefulness of physiologic dual-chamber pacing in drug-resistant idiopathic dilated cardiomyopathy. Am J Cardiol 1990;66:198–202.

42. Wish M, Gottdiener JS, Cohen AI, Fletcher RD. M-Mode echocardiograms for determination of optimal left atrial timing in patients with dual chamber pacemakers. Am J Cardiol 1988;61:317–322.

43. Mabo P, Cazeau S, Forrer A, Varin C, De Place C, Paillard F, Daubert C. Permanent DDD pacing for very long PR interval alone (abstr). PACE 1992;15:509.

44. Murgo JP. Does outflow obstruction exist in hypertrophic cardiomyopathy? N Engl J Med 1982;307:1008–1009.

45. Maron BJ, Epstein SE. Dynamic obstruction to left ventricular outflow: the case for its existence in hypertrophic cardiomyopathy. Z Kardiol 1987;76(Suppl 3):69–77.

46. McIntosh CL, Maron BJ. Current operative treatment of obstructive hypertrophic cardiomyopathy. Circulation 1988;78:487–495.

47. Spilkin S, Mitha AS, Matisonn RE, Chesler E. Complete heart block in a case of idiopathic hypertrophic subaortic stenosis: noninvasive correlates with the timing of atrial systole. Circulation 1977;55:418–422.

48. Shemin RJ, Scott WC, Kastl DG, Morrow AG. Hemodynamic effects of various modes of cardiac pacing after operation for idiopathic hypertrophic subaortic stenosis. Ann Thorac Surg 1979;27:137–140.

49. Non RO, Schenke WH, Maron BJ, Tracy CM, Leon MB, Brush JE, Rosing DR, Epstein SE. Differences in coronary flow and myocardial metabolism at rest and during pacing between patients with obstructive and patients with nonobstructive hypertrophic cardiomyopathy. J Am Coll Cardiol 1987;10: 53–62.

50. Fananapazir L, Cannon RO, Tripodi D, Panza JA. Impact of dual-chamber

permanent pacing in patients with obstructive hypertrophic cardiomyopathy with symptoms refractory to verapamil and β-adrenergic blocker therapy. Circulation 1992;85:2149–2161.

51. Choi BW, Tripodi D, Fananapazir L. Exercise induced end diastolic volume changes in obstructive hypertrophic cardiomyopathy with dual chamber pacing. J Am Coll Cardiol 1992;19:306A.

52. Jeanrenaud X, Vogt P, Goy JJ, Fromer M, Kappenberger L. Permanent pacemaker therapy for hypertrophic obstructive cardiomyopathy (HOCM). J Am Coll Cardiol 1992;19:325A.

53. McDonald K, McWilliams E, O'Keeffe B, Maurer B. Functional assessment of patients treated with permanent dual chamber pacing as a primary treatment for hypertrophic cardiomyopathy. Eur Heart J 1988;9:893–898.

54. Schroeder JS, Berke DK, Graham AF, Rider AK, Harrison DC. Arrhythmias after cardiac transplantation. Am J Cardiol 1974;33:604–607.

55. Bexton RS, Nathen AW, Hellestrand KJ, Cory-Pearce R, Spurrell RAJ, English TAH, Camm AJ. Sinoatrial function after cardiac transplantation. J Am Coll Cardiol 1984;3:712–723.

56. Payne ME, Murray DD, Watson KM, Galbraith TA, Horwanitz EP, Starling RC, et al. Permanent pacing in heart transplant recipients: underlying causes and long-term results. J Heart Lung Transplant 1991;10:738–742.

57. Miyamoto Y, Curtiss EI, Kormos RL, Armitage JM, Hardesty RL, Griffith BP. Bradyarrhythmia after heart transplantation. Incidence, time course, and outcome. Circulation 1990;82(Suppl):IV3l3–317.

58. Dodinot B, Costa AB, Godenir JP, Pinelli G, Peiffert B, Mattei MF, Villemot JP. AV block after cardiac transplantation: pacing mode selection (abstr). PACE 1991;14:692.

59. Buja G, Miorelli M, Livi U, Chiominto B, Nava A. Pacemaker indication in patients with complete AV block following orthotopic heart transplantation. PACE 1991;14:737.

60. Scott CD, Omar I, McComb JM, Dark JH, Bexton RS. Long-term pacing in heart transplant recipients is usually unnecessary. PACE 1991;14:1792–1796.

61. Heinz G, Hirschl M, Buxbaum P, Laufer G, Gasic S, Laczkovics A. Sinus node dysfunction after orthotopic cardiac transplantation: postoperative incidence and long-term implications. PACE 1992;15:731–737.

62. Ellenbogen KA, Szentpetery S, Katz MR. Reversibility of prolonged chronotropic dysfunction with theophylline following orthotopic cardiac transplantation. Am Heart J 1988;116:202–206.

63. Murali S, Uretsky BF, Reddy S, Griffith BP, Hardesty RL, Trento A. Hemodynamic abnormalities following cardiac transplantation: relationship to hypertension and survival. Am Heart J 1989;118:334–341.

64. Quigg RJ, Rocco MB, Gauthier DF, Creager MA, Hartley H, Colucci WS. Mechanism of the attenuated peak heart rate response to exercise after orthotopic cardiac transplantation. J Am Coll Cardiol 1989;14:338–344.

65. Markewitz A, Osterholzer G, Weinhold C, Kemkes BM, Feruglio GA. Recipient P wave synchronized pacing of the donor atrium in a heart transplanted patient: a case study. PACE 1988;11:1402.

66. Kacet S, Molin F, Lacroix D, Prat A, Pol A, Warembourg H, Lekieffre J. Bipolar atrial-triggered pacing to restore normal chronotropic responsiveness in an orthotopic cardiac transplant patient. PACE 1991;14:1444–1447.
67. Markewitz A, Kemkes BM, Reble B, Osterholzer G, Reichart B, Puricelii C, Feruglio GA, et al. Particularities of dual chamber pacemaker therapy in patients after orthotopic heart transplantation. PACE 1987;10:326–332.
68. Breedveld RW, van Gelder LM, Mitchell AG, Peels CV, Yacoub M, El Gamal MIH. Optimized hemodynamics by implantation of a dual chamber pacemaker after heterotopic cardiac transplantation. PACE 1992;15:274–280.
69. Raza ST, Tam SKC, Sun SC, Laurance R, Berkovitz B, Shemin R, Cohn LH. Sequentially paced heterotopic heart transplants in the left chest provides improved circulatory support for the failed left ventricle. A potential bridge to orthotopic transplantation. J Thorac Cardiovasc Surg 1989;98:266–274.
70. Pirolo JS, Tweddell JS, Brunt EM, Pyo R, Shuman TS, Cox JL, Ferguson TB. Influence of activation origin, lead number and lead configuration on the noninvasive electrophysiologic detection of cardiac allograft rejection. Circulation 1991;84(Suppl):344–354.
71. Castejon R, Cabo J, Gamallo C, Diez-Pardo JA, Cordovilla G. Electrophysiological and anatomical findings in heart transplantation: experimental study. PACE 1990;13:845–851.
72. Grace AA, Newell SA, Cary NR, Scott JP, Large SR, Wallwork J, Schofield PM. Diagnosis of early cardiac transplant rejection by fall in evoked T wave amplitude measured using an externalized QT drive rate responsive pacemaker. PACE 1991;14:1024–1031.

Index